AIDS In Africa

The Social and Policy Impact

AIDS In Africa

The Social and Policy Impact

Norman Miller and
Richard C. Rockwell
Editors

Studies in African Health and Medicine
Volume 10

The Edwin Mellen Press
Lewiston/Queenston

Published in association with:

The National Council for International Health
1701 K. St. NW
Washington, DC 20006

The African-Caribbean Institute
4 West Wheelock
Hanover, NH 03755

This is volume 1 in the continuing series
Studies in African Health and Medicine
Volume 1 ISBN 0-88946-187-2
SAHM Series ISBN 0-88946-281-X

The Edwin Mellen Press
P.O. Box 450
Lewiston, New York
USA 14092

The Edwin Mellen Press
P.O. Box 67
Queenston, Ontario
CANADA L0S 1L0

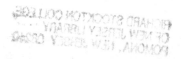

In Africa . . .

For those who suffer
For those who offer succor
For those who teach . . .
so that knowledge will overcome

TABLE OF CONTENTS

PART V
RESOURCE MATERIAL FOR
THE STUDY OF AIDS IN AFRICA

FOREWORD

AIDS IN AFRICA:
The Triple Disaster

Kenneth Prewitt*

The crisis presented by AIDS in Africa extends beyond its toll as a viral epidemic, as tragic as this toll in human lives and suffering may be. In complex ways AIDS disrupts the economic and social development of Africa -- the loss of trained personnel, the deflection of scarce resources, the strain on public health and education systems, the reduction of tourist revenue, and the potential political unrest resulting from a pressing social problem. But even these many development-related difficulties do not exhaust the harm being visited on Africa by AIDS.

The world's image of that troubled continent is linked to AIDS. Public discourse about AIDS in general, but especially about AIDS in Africa, is clouded by the persistent, pernicious presence of racial stereotypes, moralistic reasoning, and xenophobic policies. How strong is this influence? What might aggravate it? What might lessen it? What are its consequences? These questions are no less important to considering AIDS in Africa than the biomedical and epidemiological issues, or the public health and education challenges.

Let us consider first the more familiar issues. Biomedical protection against HIV is many years away, not less than five and likely more. The human immune system is exceedingly complex, and the AIDS virus is presenting challenges with which laboratory science is not yet able to cope. Following the hoped for research breakthrough in the laboratory, there still will be several years of clinical trials and field testing. With this unforgiving biomedical truth in hand, coupled with the facts about the prevalence of HIV in Africa and its known modes of transmission, agencies have turned in some

---

* Kenneth Prewitt, Ph.D., a political scientist, is vice-president of the Rockefeller Foundation, and a former president of the Social Science Research Council.

desperation to efforts focused on altering the behaviors and practices which give AIDS its pandemic energy. That is, in the absence of a vaccine capable of arresting the spread of AIDS, the effort turns elsewhere -- to alerting members of the community of practices which could place them at risk, to informing those in high-risk groups how to lessen the probability of infection, and to pleading with the already infected to cease those practices known to spread the virus.

These are difficult areas for a campaign aimed at persuading people to alter long-established practices sanctioned by cultural norms. Such campaigns are especially difficult in Africa. The international aid agencies and the national ministries of health, on which much of the burden has thus far fallen, are poorly informed about the very behavior in Africa that is the target of behavior modification efforts. The design of education efforts is still in a trial and error phase. The mainstays of a campaign, media and the schools, are ill-equipped for the task now assigned to them -- bringing complex public health messages to the African population.

Despite the difficulties, over the near term we must depend on social and educational effort rather than biomedical technology to arrest the spread of the virus. The information and analysis available in this collection of essays contribute a much needed resource to this effort. Conventional public health and education efforts, alas, are not enough. There is an even more difficult educational challenge before the world community.

The AIDS pandemic has, to be sure, provided a global stage for compassion and a far-flung effort to treat and to cure. The enormous commitment of research and public health resources, the global mobilization of private voluntary organizations, the dedicated and often courageous actions of thousands of medical and health workers, and the search for an appropriate educational response, are expressions of human compassion at its best. Africa has been a beneficiary of this internationally expressed concern.

If compassion is strongly at work, so also is fear and approbation. There is anxiety, anger, and a moralistic sub-text in public discussion about AIDS. In this sub-text, AIDS is a disease of the immoral; in the United States, of the homosexual, the prostitute, the drug user; and in Africa, of the sexually promiscuous. From this perspective a silent killer has been set loose by the self-indulgent, undisciplined habits of unclean groups. There is fear that the innocent may not be able to protect themselves, and anger at those responsible. Hints of quarantine hover -- in debates about mandatory testing, in the use of isolation wards in prisons and hospitals, in work-place segregation; in discussion about closing borders to travelers and students from high-incidence countries -- all fueled by the substantial number of citizens who erroneously believe that AIDS is spread through casual contact.

Africa, along with the U.S., is at the forefront of global attention on AIDS. As noted, this attention brings the welcome resources of international aid and public health. It also offers an unwelcome focus for the fears and angers of those all too willing to "blame the victim."

A long history, unpleasant to recall, formed in the Western imagination a view of Africa as the Dark Continent, a place of exotic, savage customs. Echoes of these images from earlier centuries can still be heard, accompanied by what Marguerite Duras calls, "the involuntary racism that inheres necessarily in all exoticism." AIDS in Africa, with its innuendo of sexual excess, gives license to those who would attribute Africa's current political and economic problems to the "backwardness" of its people. The fear of AIDS and the anger toward its carriers has the potential in some quarters to reawaken earlier and ugly ideologies.

From the perspective of Africa's development, AIDS is a triple disaster. There is the tragedy of the disease itself, the human suffering, and death. There are the multiple ways in which AIDS complicates the already daunting development problems facing the continent and threatens to reverse hard-won advances. Finally, the special characteristics of AIDS -- its mysterious origin, its resistance to biomedical treatment, its association with social deviance and its hint of exotic behavior -- provide a ready justification for those who would just as soon not be bothered by Africa, its need for international aid, and its development difficulties.

Starting from the deeply planted image of Africa as "the dark continent," strengthened by the racist ideology used to buttress slavery and then colonization (which has its final outpost in apartheid), and finding modern expression in development doctrine that treats Africa as a problem to be solved rather than a voice to be heard, there is a view of Africa which denies its dignity and ignores its accomplishments. The prevalence of AIDS in Africa raises the specter that this view may gain in currency. To be alert to this danger, and to protect against it, sets for the world community a task no less difficult, or important, than preventing the spread of the infection itself.

PREFACE

Russell Morgan
Norman Miller*

This volume brings together working papers and resource material from authors in Africa, North America and the United Kingdom. The writers are from both academic disciplines and operational organizations concerned with health and development. This diversity is a strength *and* a limitation. No single thread weaves this collection of papers together, and no over-arching theme moves them towards a common conclusion. Rather these are position reports that begin to map the social science, policy and health terrains of the disease. They are aimed not so much at the academic research world of African and international affairs, but at those who would teach about AIDS in Africa, and those African and non-African policy makers who might bring their existing expertise to bear on the problem. In this sense it is a recruiting volume, one that is produced in hopes of helping solve the dilemma of HIV/AIDS.

A few caveats are necessary. A sense of urgency surrounds this endeavor. The fact that the disease has entered so rapidly onto the world stage, and the fact that our knowledge is changing so fast, necessitated this book be brought out quickly. Although there are justifications for this haste, there are also costs. Errors of fact and of judgment will inevitably be published, style and grammatical problems will be found. We have struggled to correct the errors, but have also decided to plead *nolo contendere*. We have sacrificed consistency and fine-tuned editing in order to publish promptly.

Nor have we enforced an overview or a common departure on the authors. We have not attempted to extract comparative conclusions, nor even a common definition of Africa. Some writers refer to sub-Saharan

---

** **Russell Morgan**, Dr. P.H., served in Kenya as a Peace Corps volunteer. He is Executive Director of the National Council for International Health, and a member of the Program Board of U.S.A. for Africa. **Norman Miller**, Ph.D., serves as President of the African-Caribbean Institute, and concurrently teaches at Dartmouth College.*

Africa, others to the continent as a whole. We are also aware that important work on African AIDS is not only underway in Africa itself, but also in countries that have institutions and individuals who have been concerned with that continent for decades. This volume hints at some of these overseas efforts in North America and the United Kingdom, but we have been unable to assess parallel efforts in France, Belgium, Holland, West Germany and the Scandinavian nations, to name only the most obvious.

Although many individuals and several organizations have contributed resources and staff help in compiling this material, two organizations in particular are responsible for producing the text: The National Council for International Health and the African-Caribbean Institute.

NCIH is a professional association of some 2500 individual members and 170 institutional members. For over 15 years NCIH has served the health community by identifying various ways to improve health care, foster cooperation, offer technical assistance to agencies and help educational programs be more effective. Its concern is to develop better health care concepts and to educate its constituency on emerging issues in international health.

The Council's members come from every segment of the health and medical fields including public health, nursing, dentistry, medicine, social work, health education, health policy, pharmacy, nutrition/food, health economics and manpower, population and family planning. Its member organizations include those from voluntary agencies, professional and trade groups, government agencies, universities, corporations, hospitals, foundations, and research and consulting firms.

NCIH joined the African-Caribbean Institute in support of this book with the hope that it will provide readers with a better understanding of how the disease is transmitted, where and for whom it is most serious, and how we can arrest its spread and hence its deadly toll.

The African-Caribbean Institute is an educational, non-profit organization dedicated to the increased understanding of these two important regions. Its objective is to stimulate cross-cultural awareness through research, analysis, publications and the production of film material. The Institute has traditionally focused on environment and development issues, including environmental health. ACI sponsored the recent symposium on AIDS at the African Studies Association meeting in Denver, Colorado, from which many of the papers in this volume originated.

Both ACI and NCIH wish to acknowledge other organizations that have generously contributed to this undertaking. These include the Social Science Research Council, the American Academy for the Advancement of Science, the U.S. Bureau of the Census, the Futures Group, and the Department of Community and Family Medicine at Dartmouth Medical School. Individuals include David Sills of SSRC, who along with Judith Miller, provided editorial advice; Neil Brendan and Martin King at NCIH, who provided administrative support; and Clifford Pease, M.D., Robert Greenberg, M.D., and James Strickler, M.D., who kindly provided advice or reviewed portions of the manuscript before final publication. Nancy Schmidt, not only authored a major piece in this volume, but also undertook the organization and editing of other bibliographical materials herein. Linda Aldrich at Dartmouth and Herbert Richardson and Lois Holden at the Edwin Mellen Press have made major contributions to the book's production.

While NCIH and ACI are pleased to support this endeavor, one final caveat is important: the views of the authors and the data they present are theirs alone and do not necessarily reflect the views of NCIH, ACI, or their memberships.

GLOSSARY OF TERMS

Peter Kilmarx[*]

ABBREVIATIONS

AIDS-Acquired Immuno-Deficiency Syndrome
ARC-AIDS Related Complex
CDC-Centers for Disease Control
ELISA-Enzyme Linked Immuno-Sorbent Assay
HIV-Human Immunodeficiency Virus
HTLV-Human T-cell Lymphotrophic Virus
IFA-Indirect Fluorescent Antibody test
LAV-Lymphadenopathy Associated Virus
NGO-Non-Governmental Organization
PVO-Private Volunteer Organization
SES-Socio-Economic Status
STD-Sexually Transmitted Disease
USAID-United States Agency for International Development
WB-Western Blot
WHO-World Health Organization

GLOSSARY

ACQUIRED IMMUNO-DEFICIENCY SYNDROME (AIDS)-The severe manifestation of infection with HIV characterized by weight loss, chronic diarrhea, prolonged fever, enlarged lymph nodes, and opportunistic infections.

AIDS RELATED COMPLEX (ARC)-A symptomatic manifestation of HIV infection that does not meet the definition of AIDS.

ANTENATAL - Before birth.

ANTIBODY-A protein produced by white blood cells to combat foreign or infectious agents called antigens. Antibodies bind with the specific antigen for which they were produced and often cause the destruction and removal of the antigen.

ANTIGEN-A foreign or infectious agent, including bacteria and viruses, that stimulates white blood cells to produce antibodies.

---

[*] **Peter Kilmarx**, a medical student at Dartmouth Medical School, Hanover, New Hampshire compiled this glossary. He has studied and worked in Zaire and has written on AIDS control and prevention in rural Africa.

ANTIGENEMIC-The presence of antigen, e.g. HIV, in the blood.

CHANCROID-An infectious venereal ulcer caused by a specific bacterial infection.

CHLAMYDIA-An infectious bacteria and cause of a specific sexually transmitted disease.

CLITORIDECTOMY-Removal of the clitoris.

CONGENITAL-Existing at birth. May be genetically caused or environmentally caused, as by infection.

DOUBLING TIME-The time required for the prevalence of an infection or disease to double.

ENZYME LINKED IMMUNO-SORBENT ASSAY (ELISA)-A screening test for antibody in blood samples, e.g. antibody to HIV. Less specific than the Western Blot test, i.e. there are more false positives with the ELISA than with the Western Blot. To be considered truly positive, a blood sample must be repeatedly positive with the ELISA and then found to be positive with the Western Blot.

EPIDEMIOLOGY-The study of the prevalence and spread of disease.

FALSE NEGATIVE-A negative test for someone who actually has the condition being tested.

FALSE POSITIVE-A positive test for someone who actually does not have the condition being tested.

HORIZONTAL TRANSMISSION-Infection by direct contact with an infected individual or by contact with infected bodily fluids or tissue.

HUMAN IMMUNODEFICIENCY VIRUS (HIV)-The causative agent of AIDS. HIV I was the first discovered, and is more prevalent in central Africa and the United States, HIV II was the second discovered, and is more prevalent in Western Africa.

HUMAN T-CELL LYMPHOTROPHIC VIRUS (HTLV)-A family of retroviruses that specifically infect T-lymphocytes. HTLV-III is another name for HIV, now obsolete. Another HTLV is thought to cause leukemia.

IgM ANTIBODIES-A type of antibody that does *not* cross the plancenta. Therefore presence of IgM antibodies in the infant's serum indicates direct exposure to antigen, rather than passive in utero transfer of antibodies independent of direct exposure.

IMMUNOCOMPETENT-Having an intact, functional immune system.

INCIDENCE-The number of new cases of a disease in a population in a given period of time. For example, a city may have an incidence of three new cases of AIDS per thousand population per year.

INCUBATION PERIOD-The amount of time between exposure to a disease and the clinical or symptomatic manifestation.

INDIRECT FLUORESCENT ANTIBODY TEST (IFA)-A test for an antigen using a fluorescent antibody. If the antigen is present, the antibody will bind to it, and will be detectable by fluorescence microscopy.

LYMPHDENOPATHY-any disease affecting the lymph nodes, which may be enlarged and tender.

LYMPHADENOPATHY ASSOCIATED VIRUS (LAV)-Another name for HIV, now obsolete.

NON-SPECIFIC REACTIVITY-A cause of false positive results in a blood test.

OPPORTUNISTIC INFECTIONS-An infection by an organism that is only capable of causing disease when the host's defenses are lowered. Many of these organisms are normally present and only cause disease when one is immunosuppressed as in AIDS.

PANDEMIC- A wide-spread epidemic

PARENTERAL-By some means other than by mouth, e.g. by injection.

PERCUTANEOUS-Through the skin.

PERINATAL-Before, during, or after birth; i.e. from the 28th week of gestation through the first week after delivery.

PERIOD OF INFECTIOUSNESS-The period in the course of an infectious disease during which an infected individual may infect another individual.

PERSISTANT GENERALIZED LYMPHADENOPATHY-A manifestation of HIV infection characterized by enlarged and tender lymph nodes.

PREVALENCE-The number of cases of a disease or condition in a given population at a specific time. For example, a city may presently have a 1% prevalence of HIV seropositivity.

POLYGYNY-The practice of having more than one wife at a time.

POST-PARTUM-After childbirth.

PRURITIC DERMATITIS-An itchy inflammation of the skin.

RETROVIRUS-A family of viruses, characterized by the presence of the enzyme reverse transcriptase, which makes them uniquely able to make DNA from RNA. Other organisms can only make RNA from DNA.

SENSITIVITY-The power of a laboratory test to detect a given condition. The probability that a test will be positive when the disease is present. A highly sensitive test will have few false negatives.

SEROCONVERSION-The initial development of antibodies to an antigen, whereby someone who was seronegative becomes seropositive.

SERONEGATIVE-The absence of antibodies in one's blood serum.

SEROPOSITIVE-The presence of antibodies in one's blood serum.

SEROPREVALENCE-The number of seropositive persons in given population at a specific time. For example, patients presently in a given hospital may have a seroprevalance of 5%.

SEROSURVEYS-Studies in which a sample population is blood tested for the presence of antibody.

SPECIFICITY-The power of a laboratory test to indicate when a given condition is *not* present. The probability that a test will be negative when the disease is not present. A highly specific test will have few false positives.

T-HELPER LYMPHOCYTES-White blood cells that stimulate other white blood cells, as in the production of antibody. "The conductors of the immune symphony."

T-LYMPHOCYTES (T-CELLS)-A class of white blood cells that are produced in the thymus, including T-helper and T-suppressor cells. In AIDS, there is a decline in the number of T-helper cells relative to T-suppressor cells.

T-SUPPRESSOR LYMPHOCYTES-White blood cells that turn-off other white blood cells.

TREPONEMATOSES-Infections by treponemes, a group of bacterial organisms causing diseases including syphilis and yaws.

VERTICAL TRANSMISSION-Infection from parent to offspring as by genetic inheritance, transplacental infection, or breast milk.

WESTERN BLOT-A test for antibody in blood samples, e.g. antibody to HIV. More specific than the ELISA.

[See: Harris County Medical Society and Houston Acadamy of Medicine. AIDS: a guide for survival. August, 1987; Williams and Wilkins' Stedman's Medical Dictonary; and John Wiley & Sons' International Dictonary of Medicine and Biology.]

Africa

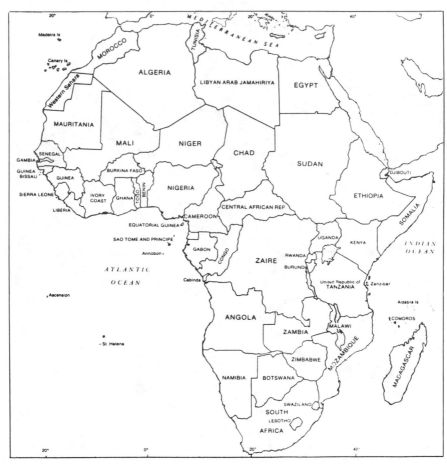

The boundaries and names on this map do not imply official
endorsement or acceptance by the United Nations

INTRODUCTION

Norman Miller

Richard C. Rockwell*

Few human tragedies in recent history have focused the world's attention as does the HIV/AIDS pandemic. For Africa the spread of the disease comes at a time when many nations are ill-equipped to respond. Crippling famines, internal strife, economic misfortunes, and shortage of resources have made AIDS potentially more serious in Africa than on any other continent of the world.

This book seeks to clarify the health and social realities in Africa, to pose questions and concepts for understanding the problem, and to provide bibliographic resources needed by instructors and researchers who would take up the AIDS challenge.

AIDS has created a problem of enormous complexity, particularly for developing nations. There is no known cure for the disease, and the only way to avoid the risk of infection is to avoid exposure. However, reducing exposure, because transmission is largely sexual in nature, means changing behavior that is driven by biological imperatives. AIDS in this sense is a behavioral illness. To change or modify sexual behavior on a broad scale may be impossible, because specific cultural mores preclude any single educational program.

These complexities are underscored when we realize there can be no panacea for a continent that is four times the size of the United States, with over 900 ethnic groups, 300 language families, and 51 countries. Each African country has a rich history and complex political chemistry that must be addressed in the search for policy solutions on AIDS.

---

* See authors' biographies at back of book.

Overview Of AIDS In Africa

In order to gain an understanding of the HIV/AIDS pandemic in Africa one must first ask a number of questions. What are the facts about the prevalence of the virus and the incidence of the disease? What are the basic social and medical characteristics of the pandemic? What are the options of prevention, education and care for the ill? What kinds of research should social and behavioral scientists be undertaking? What would be most helpful to African governments? What stereotypes and misconceptions must be eliminated?

Basic information on HIV/AIDS is woefully lacking in Africa and, to an extent, in the developed world as well. Research findings on the social impact of the epidemic are just beginning to emerge, and much of the data is still controversial. For example, Biggar and Merritt, authors in this volume, estimate that in 1987 some 1.4 to 1.8 million Africans were sero-positive, or infected with the HIV-1 virus, while the World Health Organization has released estimates ranging to 5 million. Much of the epidemiological data published about Africa in 1984-85 has been recanted and discarded because of major serum testing problems. Realizing full well that any picture drawn today in all likelihood will be changed by new data that emerge, the following points seem to be valid:

> The highest risk of infection is found among persons in the age group 20-40. For men, ages 25-29 are at special risk; for women, ages 30-34.

> The full demographic impact of the disease on women and children is unknown, but prenatal infection is occurring and the health of newborn children is a major concern.

> Because the pandemic seems largely urban in Africa, the highest risk social groups are urban dwellers and the geographically mobile (who can acquire or spread the disease to other urban centers and rural areas). Among them are commercial and government elites, military and paramilitary personnel, police, truckers, and prostitutes.

> The continent is by no means uniformly affected. Some nations seem relatively free of HIV; others seem to show levels of infection several times higher than in developed nations. Most of the available information pertains to the HIV-1 virus; much less is known about the prevalence of HIV-2 and the

incidence of disease associated with it. Little is known about the origins of the virus, except that it can be found in blood samples that were collected from all over the world at about the same time, some as early as the late 1950s.

Under current treatment regimens, a majority of those who are now infected will become ill and die. No one is sure what the conversion rate--from being infected by HIV to being ill with AIDS--really is, or when symptoms typically first appear after infection, but by the end of a 10-year period, at least 90% of the infected will likely have shown symptoms and many will have died.

There will be a great many people who develop the illness who do not understand either their symptoms or their potential role in spreading infection. Medical care systems will be inadequate to the task of caring for the ill; victims and their kinsmen will embark on desperate searches for cures, with large expenditures of savings and an aggressive search for health care and ways to finance it.

No matter how large or how small the African population of the infected and the ill is and will become, the numbers will be too large for African medical and social systems to cope with unless a significant redistribution of resources occurs or significant external aid is made available.

The Impact On African Leadership: A Hollowing Out?

The fact that AIDS is currently seen as an urban disease largely centering on the 20-40 age groups and perhaps on those who are in the middle or upper income brackets presents a particularly sobering picture for the national leadership. The process can be described as a "hollowing out" of the leadership core. It is this group of well-trained leaders who have the resources, the money, the cars and the leisure time to pursue multiple sexual liaisons if they are so inclined. Many are part of the "bachelor town syndrome," wherein a man lives in a major city in order to work, while his wife and family maintain the farm in a rural area.

Two cases, one from the commercial sector and one from the military illustrate the hollowing-out process. During 1986 in Zaire a prominent bank president, two vice presidents and the secretary with whom they were all sexually active, died of AIDS within a month. During a short period of time the bank essentially lost its entire leadership. This is the kind of loss which corporations in the west guard against with insurance policies and prohibitions against the entire executive staff flying on a single airliner. The fear is that such wholesale losses could become a common pattern in many African nations.

Second, the military leadership is also seen as being particularly at risk because salaries, cars and mobility have permitted them to maintain a sexually active social life. Laissez-faire attitudes, adventurous outlooks and quixotic lifestyles all promote taking social risks. In some African military units, higher rank is associated with higher exposure to the virus, and far more officers are reportedly ill with the disease than enlisted men. A by-product of this pattern is that key officers will be lost, which will in turn lead to an instability of command.

There is already enough evidence to merit further investigation of the hollowing-out process and its consequences. It is important to note, however, that the disease cuts across all social and economic classes, leaders as well as non-leaders. As Torrey, Way and Rowe point out in this volume the disease plays no favorites, at least among urban dwellers.

When analyzing the hollowing-out process, there is a tendency to look for factors that explain promiscuous sex lives, but in this is a serious risk of projecting age-old western sterotypes and prejudices about sexuality onto African cultures. As both Brokensha and Waite suggest there is no evidence that Africans are more likely to be sexually promiscuous than people from any other continent; it is not even essential to assume that elites are likely to be more promiscuous than others. Sexual promiscuity could produce such a hollowing-out effect in any society in which a heterosexual epidemic is not confined to small risk groups. If the elite group is small, losses from it at the same rate as from other groups could have grave consequences.

AIDS And The Economies Of Africa
Because the infection is concentrated in the 20-40 age group, AIDS is attacking the most sexually active and the most economically productive

sectors of African populations. The 20-40 age group carries an enormous economic burden in societies in which nearly 50% of the population is under 15 years of age and another segment is over 60. Both the young and the old are heavily dependent on the more productive age groups. In African societies with this kind of dependency ratio, there will be a ripple effect: as bread-winners become ill, dependent children and the aged must begin to look elsewhere for support. They, the young and the old, will not necessarily be ill themselves, but they will surely be impoverished. Such effects will be seen even if, in the long term, the dependency ratio does not change as more and more children become ill and die. For dependent people in many African nations, in which sustenance levels are often already at the margin for substantial portions of the population, this could be as fatal as the illness itself. What money bread-winners do have could easily be siphoned off in a search for cures, palliative care, and a modicum of comfort.

Reactions of governments to the spreading epidemic will have substantial effects on long-term economic and social development. Who will pay for prevention campaigns, for education and awareness programs, for condoms, for treatment, and for death and burial costs? It will cost substantial amounts of money simply to keep the prevalence of the virus at its present levels; such costs will be incurred even if no other African were ever to be infected. From what other government activities will these funds be drawn?

Many African nations spend less than $15 per capita per year on health care and the prevention of disease. Will these amounts be dramatically increased? Will these funds come from internal as well as external sources, and with what effects on other needed programs? In the most severely affected nations, one can expect governments to be compelled to spend not only much more on health but also more on police and security functions. This will mean less money for agriculture, forestry, energy, roads, water, soils, education, and other developmental costs, in nations in which such expenditures are critical to prevent further erosion of economic standing and the quality of life. Such erosion could feed the pandemic's spread and exacerbate its social consequences.

We have underscored the fact that issues about AIDS in Africa are in at least one sense more serious than they are anywhere else, because these nations have few resources to cope with the epidemic and little surplus capacity on which to draw. Nations that are already taxed by the demands they face could be woefully overextended in an effort to cope with AIDS. Given these conditions, it is unlikely that foreign aid from the developed nations can pick up a major portion of the costs.

Merritt, Lyerly, and Thomas' chapter in this volume touches on this question, posing the issue of "absorption capacity." Many donor nations already provide aid monies for African AIDS programs, as do the World Health Organization and many private voluntary organizations. These authors suggest that the effective capacity of government managers to absorb existing funds may already be stretched. New funds could exceed their capacity; if the disease itself is prevalent among them, the situation would be aggravated. But this is merely a managerial issue--a particularly ironic one when, besides African resources, it is the American staff of USAID missions that is deemed too small--and has little connection to the broader social catastrophe that could be unfolding. It may become necessary for donor nations to rethink their funding strategies and targets and to involve private voluntary organizations in their funding.

Questions For Social Analysis

Because we are in the early phases of understanding the social reality of the AIDS pandemic, this volume is more important for the questions it asks and the concepts it poses than for the data it offers. It is important that some of these questions be posed at the outset and that the authors who touch upon them in this volume be indicated. Many basic questions are addressed in several chapters.

> Down what social avenues is the disease now spreading in Africa? Which social groups are most likely to be intensely affected? What differential social impacts might be expected if the disease takes one or another path through the social structure? (Dawson, Torrey)

Is the practice of a man's having multiple sexual partners a fact in Africa, or is it part of a continuing series of Western hostile remarks about Africa? What factors are associated with the practice, not only in Africa but throughout the world? To what extent is this practice rooted not in culture and personality but in poverty and the disruption of familial and community bonds by geographic mobility? Is the solution economic rather than cultural? (Brokensha, Waite)

Many African nations have pursued a policy of clustering traditionally nomadic populations into villages. This sometimes has resulted in ecological fragility and an increase in endemic diseases such as sleeping sickness, as well as in damage to systems of social relationships and social control? Are new settlements potential foci for infections? What kinds of policy adjustments might be possible to preclude this? (Yeager)

Physicians and epidemiologists have focused on the role of other diseases in the transmission of HIV, particularly on other sexually transmitted diseases and the sores that they leave. What is the epidemiological role of cofactors rooted not in infection by other diseases but in poverty, malnutrition, and crowding? Is there evidence of higher susceptibility to infection among people living at the margin of subsistence, and is continued economic development and food assistance thus part of the solution to Africa's AIDS problems? Is the overflowing granary of the West a part of the solution to AIDS? (Haq, Torrey, et al.)

What kinds of social responses to the epidemic can be expected and what should be encouraged from different sectors of African societies, such as the individual, family, community, nation, and nongovernmental organizations, as well as the United Nations and bilateral and multilateral agencies? (Merritt, Greeley, Cowan, et al., Haslegrave)

Are African elites--who may now promote spread of the disease outside the cities by their mobility--promising targets of a focused education and prevention campaign? Given that campaigns should be designed for individual African nations and not simply as transplants of these campaigns for some developed nation, of what will these programs consist and how might they be developed and implemented by Africans for Africa? The paper by Schoepf, et al. offers some hope that intelligent and sensitive programs can be designed. (Schoepf, Merritt, et al.)

Do traditional healers, herbalists, and others who stand outside the Western medical profession have the possibility of making a singular contribution to coping with AIDS? While they are recognized as occasional agents of infection today, in the future they could equally well be mainstays of an education campaign as well as the health care system, particularly in rural areas. Western medicine's scorn and distrust of their work could undermine one of the more effective means that Africa has to cope. (Good)

What kind of information is required to permit assessment of the long-term social and economic consequences of the disease for Africa? It is clear that more is needed than records of hospital admissions and accounts of expenditures on preventions and education campaigns, but how can such data be developed for nations without substantial resources of money or personnel? Even the developed nations, with their vastly greater resources, have not been particularly successful in generating and sustaining data bases on such relatively mundane topics as the long-term effects of schooling or of unemployment. We see little sign that even the United States is developing a comprehensive social impact assessment system for its own AIDS epidemic. For a number of complicated political and cultural reasons, needed information will probably not be forthcoming in Africa either, leaving African analysts and policy makers to proceed with insufficient or even misleading information. What can be done to help Africans cope in the absence of comprehensive, reliable information and of useful forecasts of the future? (Biggar, Torrey, et al.)

How robust might African societies be in the face of losses of significant portions of the educated urban population? Are there replacements available for persons lost to the disease, or can these societies evolve different methods of filling their needs for leadership and technical skills? (Yeager)

What effects can be anticipated and what effects can be prevented concerning Africa's role in the world economy and the ability of Africans to move freely about the globe? We already hear voices urging quarantine of the entire continent and abandonment of Africa as "lost." Although such ideas derive from a fundamental lack of understanding of the scope of the pandemic in Africa, wrong ideas can carry the debate unless information is generated and effectively disseminated among policy makers. (Waite, Merritt, et al.)

Looking Ahead

This volume is designed to move from epidemiological assessments of the problem, through historic and ecological issues, to longer sections that address the management and policy questions and thereafter the social and educational questions. We have interspersed the text with a few overview pieces which set the stage and have brought in some specific case reports from Uganda and Zaire as illustrations. The final section of the book is designed as a resource guide that addresses the question "Where do we go from here?"

The language of crisis and catastrophe has permeated the discussion of AIDS in Africa. In this book the editors and contributors have tried to curb the language while not side-stepping the real problems that HIV/AIDS poses for Africa. Our hope is to stimulate interest among researchers and policy makers to confront the pandemic with greater sensitivity and more information. We would therefore consider our effort successful if, in ten years' time this set of analyses, resource guides and bibliographies has contributed in some way to improved research and an improved dialogue among Africans and between Africans and non-Africans.

PART I

Epidemiology and Current Assessment

OVERVIEW
AFRICA, AIDS, AND EPIDEMIOLOGY

Robert J. Biggar*

SUMMARY: The acquired immunodeficiency disease syndrome (AIDS) is now a well-understood disease. The clinical manifestations are due to conditions which occur in persons who are profoundly immune compromised. This suppression of the immune system is caused by a human retrovirus, the human immunodeficiency virus (HIV), and takes several years to become clinically relevant. However, in the absence of effective therapy, the condition is progressive, and no one has recovered to an immunocompetent status. We fear a very high proportion of infected persons will develop AIDS and die as a consequence. The epidemiology of AIDS and HIV in Africa is reviewed, with emphasis on the magnitude of the problem and its impact on selected population groups.

Introduction

The epidemic of acquired immunodeficiency syndrome (AIDS) has developed rapidly to involve many parts of the world and will threaten development in some areas. To understand this problem requires a brief summary of the biology and pathogenesis of this disease. As the name suggests, AIDS includes a wide range of clinical conditions that are the result of a profound suppression of the immune system. This immunosuppression is caused by infection with the human immunodeficiency virus (HIV) and is slowly progressive. Several years elapse before the immune system collapses to the point that it can no longer protect the body from common infections. At 5 years after infection, 15 to 20 percent of persons had developed AIDS illness (1,2).

*Robert J. Biggar, M.D. is the International AIDS Coordinator, Environmental Epidemiology Branch, National Cancer Institute, Bethesda, Maryland, USA. Parts of this presentation were previously published (reference 17) and are republished with the permission of the editor.

Unfortunately, however, almost all subjects in our studies who have not yet developed AIDS have clinical or laboratory evidence of immune abnormalities (3,4). Furthermore, among persons already infected with HIV when first tested (duration of infection unknown) 40 percent have developed AIDS, and the per-year risk is increasing(1). No cofactors that influence progression to immunodeficiency are known, and no one who has developed AIDS is considered to have recovered a normal immune system. Thus, we fear that a very high proportion (possibly all) of infected persons will develop AIDS given sufficient time, unless there are new breakthroughs in therapy. Recovery from the specific illness that leads to the AIDS diagnosis may occur, but the subject remains at high risk of developing second episodes or other illnesses. Survival after first AIDS diagnosis is 1 to 2 years on average (4). Drugs currently under investigation are too toxic and expensive to be considered for widespread application on a worldwide basis and their long-term efficacy remains to be proven.

HIV transmission occurs most commonly by sexual exposure or exposure to contaminated blood or blood products such as Factor VIII used to treat hemophiliacs (5). Thus, the majority of the cases have occurred in groups with lifestyles or clinical problems resulting in high risk exposures. In the United States and Europe, these have been persons with a high risk of sexual contact with an infected person (homosexual men, spouses of seropositive persons and prostitutes), intravenous drug abusers who share needles and syringes, hemophiliacs, and blood transfusion recipients. Transmission from mother to newborn also occurs. Recent data support the concept that the infectiousness of a seropositive person increases with time, being quite low initially but substantial in the period just prior to AIDS (6,7). A survey showed that among women who had regular sexual contact with a man who developed AIDS or other symptoms of immunodepression, 23 percent were seropositive (8).

AIDS In Africa

The story of the recognition of AIDS in Africa has been published elsewhere (9). When AIDS began to be recognized in Europe in 1981-82, clinicians noted that there were persons from central African countries who were coming to Europe for treatment of unusual illnesses that resembled AIDS. Subsequent on-site investigations in Africa confirmed that the AIDS-like illnesses were occurring in some areas of Africa. With the discovery of HIV, it is now clear that these cases have the same etiology. Early serological studies were confused by the presence of an unexpected high frequency of non-specific reactivity, but in studies done since 1986 this problem has been resolved by better technology.

The results of serosurveys using accurate tests have shown that HIV infection in central Africa is largely heterosexually transmitted. Evidence favoring this includes the high rate in groups at risk of venereal disease, such as prostitutes and venereal disease clinic patients (10-12), and the great concentration of HIV infected persons in the years of greatest sexual activity (15-65 year-olds) with the peak age-specific prevalence being during the years of peak sexual activity (25-29 years-old for women; 30-34 years-old for men) (12). Males and females are almost equally infected, in contrast to the usual male predominance outside of Africa. This should not be construed as evidence of equal efficiency of male-to-female and female-to-male transmission, because the data about the frequency of exposure are not available. If males were exposed much more frequently than women, the transmission rate from female-to-male would be proportionately lower than male-to-female.

Other routes of transmission certainly occur in Africa as they do elsewhere. Transfusion-transmitted AIDS must be a problem when the prevalence of HIV infection among blood donors ranges from 5 to 20 percent (12,13), and this problem will increase as the prevalence increases further, in the absence of effective donor screening programs. Likewise, where 5 to 10 percent of the antenatal clinic attendees are seropositive (12,14), a substantial amount of vertically-transmitted pediatric AIDS can be anticipated.

Needle re-use may contribute to transmission among children of seronegative mothers who are found to be seropositive (15). However, in these studies, it has been difficult to determine if the excess exposure to potentially contaminated needles was a result of treatment of AIDS-related illnesses or the cause of HIV infection. In hospital care settings in the United States, accidental percutaneous exposure to a contaminated needle rarely (perhaps 1 per 1000 episodes) results in HIV infection (16), but this is not analogous to exposure via a re-used needle through which material is being injected, which is the situation in Africa when needles are in short supply. With respect to insect-borne infection, there is no evidence that this contributes substantially to transmission, since the age distribution of HIV-infected persons is largely confined to the sexually active age groups, whereas insects bite all age groups.

The magnitude of the HIV-infection in several areas has resulted in speculation about the numbers of HIV-infected persons in Africa. All the same reservations about the dangers of extrapolating results from small and selected risk groups apply to Africa as elsewhere. But more important, in contrast to the United States and Europe, almost half of the population of Africa, both urban and rural, are children. Children over two and less than 15 years old will have a very low prevalence of HIV infection (15). The majority of those who become infected congenitally or perinatally will die with immunosuppression-related illnesses early in life, leaving only the few children who become exposed through blood products and percutaneous exposures to HIV-contaminated equipment. These will be a small fraction of all HIV-infected persons.

It is among young adults exposed through heterosexual exposure that the great majority of seropositives are found. In our survey of Lusaka, Zambia, conducted in 1985 (12), for example, HIV-antibody prevalence among healthy subsets of this population (blood donors, antenatal mothers, hospital workers) was high, reaching 25 to 30 percent in the peak 5-year age groups. However, young and middle-aged adults are only a small segment of the whole population. Adjusting the proportion of HIV-positive persons among healthy subjects to the number of persons in urban areas by that age, one can conclude that perhaps 4 to 5 percent of the urban population was HIV-infected in this central African city. If the rural prevalence is one tenth of this proportion and if Lusaka is considered representative of other urban areas of Zambia, then the total population infected in Zambia in 1985 would be less than 150,000. These calculations and a discussion of the impact of

AIDS and HIV infection on a worldwide basis have been published elsewhere (17).

By similar calculations for other central African countries in the epidemic area, I estimate that less than one million persons were seropositive in Africa in 1985. Admittedly, there are many assumptions (especially about how representative of the general population these "healthy" subjects are) in these very crude estimates, but they yield considerably less than the 20 percent of all urban residents suggested in one summary report (18). In the absence of a properly conducted random sample survey, however, there will continue to be controversy about this issue, and such surveys, not yet done in America or Europe, will be hard to do in Africa.

Projecting the future in Africa is also fraught with difficulty. The earliest serum known to be positive for HIV antibodies comes from a collection in Zaire in 1959 (19), but few large sera collections exist from any areas of Africa from the 1950's or earlier, and it cannot be certain that other areas would not have been positive as early or earlier. The most reliable longitudinal data about a population from this area come from a study of women attending an antenatal clinic in Kinshasa, Zaire. In 1970, 0.25 percent were seropositive; by 1980, 3 percent were positive and by 1986, 7 percent were positive (20). Using an exponential model, it is possible to calculate a 4.7 year doubling time (17). However, the nature of the women attending this clinic may have changed over time, which would render the accuracy of this projection suspect.

Although the numbers themselves are alarming, the type of person most likely to be HIV seropositive needs also to be considered. In particular, these are urban, young adults, more often of higher education and job rank (12). Thus, if these subjects are prematurely removed from productivity, the impact on development will be disproportionately more severe than the simple numbers indicate. On a slightly more optimistic note, however, these subjects are also the most easily reached and influenced by a public health education or intervention campaign.

In the absence of effective therapy, most of these persons will probably develop HIV-induced immunodeficiency and be at high risk of AIDS. Furthermore, in the absence of a protective vaccine that is widely distributed, HIV infection will continue to spread. The most encouraging aspect of AIDS is the international response to the problem, in which almost all countries are working together to study the illness, monitor the extent of the problem and formulate practical approaches to reducing the introduction and propagation of HIV. AIDS will continue to be a major problem, but public health and education measures have made a significant impact already and increasingly will do so in the future.

ENDNOTES

[1]Goedert JJ, Biggar RJ, Weiss Sh, *et al.*: "Three-year incidence of AIDS in five cohorts of HTLV-III-infected risk group members." *Science* 1986; 231: 992-95.

[2]Hessol NA, Rutherford GW, O'Malley PM, *et al.* "The natural history of human immunodeficiency virus infection in a cohort of homosexual and bisexual men: a 7-year prospective study." III International Conference on AIDS. Abstract M.3.1. Washington, D.C., June 1-5, 1987.

[3]Melbye M., Biggar RJ, Ebbesen P, *et al.*: "Long-term seropositivity for human T-lymphotropic virus type III in homosexual men without the acquired immunodeficiency syndrome: development of immunologic and clinical abnormalities. A longitudinal study." *Annals of Internal Medicine* 1986; 104: 496-500,

[4]Melbye M: "The natural history of human T lymphotropic virus-III infection: the cause of AIDS." *British Medical Journal* 1986; 292: 5-12.

[5]Biggar RJ: "The epidemiology of the human retroviruses and related clinical conditions." In *AIDS: Modern concepts and therapeutic challenges*, edited by S. Broder. Marcel Dekker, Inc., New York 1986; pp. 91-121.

[6]Goedert JJ, Eyster ME, Biggar RJ: "Heterosexual transmission of human immunodeficiency virus associated with severe T4-cell depletion." III International Conference on AIDS. Abstract. W.2.6. Washington D.C., June 1-5, 1987.

[7]Nzilambi N, Ryder RW, Behets F, Francis H, Bayende E, Nelson A, Mann JM *et al.*: "Perinatal HIV transmission in two African hospitals." III International Conference on AIDS. Abstract TH.7.6. Washington, D.C. June 1-5, 1987.

[8]Padian N, Marquis C, Francis DP, *et al.*: "Male-to-female transmission of human immunodeficiency virus." *Journal of the American Medical Association* 1987; 258: 788-90,

[9]Biggar RJ: "The AIDS problem in Africa." *Lancet* 1986; 1: 79-83.

[10]Kreiss JK, Koech D, Plummer FA, *et al.*: "AIDS virus infection in Nairobi prostitutes: spread of the epidemic in East Africa." *New England Journal of Medicine* 1986; 314: 414-18.

[11]Van de Perre P, Clumeck N, Carael M *et al.*: "Female prostitutes: a risk group for infection with human T-cell lymphotropic virus type III." *Lancet* 1985; 2: 525-26.

[12]Melbye M, Njelesani EK, Bayley A *et al.*: "Evidence for heterosexual transmission and clinical manifestations of human immunodeficiency virus infection and related conditions in Lusaka, Zambia." *Lancet* 1986; 2: 1113-15.

[13]Clumeck N. "Antibody to HTLV-III in blood donors in Central Africa." *Lancet* 1985; 1: 336-37.

8

[14]Quinn TC, Mann JM, Curran JW, *et al.*: "AIDS in Africa: an epidemilogic paradigm." *Science* 1986; 234: 955-63.

[15]Mann JM, Francis H, Davachi F, *et al.*: "HTLV-III/LAV seroprevalence in pediatric inpatients 2-14 years old in Kinshasa, Zaire." *Pediatrics* 1986; 78: 673-77.

[16]Weiss SH, Biggar RJ: "The epidemiology of human retrovirus-associated illnesses." *Mt. Sinai Journal of Medicine* 1986; 53: 579-91.

[17]Biggar RJ: "AIDS and HIV infection: estimates of the magnitude of the problem worldwide (1985-86)." *Clinical Immunology and Immunopathology* 1987; 45: 297-309.

[18]*The Panos Dosier: AIDS and the Third World.* The Panos Institute and the Norwegian Red Cross. London, 1986.

[19]Nahmias AJ, Weiss J, Yao X, *et al.*: Evidence of human infection with an HTLV-III/LAV-like virus in central Africa, 1959. *Lancet* 1986; 1: 1279-80.

[20]Desmyter J, Goubau P, Chamaret S, *et al.*: "Anti-LAV/HTLV-III in Kinshasa mothers in 1970 and 1980." Presented at the International Conference on AIDS, 23-25 June, 1986 (Abstract number 110).

DATA ON AIDS IN AFRICA: AN ASSESSMENT

Cynthia Haq*

SUMMARY: This survey covers selected data available at the beginning of 1988 on the epidemiology of AIDS in Africa. It is presented in tabular and graphic form, and is preceded by a brief discussion on the problem of defining AIDS.

Introduction

Accurate estimates on the scope and prevalence of AIDS in Africa are restricted by several factors. Epidemiologic research data are still primarily confined to urban areas, and research has little explored rural areas, where the majority of Africans live. AIDS is occurring in some areas where health services are unavailable, in low income areas of cities and in fringes of urban areas where many cases escape diagnosis. Finally, serologic surveys performed prior to 1985 are inaccurate due to a high incidence of false positivity.**

In spite of these limitations a broad picture of AIDS in Africa is emerging. The information below is presented in seven parts:

1. Issues of Defining AIDS and Natural Disease Progression

2. WHO Clinical Definition of AIDS

3. Prevalence of AIDS World Wide

---

*Cynthia Haq, MD is Assistant Professor of Community and Family Medicine at Dartmouth Medical School in Hanover, NH. She is a family physician and medical school instructor, and has worked in Uganda with AIDS patients.

**The specificity of HTLVIII or HIV seropositivity on ELISA testing has been questioned because 5-20% of sera collected from healthy Africans in the 1960's and early 1970's revealed positive ELISA tests with normal levels of T-helper lymphocytes. Reactivity may be affected by recurrent malaria and other parasitic diseases, or previous pregnancies. Western blot studies used to confirm these positive ELISA tests have failed to reveal specific banding patterns confirming true HIV infection. Thus while AIDS is significantly underreported from many areas, serologic surveys, inadequately confirmed in some earlier studies, may overestimate the number of HIV infected individuals.

Issues Of Definition And Disease Progression

Infection with the Human Immunodeficiency Virus (HIV), a human retrovirus, can result in a spectrum of illnesses, the end stage of which is AIDS. The major problem in AIDS is progressive immune suppression which results in increasing susceptibility to opportunistic infections, malignancies, and eventual death.[2]

Infection with HIV virus does not necessarily result in AIDS. It can range from an absence of symptoms, through mild illness to fatal disease. Most people presently infected with the HIV virus show an absence of symptoms. (Figure 1)[3]

The Centers for Disease Control (CDC) in the United States has classified the clinical features of HIV infection into four categories:

I.   Initial infection with the virus and development
            of antibodies
II   Asymptomatic carrier state
III.   Persistent generalized lymphadenopathy
IV.   Other HIV-related disease including AIDS[4]

The majority of people infected with the virus develop antibodies (seropositivity) within 2-8 weeks of initial infection. A minority develop an acute, short-term illness within weeks of initial infection, with rare neurological symptoms. During the asymptomatic carrier state a reduced number of T-helper lymphocytes may be present. Various terms have been used for the stage of development of symptoms, including persistent generalized lymphadenopathy, AIDS-prodrome, AIDS related conditions, and AIDS related complex (ARC). Persistent generalized lymphadenopathy is defined as swollen lymph glands in two sites other than the groin for more than three months. It may or may not be associated with symptoms of night sweats, fever, diarrhea, or infections with oral candidiasis (Thrush) or herpes zoster (Shingles).[5]

Figure 1

Natural History of Infection with HIV

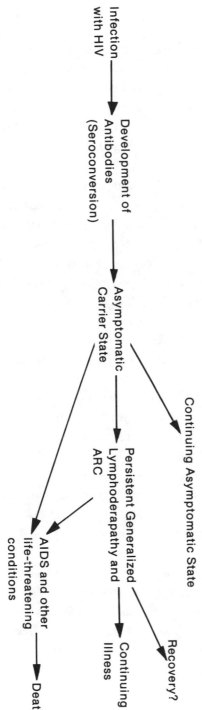

Infection with HIV ⟶ Development of Antibodies (Seroconversion) ⟶ Asymptomatic Carrier State

Continuing Asymptomatic State ⟶ Recovery?

Persistent Generalized Lymphoderapathy and ARC ⟶ Continuing Illness

AIDS and other life-threatening conditions ⟶ Death

SOURCE:
Adapted from Bartlett.[3]

Patients with ARC show symptoms, signs and immunologic defects similar to patients with AIDS, but less severe. Neither opportunistic infection nor malignant lesion can be diagnosed in ARC patients. Signs and symptoms in ARC patients include malaise, anorexia, abdominal pain, fever, headache and lymphadenopathy. Persistent diarrhea is one of the major complaints. Weight loss is found in all patients and is generally progressive. Skin lesions are common.[6]

The rate of progression from the asymptomatic carrier state to persistent generalized lymphadenopathy, ARC or AIDS, has not been extensively studied, but rates in Africa seem to be similar to or lower than reports from the United States. Rates of progression over one year in 125 asymptomatic seropositive hospital personnel in Kinshasa, Zaire showed generalized lymphadenopathy or ARC developed in 10% and AIDS in 1%.[7] Other studies in Africa as well as the United States have shown that per year AIDS develops in 2-5% of HIV-infected persons, regardless of rate of infection or lifestyle.[6]

AIDS is the end stage of HIV infection. It is characterized by life-threatening opportunistic infections and/or cancers without other explanations for immunodeficiencies and eventual death. The spectrum of symptoms and opportunistic infections varies geographically. In Africa the most common opportunistic infections are tuberculosis, cryptococcal meningitis, herpes simplex infection, oral or esophageal candidiasis, cryptosporidiosis, central nervous system toxoplasmosis, and skin rashes. Chronic diarrhea and weight loss are quite common. Pneumocystis carinii pneumoni is less common than the United States. Kaposi's sarcoma is the most common malignancy occurring in patients with AIDS, and in Africa occurs in 2-20% of patients.[5]

AIDS has been defined by the CDC and the World Health Organization (WHO) by strict serologic and clinical criteria. The CDC definition briefly consists of serologic evidence of HIV infection, one or more opportunistic infections (protozoal, fungal, bacterial, viral infections or cancers are specified) with exclusion of known causes of immune suppression.[8]

Figure 2

Provisional WHO Clinical Case Definition of AIDS
(Bangui Workshop Criteria)[8]

Adults

AIDS in an adult is defined by the existence of at least 2 of the major signs associated with at least one minor sign, in the absence of known causes of immunosuppression such as cancer or severe malnutrition or other recognized etiologies.

1. Major signs
   (a) weight loss > 10% of body weight;
   (b) chronic diarrhea >1 month;
   (c) prolonged fever >1 month (intermittent or constant)

2. Minor signs
   (a) persistent cough for >1 month;
   (b) generalized pruritic dematitis;
   (c) recurrent herpes zoster;
   (d) oro-pharyngeal candidiasis;
   (e) chronic progressive and disseminated herpes simplex infection;
   (f) generalized lymphadenopathy.

The presence of generalized Kaposi's sarcoma or cryptococcal meningitis are sufficient by themselves for the diagnosis of AIDS.

Children

Pediatric AIDS is suspected in an infant or child displaying at least 2 of the following major signs associated with at least 2 of the following minor signs in the absence of known cases of immunosuppression such as cancer or severe malnutrition or other recognized etiologies.

1. Major signs
   (a) weight loss or abnormally slow growth;
   (b) chronic diarrhea >1 month;
   (c) prolonged fever > 1 month.

2. Minor signs
   (a) generalized lymphadenopathy;
   (b) oro-pharyngeal candidiasis;
   (c) repeated common infections (otitis, pharyngitis, etc.);
   (d) persistent cough;
   (e) generalized dermatitis;
   (f) confirmed maternal LAV/HTLV-III infection.

For use in areas where diagnostic resources are limited, the WHO developed a provisional case definition for AIDS at a workshop in Bangui, Central African Republic. (Figure 2)[8]

Studies in Zaire have shown that only about 59% of the persons identified by the Bangui definition, as having AIDS do have HIV infection, but that the definition picks up about 90% of infected ill persons. False positives with the clinical case definition are often due to the presence of tuberculosis which coexists in many areas of Africa and may occur with similar symptoms.[9] Due to the lack of diagnostic facilities, clinical case reports of AIDS by CDC-WHO criteria tend to be much less frequent than reports of AIDS based on the Bangui clinical case definition. A study of patients in the Central African Republic revealed that cases of AIDS based on HIV seroprevalence rates were severely underreported (only 13% of predicted) when strict CDC-WHO criteria were used. When the clinical case definition was used the majority (80%) of predicted cases were diagnosed.[10] The low numbers of AIDS cases diagnosed on the basis of CDC criteria may partly explain the low numbers of AIDS cases reported from countries where HIV seroprevalence is relatively high.

Prevalence Of AIDS World Wide

The WHO has estimated that world wide 5-10 million people are infected with the HIV, and that 1-2 million may be infected in Africa alone.[11] Estimates of numbers infected with HIV vary widely however, and documented global cases of AIDS are much lower. (Table 1)[12] Reported cases of AIDS represent only the tip of the iceberg of people currently infected with HIV. (Figure 3)[11]

Reported AIDS Cases And Incidence Rates, Africa, 1988

The number of reported cases of AIDS from African countries as of January, 1988 is shown in Table 2 with total and urban populations and rate per 100,000 population. AIDS case reports to WHO are based on physician diagnosis, CDC/WHO definition and Bangui definition. Not all countries

Table 1

AIDS Cases Reported by Year to WHO
(as of October, 1987)[12]

CONTINENT	?	1979	1980	1981	1982	1983	1984	1985	1986	1987	TOTAL
Africa	0	0	0	0	3	14	82	185	3,111	2,435	5,830
Americas	172	14	55	273	1,053	3,183	6,236	10,893	15,559	10,819	48,257
Asia	0	0	1	0	1	8	4	29	54	108	205
Europe	14	0	3	13	69	215	573	1,341	2,477	2,770	7,475
Oceania	0	0	0	0	1	6	45	124	239	263	678
TOTAL	186	14	59	286	1,127	3,426	6,940	12,572	21,440	16,395	62,445

Figure 3

Estimated Numbers of Persons with AIDS,
with Other Symptomatic HIV Infection, and of
Asymptomatic HIV Carriers, World, 1987

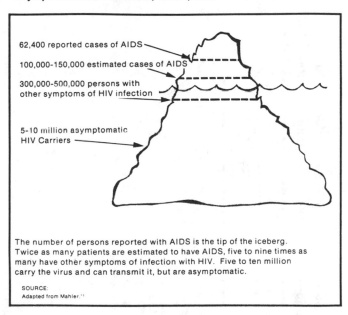

62,400 reported cases of AIDS

100,000-150,000 estimated cases of AIDS

300,000-500,000 persons with other symptoms of HIV infection

5-10 million asymptomatic HIV Carriers

The number of persons reported with AIDS is the tip of the iceberg.
Twice as many patients are estimated to have AIDS, five to nine times as
many have other symptoms of infection with HIV. Five to ten million
carry the virus and can transmit it, but are asymptomatic.

SOURCE:
Adapted from Mahler.[11]

Table 2

Reported AIDS Cases and Incidence Rates, National and Urban, for African Countries: 1987

Country	Reported AIDS Cases	1987 Population (in thousands)	National Incidence Rate (per 100,000 population)	1987 Urban Population (in thousands)	Urban Incidence Rate (per 100,000 population)
Algeria	5	23,461	.02	11,731	.04
Angola	6	7,950	.08	2,100	.29
Benin	3	4,339	.07	1,676	.18
Botswana	13	1,149	1.13	246	5.29
Burkina Faso	0	8,276	.00	699	.00
Burundi	569	5,006	11.37	322	176.91
Cameroon	25	10,255	.24	4,709	.53
Cape Verde	4	344	1.16	19	21.12
Central African Rep.	254	2,669	9.52	1,188	21.39
Chad	1	4,646	.02	1,401	.07
Comoros	0	415	.00	110	.00
Congo	250	2,082	12.01	850	29.39
Djibouti	0	312	.00	247	.00
Egypt	1	51,930	.00	24,703	.00
Ethiopia	5	46,709	.01	5,717	.09
Gabon	13	1,044	1.25	452	2.88
Gambia	14	760	1.84	162	8.66
Ghana	145	13,949	1.04	4,501	3.22
Guinea	4	6,738	.06	1,611	.25
Guinea Bissau	16	928	1.72	268	5.96
Ivory Coast	250	10,767	2.32	4,769	5.24

Kenya	964	22,378	4.31	4,837	19.93
Lesotho	1	1,622	.06	300	.33
Liberia	2	2,384	.08	996	.20
Madagascar	0	10,731	.00	2,511	.00
Malawi	13	7,438	.17	997	1.30
Mali	0	8,423	.00	1,564	.00
Mauritania	0	1,863	.00	715	.00
Mauritius	1	1,080	.09	456	.22
Mozambique	1	14,536	.01	3,212	.03
Nigeria	5	108,620	.00	26,655	.02
Reunion	1	550	.18	340	.29
Rwanda	705	6,811	10.35	473	149.04
Sao Tome & Principe	0	114	.00	46	.00
Senegal	27	7,064	.38	2,641	1.02
Seychelles	0	68	.00	36	.00
South Africa	84	34,313	.24	19,625	.43
Sudan	12	23,525	.05	5,017	.24
Swaziland	7	715	.98	212	3.30
Tanzania	1,608	23,502	6.84	6,061	26.53
Togo	0	3,229	.00	773	.00
Tunisia	2	7,562	.03	4,447	.04
Uganda	2,369	15,909	14.89	1,601	147.95
Zaire	335	32,343	1.04	12,307	2.72
Zambia	395	7,282	5.42	3,825	10.33
Zimbabwe	380	9,372	4.05	2,442	15.56

SOURCES:

AIDS Cases: Cases of AIDS reported to the World Health Organization as of December 22, 1987.
Population: U.S. Bureau of the Census, World Population Profile: 1987, TAble WP70176— ;
Estimated and Projected Population and Growth Rates: Selected Years, 1982 to 1990, forthcoming.

Table 3

Incidence of HIV: Selected African Sites

Country	Year of Study	Geographic Area	Population Subgroup	Sample Size	Number of Cases	Incidence Rate	Type of Test	Comments	Source
Central African Rep.	1987	Bangui	Random	383	30	7.83	ELISA,WB		13
Central African Rep.	'84-'87	Labaye, Sangha	Pygmy	782	1	0.1	ELISA,WB		14
Congo	1986	Brazzaville	Randomly Selected Citizens	368	18	5	Unknown		15
Ethiopia	'85-'86	National	Recruits and Outpatients	5606	4	0.07	ELISA,WB		16
Gabon	1986	Idgodue-Ivind	Symptomless Subjects	360	0	0	ELISA,WB	Rural North	17
Gabon	1986	Libreville	Symptomless Subjects	383	7	1.80	ELISA,WB		17
Ghana	1987	National	Blood Donors Sickle Cell Anemia Pts. and others	771	36	4.67	ELISA,WB IFA	Excludes Prostitutes	18
Ghana	1987	National	Prostitutes	226	57	25.22	ELISA,WB IFA		18
Kenya	1986	Nairobi	Medical Personnel	42	1	2.38	ELISA,WB		19
Kenya	1986	Nairobi	Prostitutes	90	50	56.6	ELISA,WB		19
Mauritania	1986	Nouakchott	Hospital Adults and Patients	356	2	0.56	ELISA,WB		20

Country	Year	Location	Group	N	Positive	%	Test	Ref
Nigeria	1986	Lagos	Blood Donors	124	8	6.4	ELISA	21
Nigeria	1986	Lagos	School Children	52	0	0	ELISA	21
Rwanda	1985	Kigali	Young Adults	302	53	17.5	ELISA	22
Rwanda	1985	Rural Area	Young Adults	206	6	3	ELISA	22
Rwanda	1985	Kigali	Prostitutes	84	67	80	ELISA,WB	23
Tanzania	1986	Dar Es Salaam	Pregnant	192	7	3.6	ELISA,WB	24
Tanzania	1986	Bukoba	Pregnant	100	16	16.00	ELISA,WB	24
Tanzania	1986	Bukoba	Blood Donors	36	5	14.00	ELISA,WB	24
Uganda	1985	Rakai District	Healthy Controls	410	41	10	ELISA	25
Uganda	1986	Kampala	Pregnant	1000	130	13.00	ELISA,WB	26
Uganda	1987	Kampala	Pregnant	170	41	24	ELISA,WB	26
Uganda	1987	National	Prostitutes	226	57	25.22	ELISA,WB	26
Zaire	1986	Kinshasa	Mothers	529	32	6	ELISA,IFA	27
Zaire	1986	Kinshasa	Pediatric Hospitalized Patients	368	40	11	ELISA,WB	28
Zambia	1986	Lusaka	STD Clinic Patients	144	42	29.2	ELISA,WB	29
Zambia	1986	Lusaka	Skin Clinic Patients	56	15	26.8	ELISA,WB	29
Zambia	1986	Lusaka	Antenatal Clinic	184	16	8.7	ELISA,WB	29
Zambia	1986	Lusaka	Surgery Pts.	111	23	20.7	ELISA,WB	29
Zambia	1986	Lusaka	Medicine Pts.	233	32	13.7	ELISA,WB	29
Zambia	1986	Lusaka	Blood Donors	207	38	18.4	ELISA,WB	29
Zambia	1986	Lusaka	Hospital Workers	100	19	19	ELISA,WB	29

report AIDS to the WHO, and in many cases AIDS reporting is incomplete due to limited access to health care. Countries reporting zero cases of AIDS may be reflecting these factors, rather than an absence of AIDS. Limitations of surveillance, clinical definitions and underreporting contribute to the underestimation of AIDS in Africa.

The greatest number of AIDS cases currently reported exist in Central and East Africa, with significant numbers also present in West Africa. Reported cases from North and South Africa currently are low.

Incidence Of HIV, Selected African Sites

Incidence rates of HIV seropositivity from selected sites are illustrated in Table 3.[13-29]

While several population based studies have been performed, it is important to keep in mind the limitations of these data. Most surveys have occurred in urban areas where HIV prevalence rates are felt to be much higher than in rural districts. Many have been performed only in high risk populations. Extrapolation of these figures to general prevalence rates for regions of Africa is difficult if not impossible. For a more detailed analysis of prevalence rates see the following article by Barbara Torrey, *et al*.

The selected incidence data again show a higher rate of HIV infection in Central and East Africa, roughly corresponding to prevalence rates of AIDS reported from these countries. Rates are much lower in rural populations that are relatively isolated, such as the pygmy in the Central African Republic. In most countries where incidence rates can be compared between urban and rural populations (i.e., Rwanda), HIV incidence is higher in urban regions. Rates are also greater among high risk populations such as prostitutes, clients of sexually transmitted disease clinics, and hospitalized patients. Lower rates are seen in school-aged children.

Risk Factors For HIV Infection

In Africa, as in the rest of the world, HIV is transmitted primarily through sexual activity and exposure to contaminated blood. Heterosexual transmission is the primary route of transmission in Africa (see the previous article by Biggar). Incidence rates reported are highest in sexually active adults and in groups with multiple sexual partners (prostitutes and male clients). A nearly equal male and female incidence rate confirms heterosexual transmission. Heterosexual risk factors include having a number of sexual partners, being a prostitute, having sex with a prostitute, and being the sexual partner of an infected person. Seropositivity among Nairobi prostitutes has been found to be significantly associated with sexually transmitted diseases such as gonorrhea, genital ulcers, and syphilis. Seropositivity among men in Zambia has also been correlated with the presence of genital ulcers.[30] Homosexual activity and oral intercourse is rarely reported in most geographic areas of Africa. Supporting these observations is the fact that if homosexual transmission played an important role a higher male prevalence would be expected.

The HIV seroprevalence rate among male and female patients by age group is seen in Table 4 for Kinshasha, Zaire[29] and Lusaka, Zambia.[30] Both of these studies were performed in urban areas and illustrate similar patterns of infection. The prevalence among men and women is similar, with peak prevalence at an earlier age among women, corresponding with a younger age of peak sexual activity. An older age of peak prevalence is seen in males. The prevalence rate seen in infants (8%) is similar to that seen in women during their reproductive years (6-10%). A low prevalence exists in children age 1 to 15 and adults over age 50.

The proportion of estimated seropositive subjects in Zambia is contrasted with the total population distribution in Figure 4.[31] One can see from the figure that even though a substantial proportion of the population of Zambia is estimated to be infected with HIV, infected individuals are primarily adults and a minority of the overall population distribution. In Zambia, as in most African populations, nearly half of the population is under 15 years of age and at low risk of AIDS through heterosexual contact. Elderly persons comprise only a small segment of HIV infected individuals.

Transmission through contaminated blood has been confirmed following blood transfusions in multiple African sites. The high prevalence of HIV infection in blood donors and lack of effective screening programs

Table 4

HIV Prevalence Rate Among "Low Risk" Groups, by Age and Sex for Kinshasa and Lusaka

City, Year, and Age	HIV Prevalence Rate (percent)	
	Male	Female
Kinshasa, 1984-85[29]		
0 to 0.9 years	8.1	8.1
1 to 1.9 years	0.9	1.8
2 to 14 years	1.0	1.5
15 to 19 years	3.7	9.8
20 to 29 years	4.4	10.3
30 to 39 years	6.8	6.1
40 to 49 years	5.0	6.3
50 years and over	5.0	1.6
TOTAL, all ages	5.0	6.9
Lusaka, 1985[30]		
15 to 19 years	0.0	0.0
20 to 24 years	16.1	27.8
25 to 29 years	17.9	25.0
30 to 34 years	25.0	16.7
34 to 44 years	16.7	7.7
45 to 54 years	0.0	0.0
55 to 64 years	0.0	0.0
TOTAL, 15 years and over	17.2	21.2

Figure 4

Population Distribution of Zambia and HIV Infection

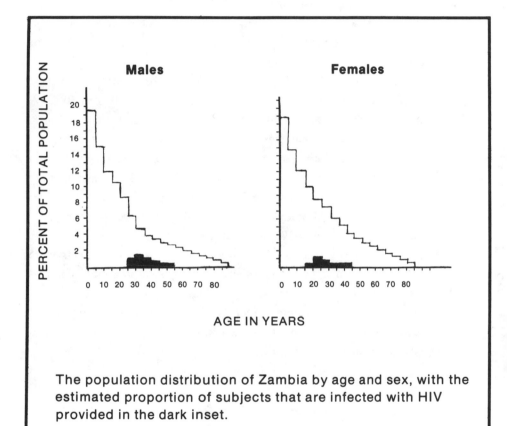

The population distribution of Zambia by age and sex, with the estimated proportion of subjects that are infected with HIV provided in the dark inset.

SOURCE:

Adapted from Biggar[31]

contribute to high prevalence rates in hospitalized patients. The re-use of contaminated needles and other medical equipment has also been associated with HIV infection. A survey of 368 pediatric hospitalized patients in Kinshasha, Zaire revealed an 11% seroprevalence rate. Seropositivity of children with seronegative mothers was found to be significantly associated with receipt of a blood transfusion, receipt of medical injections, and previous hospitalization.[28] There has been no demonstration of transmission of HIV by immunizations.

Transmission rates of HIV infection from infected mothers to their infants are not precisely known but estimated to range from 20 to 50%. A study of 191 children 2-24 months of age in Kinshasha, Zaire revealed 61% of seropositive children had seropositive mothers.[32] The majority of maternal to infant transmissions are believed to occur prenatally, though transmission at the time of delivery and through breast milk may also occur.

Casual contact or even close family contact has not been shown to transmit HIV infection. A study of 46 patients with AIDS and 204 household contacts in Zaire revealed 61% of spouses of patients with AIDS to have HIV seropositivity, but only 4.8% of nonspouse household contacts were infected. The rate of HIV seropositivity in nonspouse household contacts was not elevated when compared to seroprevalence rates of control subjects.[33] Age and sex prevalence rates do not support any insect transmission of HIV infection. There is also no evidence of spread through food, beverages or shared living spaces.

Longitudinal Prevalence Rates

Serial serological surveys of HIV infection have been performed in few African sites. Data shown in Table 5 show evidence of rapid increase in infection, particularly in high risk populations.[10,30,34,35] The increase in HIV seroprevalence in randomly selected adults in the CAR from 2% in 1985 to nearly 8% in 1987 demonstrates the rapid dissemination of HIV infection among an urban population. The increase in HIV seroprevalence among Nairobi prostitutes from 4% in 1981 to 61% in 1985 demonstrates the increase in a high risk population group.

Table 5

Prevalence of Antibody to HIV in Selected Populations Between 1980 and 1987, Number Positive/Number Tested, (%)

COUNTRY	SITE	POPULATION	1980	1981	1982	1983	1984	1985	1986	1987	SOURCE
Central African Republic	Bangui	Randomly Selected Adults						7/323 (2.1)	36/941 (3.8)	30/383 (7.8)	10
Kenya	Nairobi	Prostitutes		5/116 (4)		32/39 (82)	45/76 (59)	174/286 (61)			34
Kenya	Nairobi	Men with STDs	0/118	2/170 (3)	4/168 (6)	13/93 (14)		29/194 (15)			34
Kenya	Nairobi	Pregnant Women	0/111					22/1,110 (2)			34
Zaire	Kinshasha	Pregnant Women		15/500 (3)					36/449 (8)		30
Zaire	Equateur	Rural Randomly Selected Adults	1976 5/659 (0.8)						1986 3/388 (0.8)		35

By contrast, serial surveys performed in rural Zaire show no increase in HIV seroprevalence among randomly selected adults over a period of 10 years. HIV infection and AIDS may have existed and remained stable in Africa for a long period of time.[35]

Sequential serosurveys have revealed a possible mechanism of heterosexual spread in Africa. In traditional rural areas HIV seroprevalence rates have remained stable. In urban areas, however, seroprevalence rates have risen as much as 1% per year. Several African studies have shown that seropositive results are often first documented in female prostitutes, especially those in contact with men from other HIV-endemic areas. After rates in prostitutes rise, seropositivity rates in male patients of sexually transmitted disease clinics rise. Subsequently, rates begin to rise in pregnant women, and the general population.[9]

Conclusion

The data presented illustrate the complexity of clearly defining the epidemiology of AIDS in Africa. Marked underreporting, shifting definitions, and incomplete serological surveys leave many unanswered questions. Improved disease surveillance systems are needed to accurately assess the number of HIV infected individuals and persons with AIDS, to record the natural history of the disease and monitor the impact of prevention programs. More information is needed on the accuracy and practicality of diagnosing AIDS based on CDC/WHO and Bangui clinical criteria. The importance of risk factors such as sexually transmitted diseases, and possible co-factors for HIV infection over time in low, intermediate and high risk population groups is just beginning to emerge. As the picture of AIDS in Africa becomes more clearly defined, the numbers will continue to grow and change.

ENDNOTES

[1]Biggar Robert J.: "The AIDS problem in Africa," *The Lancet*, 1(8472):79-83, January 11, 1986.

[2]Fischinger P, "AIDS," *Current Probs CA*, Vol. 9, p. 4-36, January, 1985.

[3]Bartlett JG: "HTLV-III infection: medical management." Presented at symposium, Clinical Update on AIDS, Johns Hopkins Medical Institutions, November 18, 1985.

[4]United States Centers for Disease Control, "Classification system for human T-lymphotropic virus type III/lymphadenopathy-associated virus infections." *Morbidity and Mortality Weekly Report* 35(20):334-39, May 23, 1986.

[5]*Population Reports*: "AIDS--A Public Health Crisis," Series L, Number 6, Vol. XIV:3, L193-L228, July-August, 1986.

[6]Piot P and Colebunders R: "Clinical Manifestations and the Natural History of HIV infection in Adults," *Western Journal of Medicine*, 147(6)709-712, December, 1987.

[7]Mann JN, Colebunders RL, *et al*.: "Natural History of human Immunodeficiency Virus Infection in Zaire," *The Lancet*, Vol. 8509:11, p. 707, September 27, 1986.

[8]*Weekly Epidemiology Record*: "Acquired Immunodeficiency Syndrome (AIDS)." World Health Organization, 61(10):69-73, 7 March 1986, No. 10.

[9]Van Reyn CF and Mann JM: "Global Epidemiology, AIDS A Global Perspective." *Western Journal of Medicine*, 147(6)694-701, December, 1987.

[10]Georges AJ, *et al*.: "HIVI Seroprevalence and AIDS Diagnostic Criteria in Central African Republic," *Lancet*, Vol. 8571.11, 1332-33, December 5, 1987.

[11]Mahler H. Opening speech. Presented at International Conference on AIDS, Paris, p. 5, June 23-25, 1986.

[12]AIDS Cases Reported to WHO, Appendix 2, "AIDS: a Global Perspective", *Western Journal of Medicine*, 147(6)738, December, 1987.

[13]Martin PWV, Georges-Courbot MC and Georges AJ: "Tentative Determination of AIDS Incidence and Risk Factors in the CAR," Second International Symposium on AIDS in Africa, Naples, Italy, October 7-9, Abstract, TH-26, 1987.

[14]Gonzelez, JP, *et al*.: "True HIV-I Infection in a Pygmy," *The Lancet*, Vol. 8548:1, 1499, June 27, 1987.

[15]Blaine H.: "AIDS Seen as Threat to Africa's Future," *The Washington Post*, p. A1 and A18, May 31, 1987.

[16]Butto S., Hailu K, Bekura D. *et al.* "Serological Study on the Presence of HIV in Ethiopia," Second International Symposium on AIDS in Africa, Naples, Italy, Abstract, TH-90, October 709, 1987.

[17]Delaporte E. Dupont A, Merlin M, *et al.* "Prevalence Rates on Antibodies to HIV1 and HIV2 in Population Samples From Gabon", Second International Symposium on AIDS in Africa, Naples, Italy, Abstract, TH-29, October 7-9, 1987.

[18]Mingle JAA, Hayami M. Osei-Kwasi M, *et al.* "Reactivity of Ghanaian Sera to Human Immunodeficiency Virus, and Simian T-Lymphotropic Virus III," III International Conference on AIDS, Washington, DC, Abstract, p. 25, June 1-5, 1987.

[19]Kreiss JK, Koegh D, Plummer FA, *et al.* "AIDS Virus Infection in Nairobi Prostitutes," *The New England Journal of Medicine*, Vol. 314(7):414-18, February 13, 1986.

[20]M'Boup S, Ricard D, Danki P, *et al.* "HIV Seroprevalence in Nouakchott (Islamic Republic of Mauritania)", Second International Symposium on AIDS in Africa, Naples, Italy, Abstract, TH-4, October 7-9, 1987.

[21]Williams CK: "AIDS and Cancer in Nigeria," Vol. 8471:1,36-37, *The Lancet*, January 4, 1986.

[22]Van de Perre P, Kanyamupira JB, Carael M, *et al*.: "Urban Sexuality Changing Patterns in Central Africa: Social Determinants of HTLV-III Transmission," Unpublished, 1986.

[23]Clumeck N, Robert-Guroff M, Van de Perre P, *et al*.: "Seroepidemiological Studies of HTLV-III Antibody Prevalence Among Selected Groups of Heterosexual Africans," *JAMA*, Vol. 254, No. 18, pg. 2599-2602, November 8, 1985.

[24]Mhalu F, Mbena E, Bredberg-Raden U, *et al*.: "Prevalence of HIV Antibodies in Healthy Subjects and Groups of Patients in Some Parts of Tanzania 1987," III International Conference on AIDS, Washington, DC, Abstract, p. 76, June 105, 1987.

[25]Serwadda D., Sewankambo RK, Carswell JW, *et al*.: "Slim Disease: A New Disease in Uganda and Its Association With HTLV-III Infection," *The Lancet*, Vol. 8571:11,849-52, Saturday, 19 October 1985.

[26]Blain H: "AIDS Seen as Threat To Africa's Future," *The Washington Post*, p. A1 and A18, May 31, 1987.

[27]Desmyter J, *et al*.: "Anti-LAV/HTLVIII in Kinshasha Mothers in 1970 and 1980." Presented at the International Conference on AIDS, Paris (notes) June 23-25, 1986.

[28]Mann J and Francis H, *et al*.: "Human Immunodeficiency Virus Seroprevalence in Pediatric Patients 2 to 14 Years of Age at Mena Yemo Hospital, Kinshasha, Zaire." *Pediatrics*, Vol. 78(4)p. 673-677, October 1986.

[29]Melbye, Bayle, Manuwele, *et al*.: "Evidence for Heterosexual Transmission And Clinical Manifestations of Human Immunodeficiency Virus Infection And Related Conditions In Lusaka, Zambia," *The Lancet*, Vol. 8516:11; 1113-15, Saturday, 15 November 1986.

[30]Quinn TC: "AIDS in Africa: An Epidemiologic Paradigm," *Science*, (234), 955-63, November, 1986.

[31]Biggar RJ: "AIDS and HIV Infection: Estimates of the Magnitude of the Problem Worldwide in 1985/1986," *Clinical Immunology and Immunopathology*, 45, 297-309 (1987).

[32]Mann JM, *et al*: "Risk Factors for Human Immunodeficiency Virus Seropositivity Among Children 1-24 Months Old in Kinshasha, Zaire," *Lancet*, Vol. 654-56, September 20, 1986.

[33]Mann JM, *et al*.: "Prevalence of HTLVIII/LAV in Household Contents of Patients with Confirmed AIDS and Controls in Kinshasha, Zaire," *JAMA*, 256:6, 721-24, August 8, 1986.

[34]Piot P, *et al*.: "Retrospective Seroepidemiology of AIDS Virus Infection in Nairobi Populations," *Journal of Infectious Diseases*, 115:6, 1108-12. June, 1987.

[35]Nzilambi N, *et al*.: "The Prevalence of Infection with Human Immunodeficiency Virus over a 10-Year Period in Rural Zaire," *New England Journal of Medicine*, 318:276-79, February 4, 1988.

EPIDEMIOLOGY OF HIV AND AIDS IN AFRICA: EMERGING ISSUES AND SOCIAL IMPLICATIONS

Barbara Boyle Torrey

Peter O. Way

Patricia M. Rowe*

SUMMARY: Although no nationally representative sample survey of HIV seroprevalence yet exists in Africa, the combined results of many small-scale surveys do indicate a number of patterns. In Africa, men and women have similar HIV seroprevalence rates, although the women tend to be somewhat younger; HIV seroprevalence is much higher in urban than in rural areas and prostitutes have much higher rates than other adults. These differential infection rates raise a number of issues that social scientists need to address. This essay surveys many of the basic findings of epidemiological studies and concludes with a focus on some of these issues from a social science perspective.

Introduction

Most of the great plagues of world history ran their course only after the vulnerable population had been infected and the rest of the population had developed immunity. Epidemiological information needed to identify and contain an infectious disease was rarely used until the 19th century when John Snow plotted the cholera epidemic in London. By the 20th century the understanding of the epidemiology of smallpox and other infectious diseases helped lead to their containment or eradication. Now the emergence of AIDS poses a new epidemiological challenge that is particularly acute in Africa.

---

  * **Barbara Boyle Torrey**, M.A., Chief, Center for International Research, U.S. Bureau of the Census, specialized in Economic Development at Stanford University. **Peter O. Way,** Ph.D., Chief, Africa and Latin America Branch, Center for International Research, U.S. Bureau of the Census, was trained in sociology at the University of Chicago. **Patricia M. Rowe,** M.A., Section Chief, Africa and Latin America Branch, Center for International Research, U.S. Bureau of the Census specialized in demography at Georgetown University. The views herein are those of the authors and do not necessarily represent the views of the U.S. Bureau of the Census.

Containing the HIV virus, which causes AIDS, will depend in part on an accurate understanding of its distribution among various populations. The present data are so fragmentary that a comprehensive epidemiological description is not yet possible. However, this chapter uses the existing data on HIV to begin to sketch the outlines of its epidemiology in Africa. Comparisons of the incidence of reported AIDS cases with the seroprevalence of HIV in healthy adults in urban areas indicate that the reported AIDS cases are telling us far less about the future than we need to know today.

The chapter compares estimated seroprevalence rates with regard to:

–differences between the genders by age;
–differences between urban and rural areas; and
–differences among different risk groups in a geographic area.

It concludes with a focus on the social issues that the present data raise.[1]

Reported AIDS Cases And Estimated HIV Prevalence:
Limitations And Comparisons

Following an initial period of sensitivity and reluctance, information on cases of AIDS is now being reported to the World Health Organization (WHO) by nearly all countries. However, for a number of reasons these reports should not be considered complete, nor even representative of the actual situation in particular countries. Among the reasons for caution are the following:

–As Cynthia Haq notes, in this volume, AIDS presents itself in a variety of ways, and the disease may go unrecognized, even by trained medical personnel.
–In most African countries, systems for reporting diseases and deaths are severely lacking--the majority of cases are probably not reported.
–The reported numbers of cases are not reflections even of the cases diagnosed because of internal reporting delays and because some countries report to WHO only infrequently.
–Care should be taken in comparing reported cases for African countries with numbers for the United States or European countries due to differences in the diagnostic criteria used. A recent report from the Central African Republic suggested that only 17 percent (99 cases) of the 587 AIDS cases reported in Bangui would have been diagnosed as AIDS had the more

restrictive U.S. Centers for Disease Control (CDC) criteria
been used, rather than the Bangui Workshop African Criteria.[2]
The total extent of the underreporting of AIDS cases is unknown but will
presumably decrease with time as the medical establishments in every
country focus on this epidemic. However, even if the reporting of AIDS
improves greatly, incidence estimates only reflect the present medical
situation in a country. The long average incubation period between initial
HIV infection and the development of AIDS means that the patterns of HIV
infection in a population provide a window on the future of the epidemic.

No single number can adequately represent the widely variant
patterns of HIV infection that currently exist in many African populations.
As with any epidemic, the disease is transmitted from the infected to the
susceptible population. The WHO has characterized three patterns of HIV
transmission, based on available epidemiological studies.[3]

Pattern 1--Most cases of AIDS occur among homosexual and
bisexual males and intravenous drug users. Heterosexual
transmission is responsible for only a small but increasing
proportion of the total. As a result, the infected are
overwhelmingly male and perinatal transmission is limited.
National seroprevalence overall is probably less than 1 percent,
but may exceed 50 percent among some groups practicing high-
risk behaviors. The United States, most European countries,
and some Latin American countries appear to follow this
pattern.
Pattern 2--Most cases of AIDS occur among heterosexuals.
The male-to-female ratio is approximately 1, and perinatal
transmission is common. Infections related to intravenous
drug abuse or homosexual contact are rare. National
seroprevalence may be above 1 percent, and in some urban
areas up to 15 percent of the sexually active young adult
population is infected. Most African countries and several
Latin American countries appear to follow this pattern.
Pattern 3--HIV has only recently been introduced to these
countries. The majority of cases originate outside the country,
and a strong homosexual or heterosexual pattern has not
emerged. The majority of Asian countries, countries in
northern Africa, and most countries in Oceania currently fall
into this pattern.

In Africa today, heterosexual contact is almost certainly the most
important form of HIV transmission. Consequently, population subgroups
characterized by multiple sexual partners (for example, prostitutes and their

Table 1

Comparison of AIDS Incidence Rates and HIV Seroprevalence Rates for Selected African Countries

Country	AIDS Urban Incidence Rate (per 100,000 population)	HIV Seroprevalence Rate for Healthy Adults in the Capital City (percent)	Source For Prevalence Data
Rwanda	149.0	17.5 (1985)	V0001
Uganda	148.0	13.6 (1986)	H0003
Congo	29.4	7.6 (1986-87)	C0009
Tanzania	26.5	3.6 (1986)	M0014
Kenya	19.9	2.6 (1987)	K0010
Zambia	10.3	18.6 (1985)	M0003
Guinea Bissau	6.0	3.7 (1987)	C0011
Ivory Coast	5.2	2.6 (1987)	V0002
Ghana	3.2	4.7 (1987)	M0018
Gabon	2.9	1.8 (1986)	D0005
Zaire	2.7	5.7 (1987)	N0008

NOTE:

AIDS urban incidence rate— based on number of AIDS cases reported to the World Health Organization and an urban population for 1987 estimated at the U.S. Bureau of the Census.

HIV1 prevalence rate— Information comes from various sources; see Sources for full citation.

SOURCE:

Okie, Susan 1987. "71,000 AIDS Cases Reported," *The Washington Post*, December 22, 1987, p. A4; United Nations, 1986 World Population Prospects: Estimates and Projections as Assessed in 1984, ST/ESA/SER.A/98, New York; and U.S. Bureau of the Census, 1988, World Population Profile: 1987 forthcoming. For prevalence data see Sources.

clients) are the focus of much attention. Urban areas, typically characterized by more of this behavior than rural villages, generally also have higher HIV seroprevalence rates, although there are important variations, as will be shown below. Important differences may exist in HIV seroprevalence among the various age cohorts and between gender groups. These variations have implications for the future spread of HIV infection and of AIDS as well as for the appropriate measures to take in combating the disease.

At the present time, no results are available from representative sample surveys of the seroprevalence of HIV in national populations in Africa, (nor elsewhere). Several national surveys, such as one in Uganda, are underway or planned. In the absence of data from representative surveys, present information on the seroprevalence of HIV infection is based on a large and rapidly growing number of small-scale surveys. Typically, participants in these surveys are drawn from particular population subgroups such as blood donors, prostitutes, women attending clinics, or patients in hospitals. None are representative of the total population with respect to age/sex composition, geographic dispersion, level of sexual activity, or other basic indicators.[4]

To illustrate how unclear the epidemiology of this disease still is, Table 1 compares the rates of AIDS to the estimates of HIV seroprevalence surveys of healthy adults in capital cities. Most countries in Africa are now reporting AIDS cases to WHO, although all reporting have the problems mentioned above. The cumulative incidence rates vary considerably--from 14 per 100,000 population in Uganda to virtually zero in such places as Algeria or Mozambique. When these rates are compared, however, to the results of some of the HIV seroprevalence studies, a somewhat different pattern develops. The sources of these seroprevalence data are given in the references, and the surveys themselves are compared in more detail with other surveys in the following sections. Although Uganda nominally has the highest cumulative incidence rate of AIDS as reported to WHO, surveys suggest that the HIV seroprevalence rate may be higher in Lusaka, Zambia than in Kampala, Uganda. The Congo, which has a high rate of reported AIDS, in fact, has a much lower seroprevalence of the virus in selected surveys relative to some of the other capital cities. The seroprevalence

36

surveys, of course, have all of the problems mentioned above. The discrepancy in the incidence of the reported cases of AIDS versus the estimated seroprevalence of the virus in healthy adults in capital cities should make everyone cautious about using either set of data until we have more complete descriptions of this disease.

Comparisons of the estimated seroprevalence of HIV by gender and age, in urban and rural communities, and for different high and low risk groups among these communities show discrepancies as large as those between reported AIDS cases and estimated HIV seroprevalence.

HIV PREVALENCE BY AGE AND GENDER

Like most pathogens, HIV does not infect everyone equally. As noted above, in most industrial countries AIDS is predominantly a male disease. In Africa, however, HIV has infected men and women almost equally; in some age groups women in fact have a higher estimated seroprevalence rate than men. The virus' impact is differentiated much more by age than by sex.

Two studies provide detailed descriptions by age and gender of the seroprevalence impact of HIV among healthy people. Table 4 in Cynthia Haq's preceding article summarizes the reported results of these studies in Zambia and Zaire. The pattern of infection among these African countries is similar:

–a similar overall seroprevalence among men and women;
–a higher seroprevalence in young adult women than men;
–a higher seroprevalence in older adult men than women; and
–very low seroprevalence (1.3 percent) among children from ages 1 to 14 and above the age of 50 for women and 45 for men (1.6 and 0.0 percent, respectively).

The age data point out the importance of examining population subgroups as well as looking at the population in general. Substantial proportions of the young adult populations in the two above studies were seropositive, while the seroprevalence rates for the total population would not be so alarming.

An anomaly in comparison of the two studies perhaps can be traced to the issues of sample size and sample selection discussed in the endnotes. The seroprevalence rates for both men and women ages 20 to 44 in Lusaka are much higher than those in Kinshasa, while none of the older adults in Lusaka were infected. This may be attributable to the sample in Lusaka being composed of blood donors and hospital workers. As a result the sample size for older persons in Lusaka is quite small, and may be unrepresentative.

This age and sex pattern of infection is very different from that found in Europe and the United States. In the United States, 93 percent of the AIDS cases have been men. The age pattern among adult U.S. men is similar to the distribution among men in Africa. But the rate of infection among infants is much higher in Africa than in the United States. Since many more young women are seropositive in Africa, they are passing on their antibody and often the virus to their newborn children. However, the very low infection rate among children ages 2 to 15 suggests that some of the proposed transmission vectors, such as insect bites or casual contact with infected family members, are unlikely. Children between the ages of 2 and 15 are as susceptible, or more so, to insects in Africa as anyone else. And children are objects of affection and attention in Africa. Their low level of seropositivity reinforces the strong correlation of transmission by sexual behavior and by in-utero transmission from mother to child.

Comparisons Of Urban And Rural Estimates Of HIV Seroprevalence

The estimates of HIV seroprevalence in Table 1 and in Table 4 of Dr. Haq's article are for healthy individuals in urban areas, usually the capital city. These are the areas that have been studied first by researchers because they are most accessible to the large urban hospitals that have the facilities and the staff to perform the tests. But most African countries have only a small proportion of their populations living in urban areas. Therefore, we know that the results of these surveys are not representative of the general population in the countries and are likely to overstate vastly the infection rate of the national population.

Fortunately, surveys that have been done in rural areas show a much lower HIV seroprevalence than in the urban areas (Table 2). For instance, the HIV seroprevalence rate for similar kinds of people who live only 15

Table 2

Comparison of HIV Seroprevalence Rates for Healthy Adults in Capital City Versus Less Urban Areas for Selected African Countries

Country	Area	HIV Seroprevalence Rate (percent)	Source
Angola	Luanda (1986)	0.4	B0005
	Cabinda (1986) border village	0.0	B0005
Cameroon	Yaounde (1987)	0.5	K0011
	Maroua (1987) semirural	0.5	G0002
	Mora (1985) rural	0.0	G0002
Central African Republic	Bangui (1987)	7.8	M0017
	Bambari (1987) semirural	3.7	G0002
Congo	Brazzaville (1986)	5.0	H0002
	Brazzaville (1986-87)	7.6	C0009
	Pointe Noire (1985) semirural	0.0	G0002
Gabon	Libreville (1986)	1.8	D0005
	Franceville (1986) Western Province	0.3	D0005
	Haut Ogone Province (1986)	0.0	D0002

Kenya	Nairobi (1985-86)	2.4	K0002
	15k outside Nairobi (1985)	0.9	M0012
	Sololo (1986) NE Kenya	0.9	S0012
Rwanda	Kigali (1985)	17.5	V0001
	2 remote rural areas (1985)	4.5	V0001
Senegal	Dakar (1986)	0.3	S0007
	Casamance (1986-87)	0.0	R0002
Tanzania	Dar es Salaam (1936)	3.6	M0014
	Bukoba (1986) rural towns	16.0	M0014
	Arusha (1986) rural towns	0.7	M0014
Zaire	Kinshasa (1987)	5.7	N0008
	Remote village (1986)	1.0	H0002
	Aru (1987) NE Zaire	5.3	A0006
	Ndedu (1986-87) NE village	0.5	S0011

NOTE:
Kenya— HIV seroprevalence rate for the area 15k from Nairobi is based on test of outpatients. The data for Sololo is based on patients.

SOURCE:
See Table of Sources.

kilometers away from each other can be dramatically different (outpatients in a clinic 15 K from Nairobi have a seroprevalence rate of 0.9 percent as compared with medical students and hospital personnel in Nairobi who have reported seroprevalence rates ranging from 2.4 to 4.8 percent). The seroprevalence rate in Rwanda's capital of Kigali (17.5 percent) is almost six times higher than that found in a sample in one rural area (3.0 percent).

The capital city, however, may not always have the highest seroprevalence rates. In Tanzania, for example, a survey of pregnant women in the capital city of Dar-es-Salaam estimated a seroprevalence rate of 3.6 percent in 1986, and in Arusha, in the north, pregnant women had a seroprevalence rate of 0.7 percent. However, a survey of pregnant women in Bukoba (a large Tanzanian town near the Ugandan border) estimated a rate of 16 percent. This suggests that as the disease spreads in Africa, national boundaries will become less important in determining national seroprevalence, and the movement of people within and across those boundaries will become more important.

The large differentials in the seroprevalence of HIV within countries offer an opportunity to contain the disease and prevent it from spreading to the less infected areas. Many people in the highly infected areas of the urban towns are from rural areas. The migration back and forth among the various regions of the country, especially of the young adult population, is often quite extensive. If the virus moves back to the villages as urban people go home to visit, the problems of containing the disease will be compounded.

In a recent study of rural Zaire the seroprevalence rate in 1986 is similiar to the rate in 1976.[5] This reenforces the observation that the rapid increases in seroprevalence rates are an urban phenomena. Unfortunately, the urban areas in Africa are the fastest growing areas in the world. Many of the larger cities, such as Lagos and Kinshasa, are projected to grow at a rate of almost 5 percent a year for the rest of the century. Unless this growth is slowed, the areas that are now most infected by HIV will be growing at an almost unprecedented rate, compounding the opportunity for the spread of infection.

Differences In HIV Seroprevalence Among Groups In The Same Regions

The differences in HIV seroprevalence between urban and rural areas in Africa are substantial. The differences in seroprevalence among specific groups within urban areas are even more so. Table 3 compares some survey estimates of HIV seroprevalence in high risk groups such as prostitutes, outpatients at sexually transmitted disease (STD) clinics, and inpatients at general hospitals. In general, we are defining low risk groups as groups that would have no reason to have more than an average risk of contacting an infection in the general population, such as pregnant mothers, blood donors, and healthy adults with no known illness. The differences in seroprevalence between the low risk and high risk groups are large (and within each group are even larger).

Prostitutes and their customers in all countries appear to have among the highest HIV seroprevalence rates of any group studied. Prostitutes in Ghana are estimated in one survey to have five times the seroprevalence rates of nonprostitutes. In Rwanda, men who were customers of prostitutes have a seroprevalence rate of 28 percent; males who did not frequent prostitutes had a rate of 8 percent.[6] In Nairobi, there are even considerable differences between high socioeconomic status prostitutes who, in general, come from Kenya, and low socioeconomic status prostitutes who often come from Tanzania. The lower status prostitutes had twice the estimated seroprevalence rate of the high status prostitutes in 1985 (see Table 3).

The estimated seroprevalence rates of outpatients at STD clinics also suggest that they are at high risk for HIV infection. Although their estimated infection rate is not as high as prostitutes, it is considerably higher than that of healthy adults or of medical personnel at hospitals.

Estimated HIV seroprevalence rates in high risk groups clearly can not be extrapolated to the general population, but analysts must also be cautious in using estimated seroprevalence rates among "low risk" groups as indicative of a rate in the general population. For instance, the seroprevalence rate of one low risk group, pregnant women, is itself known to be unrepresentative. In Uganda, women ages 15 to 49 are 22 percent of the total population. Pregnant women are approximately 4 percent of the

Table 3

Comparison of HIV Seroprevalence Rates Among Various Population Subgroups for Selected African Countries

Country	Population Subgroup	HIV Seroprevalence Rate (percent)	Source
Ghana (1987)	Blood donors and patients, no prostitutes	4.7	M0018
	Prostitutes	25.2	M0018
Ivory Coast (1987)	Pregnant women	2.6	V0002
	Prostitutes	17.1	V0002
Kenya (1985)	Pregnant women	2.0	Q0002
	STD Clinic patients	7.5	K0002
	High SES prostitutes	30.8	K0002
	Low SES prostitutes	65.6	K0002
Rwanda (1985)	Married blood donors	6.5	C0001
	Single blood donors	20.2	C0001
Tanzania (1986)	Pregnant women	3.6	M0014
	Blood donors	7.3	B0011
	Bar maids	28.8	M0014
Uganda (1986)	Blood donors	10.8	H0003
	Pregnant women	13.6	H0003
	Prostitutes	80.0	H0003
Zaire (1985-87)	Pregnant women (1987)	5.7	N0008
	Blood donors (1985)	12.0	Z0003
	Prostitutes (1985)	27.0	J0001
Zambia (1985)	Male blood donors and hospital workers	17.2	M0003
	Male STD clinic patients	26.2	M0003

SOURCE:
See Table of Sources.

population. Although women can become pregnant between the ages of 14 and 49, most pregnant women are between the ages of 20 and 30, the years when they are most sexually active and, therefore, most at risk for contacting the HIV virus even though they may be in a low risk group. Therefore, the estimated HIV seroprevalence rate of pregnant women is not necessarily a good proxy for the rate of healthy adults in a society, but the rate for only the most sexually active healthy adults, a smaller and more vulnerable group than the adult population in general. A similar caveat also may apply to blood donors, who may be disproportionately drawn from the young adult population.

Social And Economic Issues Raised By The HIV Epidemic

The patterns of HIV seroprevalence raise a number of immediate questions for African governments, donor organizations, and social analysts. They involve not only the magnitude of the general problem, but the effects of infection on specific groups and areas. Some of the most immediate issues are:

–How will the AIDS epidemic affect general population growth in Africa?
–How will the increase in disease affect the distribution of already scarce public resources?
–How will the geographic disparities in seroprevalence affect short-term economic urban progress?
–How will the disparities in seroprevalence by age affect generational relations?
–How will the epidemic affect the labor forces in general and labor productivity in particular?

We do not know enough to answer these questions fully although the data in hand allow some preliminary insights.

Population Growth Issues. Some have speculated that the AIDS epidemic will eliminate Africa's population growth in the future. No detailed transmission models of the AIDS virus in Africa yet exist, but several simple models have been used to project the effect of AIDS on future African growth. If the national seroprevalence rate would ever reach the extremely high level of 10 percent (current national rates are far below 10 percent today given the low estimates for rural areas where most of the population lives), future annual African population growth rates are estimated to decline from the current 3 percent to about 2 percent. Africa would still be one of the fastest growing regions in the world. These estimates of the effects of AIDS on growth rates should be considered neither definitive nor sophisticated. But they provide an estimated order of magnitude that suggests that the problems of population growth and the epidemic of AIDS will coexist rather than substitute for each other. From what we now know, more important issues are the differential impact on various population sectors and the ability of governments to deal with the rapidly rising number of AIDS cases and deaths.

Resource Allocation Issues. The lack of public resources with which to fight the AIDS epidemic will force public sector trade offs in African countries that no developed country will have to face. African countries are already beginning to see AIDS patients preempting their scarce beds in hospitals and TB sanatoriums. The average annual per capita expenditure for health care in African countries today is about $5. African countries simply do not have resources to fight this epidemic. What resources exist may, at the margin, be diverted to fight AIDS. But considerable resources to fight the epidemic must come from international donors and organizations.

Urban Issues. The disproportionately high HIV seroprevalence in urban areas in Africa and other countries throughout the world suggests that these areas will suffer the greatest effects of the disease. Urban areas are also the centers for economic development and, therefore, have attracted the better educated people in most countries. They are the people who are running the emerging modern sector of the economy. Therefore, if they are disproportionately infected by HIV, the modern economy will suffer disproportionately. It may be too facile to assume that the best educated will have the highest seroprevalence rates. A study of the hospital personnel in Kinshasa suggested that the highest seroprevalence rates were not in the doctors, who had the highest education, but in the nurses and orderlies. More detailed surveys are needed to estimate the HIV seroprevalence by education, occupation, and income class. More research will be needed to estimate the effect of this infection pattern on the social and economic infrastructures of the countries.

A more immediate geographic issue is how to prevent the spread of HIV from the high-seroprevalence areas in urban towns to the low-seroprevalence areas in rural villages. Fear of contagion may reinforce the isolation of rural areas. Could fears create an implosion of activities in rural areas helping to retard the spread of infection but also economic development and social progress?

Generational Issues. Often the catastrophes of the past, such as famine and other disease epidemics, disproportionately affected the young and the old in a population. In contrast, the HIV epidemic affects the adults most severely. These are the people in every society who are the parents of the new generation, the most productive workers in the labor force, the sources of manpower for the military. This also is the group that is the source of support for their parents.

What happens to the social patterns of responsibility when not only the parents of young children die, but their aunts and uncles? Who supports the elderly in the villages when their children die? How will the dependency ratio, the ratio of the number of working-age adults to the number of young and old, be altered by AIDS. How will the extended families of Africa and the traditional village societies adjust to the shift in the responsibilities for the young and the old?

Labor Force Issues. The modern sector labor forces and the military are also dependent on young adults who are most at risk of HIV infection. The actual number of AIDS deaths in most countries is still very small and the effect of these deaths on the economy or military is presumably negligible. But, the infection itself may affect the productivity of the workers long before the symptoms of AIDS appear. Subsequent deaths of many young and mature adults would result in a serious loss of trained and experienced workers who are, in general, the ones who are most productive in all economies.

These are only a few of the social and economic issues raised by this epidemic. Subsequent chapters in this volume will explore in more depth some of these specific issues. As we learn more about the epidemiology of HIV we will be able to answer many of our initial questions.

As noted in the introduction, the HIV virus will not wait for good data, and we must, therefore, use carefully what data are available. The mosaic of small surveys throughout the continent, when collected and pieced together, will help show the patterns and trends of this disease. While individually these studies are of limited utility for national assessment purposes, together they can be used to form a composite picture of the local situation. This picture will, naturally, vary in completeness from one location to another. In the absence of representative sample surveys a systematic inventory of results is extremely important. If these results are interpreted skillfully they will help African governments intervene and challenge the disease.[7]

ENDNOTES

[1]The data used in this paper come from the published and unpublished reports of researchers in the field. Often there are several conflicting estimates of HIV prevalence in a specific city or group. In general,the data presented are as current as possible and come from the largest available samples, although considerably more data exist for earlier years and for small samples. The Center for International Research at the U.S. Bureau of the Census is collecting epidemiological data on AIDS and HIV for the U.S. Agency for International Development. A more detailed description of the data base and the data used are provided in Appendixes I and II. All references to HIV in this chapter are to HIV1. The AIDS data base includes epidemiological data on HIV2, but its clinical expression is not yet fully defined.

[2]Georges, Alain J., et al., "HIV-I Seroprevalence and AIDS Diagnostic Criteria in Central African Republic," The Lancet, December 5, 1987, pp. 1332-33.

[3]World Health Organization, Special Programme on AIDS, 1987, "The Global Surveillance of AIDS," unpublished.

[4]Surveys on nonrepresentative samples pose special problems of interpretation. Each nonrepresentative sample of HIV infection has specific biases that can only be determined when the researcher knows how the target group is related to the broader population base. HIV prevalence rates vary so much by region within the country and among population groups that a survey that would allow statistically valid conclusions at these levels would be both large and expensive. Yet, given the important role of certain groups in spreading HIV infection, information is needed on population subgroups (for example, prostitutes and their clients). National surveys cannot provide the detail for examining such groups. The challenge, therefore, is to use carefully what imperfect data we have to form a composite picture of the situation for use in strategic planning against the disease. In order to do this we need to understand the limitations of the present data without being crippled by them. Ultimately we must hope that the disease will be contained before the data are perfected.

The sample size may be a critical variable in the estimation of HIV seroprevalence. The figures below show several instances where there are two surveys of similar population in approximately the same time period. In these cases the seroprevalence estimate from the smaller sample is higher than that from the larger sample. Such findings of course are not conclusive, but should serve as a warning about small samples. Small samples are not necessarily biased toward higher prevalence levels, but in this setting it may be that small samples are more often "samples of convenience," which are made likely to include infected persons.

[5]Nzilambi, Naila, Kevin M. De Cock, Donald N. Forthal, Henry Francis, Robert W. Ryder, Ismey Malebe, Jane Getchell, Marie Laga, Peter Piot, and Joseph B. McCormick, "The Prevalence of Infection With Human Immunodeficiency Virus Over A 10-Year Period in Rural Zaire," The New England Journal of Medicine, Vol. 318, February 4, 1988, No. 5 pp. 276-79.

[6]Van de Perre, P., J. B. Kanyamupire, M. Carael, *et al.*, 1985, "HTLV-III/LAV Infection in Central Africa," International Symposium on African AIDS, Brussels, Nov. 22-23 (Abstract).

Relationship of Sample Size
to HIV Seroprevalence Rate for Selected African Countries

Year	City	Group	Sample Size	HIV Seroprevalence Rate (percent)	Source
1987	Nairobi	Hemophilia	40	30.0	K0004
			51	23.5	K0004
1987	Kinshasa	Pregnant women	2574	6.0	B0010
			6000	5.7	N0008
1986-87	Kampala	Pregnant women	170	24.0	H0002
			1000	13.6	H0003

NOTE:
These are not enough cases to determine the relationship of sample size to estimated HIV prevalence rate. It should be enough, however, to make people cautions about using estimates from small sample sizes.

SOURCE:
For full citation see Sources.

[7]There are considerable published data on HIV seroprevalence in Africa that we have not included in this chapter, some because it is out of date, some because the sample size was not specified or the sample was not described carefully, and some because the sample was just too small. African countries cannot afford to have HIV surveys collected and then go unused. Every survey should add a piece to the larger puzzle of this disease. In order for that to be true, however, survey reports should specify:

> --the characteristics of the sample survey as carefully as possible. For instance, the age and sex of the respondents, the group identification, etc. A number of surveys are not very usable because not enough is known about the sampled population;
> --the virus being tested, and the particular test(s) used (e.g., ELISA confirmed with a Western Blot); and
> --the sample size of the survey and details about the sample selection method.

WHO's Special Programme on AIDS is developing standard procedures and survey instruments for seroprevalence surveys. Attention to these standards should increase the quality and utility of the studies being done.

APPENDIX I

AIDS/HIV STATISTICS DATA BASE
Center for International Research
U.S. Bureau of the Census

This information presented in this chapter is drawn from the initial release of the AIDS/HIV Statistics Data Base developed at the Center for International Research (CIR), U.S. Bureau of the Census, for use on IBM (and compatible) microcomputers. Support for the development of this data base was provided by the U.S. Agency for International Development.

The purpose of this data base is to allow the systematic organization and retrieval of information related to HIV infection and AIDS cases in populations in developing countries. Information from clinical studies, scientific samples, and official statistics has been compiled for this data base at the smallest available aggregate level and has been coded by the age, sex, and particular population group sampled. Also included is information on the method of testing, sample size, etc. A fuller description of the data fields, record layout, etc., is available.

A menu-driven user interface has been written to facilitate the retrieval of information. Through a series of menus the program determines the appropriate selection criteria for presentation of the data. Although the data base was developed using the dBase III Plus program, no familiarity with the program is required for use of the table retrieval program, and in fact, the dBASE III Plus program is not required for the use of the data base.

As mentioned above, this is the initial release of the data base, and it is by no means complete. Information included at this time emphasizes recent data from Africa. Material for inclusion was drawn from the scientific literature, conference papers and presentations, and the like. The CIR plans to continue work on the compilation, coding and entry of additional data, not only from Africa, but for all developing countries. Periodic updates of the data base are planned. Comments, suggestions, and additional material for inclusion in the data base are welcome. Correspondence should be addressed to:

> AIDS/HIV Statistics Data Base
> Center for International Research
> Scuderi Building, Room 407
> U.S. Bureau of the Census
> Washington, D.C. 20233
> U.S.A.

APPENDIX II

U.S. Bureau of the Census, Center for International Research
AIDS/HIV Statistics Data Base: Seroprevalence of Human Immunodeficiency Virus I (HIVI)

Country	Geographic Area	Date	Population Subgroup	Sex and Age Group	Size of sample	Type of Test	HIV Prevalence Rate	Source
Angola	Cabinda	1986	Border village	B 18-62	40	ELISA	0.0	B0005
	Luanda	1986	Blood donors	M 18-62	452	ELISA, WB	0.4	B0005
Cameroon	Maroua	1986	Random sample	B 15-44	364	ELISA, WB	0.5	G0002
	Mora	1985	Random sample	B 5-64	322	ELISA, WB	0.0	G0002
	Yaounde	1987?	Blood donors	B All	2,475	ELISA, WB	0.5	K0011
Central African Republic	Bambari	1987	Random sample	B 15-44	374	ELISA, WB	3.7	G0002
	Bangui	1987	Random sample	B 15-44	383	ELISA, WB	7.8	M0017
Congo	Brazzaville	1986-87	Blood donors	B All	8,009	ELISA	7.6	C0009
	Brazzaville	1986	Random sample	B All	368	Unknown	5.0	H0002
	Pointe Noire	1985	Random sample	B 15-44	360	ELISA, WB	0.0	G0002
Gabon	Franceville	1986	Random sample	B 15-44	371	ELISA, WB	0.3	D0005
	Haut-Ogone province	1986?	Pregnant women & young mothers	F All	488	ELISA, WB, RIPA	0.0	D0002
	Libreville	1986	Random sample	B 15-44	383	ELISA, WB	1.8	D0005
Ghana	National	1987?	Prostitutes	F All	266	ELISA, IFA, WB	25.2	M0018
	National	1987	Patients, blood donors, no prostitutes	B All	771	ELISA, IFA, WB	4.7	M0018
Guinea-Bissau	National	1987	Blood donors	B All	54	ELISA, WB, RIPA	3.7	C0011
Ivory Coast	National	1987?	Pregnant women	F All	268	ELISA, WB	2.6	V0002
	National	1987?	Prostitutes	F All	105	ELISA, WB	17.1	V0002

Country	Location	Year	Population group	Age/Sex	N	Test	%	Ref
Kenya	Nairobi	1987?	Women in labor	F All	2,910	ELISA, WB	2.6	K0010
	Nairobi	1985	Medical students	B All	42	ELISA, WB	2.4	K0002
	Nairobi	1985	Low SES prostitutes	F All	64	ELISA, WB	65.5	K0002
	Nairobi	1985	High SES prostitutes	F All	26	ELISA, WB	30.8	K0002
	Nairobi	1985	STD patients	M All	40	ELISA, WB	7.5	K0002
	Kiambu District	1985	Outpatients	B All	115	ELISA, WB	0.9	M0012
	Sololo Isiolo	1986	Hospital patients	B 12-70	103	ELISA, WB	1.0	S0012
Rwanda	2 remote rural areas	1985	Blood donors	B All	NA	ELISA	4.5	V0001
	Kigali	1985	Young adults	B All	302	ELISA	17.5	V0001
	Kigali	1985	Married blood donors	M 19+	77	ELISA, WB	6.5	C0001
	Kigali	1985	Single blood donors	M 19+	104	ELISA, WB	20.2	C0001
Senegal	Casamance	1986-87	Health workers	B All	85	WB	0.0	R0002
	Dakar	1986	Hospital workers	F All	301	ELISA, IMMUNOBLOT	0.3	S0007
Tanzania	Arusha	1986	Pregnant women	F 15-44	144	ELISA, WB	0.7	M0014
	Bukoba	1986	Pregnant women	F All	100	ELISA, WB	16.0	M0014
	Dar es Salaam	1986	Pregnant women	F All	192	ELISA, WB	3.6	M0014
	Dar es Salaam	1986	Blood donors	B All	535	ELISA, WB, RIPA	7.3	B0011
	Dar es Salaam	1986	Bar maids	F All	225	ELISA, WB	28.8	M0014
Uganda	Kampala	1986	Blood donors	B All	370	Unknown	10.8	H0003
	Kampala	1986	Pregnant women	F All	1,011	Unknown	13.6	H0003
	National	1986	Prostitutes	B All	NA	Unknown	80.0	H0003
Zaire	Aru	1987?	Total	B 17-75	319	ELISA, WB	5.3	A0006
	Kinshasa	1987?	Pregnant women	F 15-44	6,000	Unknown	5.7	N0008
	Kinshasa	1985	Blood donors	B All	25	Unknown	12.0	Z0003
	Kinshasa	1985	Prostitutes	F All	376	ELISA, WB	27.0	J0001
	Ndedu	1986-87	Random sample	B All	222	Unknown	0.5	S0011
	Village	1986	Unknown	B All	NA	Unknown	1.0	H0002
Zambia	Lusaka	1985	Blood donors and hospital workers	B 15-64	307	ELISA, WB	18.6	M0003
	Lusaka	1985	Blood donors and hospital workers	M 15-64	203	ELISA, WB	17.2	M0003
	Lusaka	1985	STD patients	M 15-64	122	ELISA, WB	25.2	M0003

52

TABLE SOURCES

A0006   Aktar, L., B. Larouze, S. Mabika Wa Bantu, *et al.*, 1987, "Distribution of Antibodies to HIV1 in an Urban Community (Aru, Upper Zaire)," Second International Symposium on AIDS and Associated Cancers in Africa, Naples, Italy, October 7-9, Abstract, TH-34.

B0005   Bottiger, B., I. Berggren;, J. Leite, *et al.*, 1987, "Prevalence of HIV and HTLV-IV Infections in Angola," Second International Symposium on AIDS and Associated Cancers in Africa, Naples, Italy, October 7-9, Abstract, TH-35.

B0010   Baende, E., R. Ryder, F. Behets, *et al.*, 1987, "Congenital HIV Transmission at an Upper Middle Class Hospital and Kinshasa," Second International Symposium on AIDS in Associated Cancers in Africa, Naples, Italy, October 7-9, Abstract, F-2.

B0011   Bredberg-Raden U., E. Mbena, J. Kiango, *et al.*, 1987 "Comparison of Commercial ELISA's for Detection of HIV in East African Sera," Second International Symposium on AIDS and Associated Cancers in Africa, Naples, Italy, October 7-9, Abstract, F-39.

C0011   Canas Ferreira, Wanda F., Kamal Mansinko, *et al.*, 1987, "Prevalence of Antibodies to HIV-1 and HIV-2 among Blood Donors in Guinea Bissau (West Africa)," Second International Symposium on AIDS and Associated Cancers in Africa, Naples, Italy, October 7-9, Abstract, TH-10.

C0001   Carael, M., P. Van de Perre, N. Clumeck, *et al.*, 1986, "Urban Sexuality Changing Patterns in Central Africa: Social Determinants of HTLV-III Transmission," Unpublished.

C0009   Copin, N., P. M'Pele, F. Yala, *et al.*, 1987, "Sero-Prevalence of Anti-HIV Antibodies in Blood Donors, Brazzaville (Congo)," Second International Symposium on AIDS and Associated Cancers in Africa, Naples, Italy, October 7-9, Abstract, TH-32.

D0002   Delaporte, Eric, B. Ivanoff, F. Brun-Vezinet, *et al.*, 1986, Antibodies to LAV/HTLV-III in a Rural Population in Gabon, International Conference on AIDS, Paris, June 23-25, Abstract.

D0005   Delaporte, E., A. Dupont, M. Merlin, *et al.*, 1987, "Prevalence Rates of Antibodies to HIV1 and HIV2 in Population Samples from Gabon," Second International Symposium on AIDS and Associated Cancers in Africa, Naples, Italy, October 7-9, Abstract, TH-29.

G0002 Georges-Courbot, M.C., M. Merlin, P.M.V. Martin, *et al.*, 1987, Serological Surveys of HIV Antibodies in Central and East Africa, Second International Symposium on AIDS and Associated Cancers in Africa, Naples, Italy, October 7-9, Abstract, TH-27.

H0002 Harden, Blaine, 1987, AIDS Seen as Threat to Africa's Future, *The Washington Post*, May 31, pp. A1 and A18.

H0003 Harden, Blaine, 1986, "Uganda Battles AIDS Epidemic," *The Washington Post*, June 2,.pp. A1 and A18.

J0001 Johns Hopkins University, Population Information Program, 1986, "AIDS -- A Public Health Crisis, Issues in World Health," *Population Reports*, 7, Series L, No. 6.

K0011 Kaptue, L., L. Zekeng, J. P. Tagu, *et al.*, 1987, "HIV Antibody Prevalence in Blood Donors and Blood Recipients in Yaounde, Cameroun," Second International Symposium on AIDS and Associated Cancers in Africa, Naples, Italy, October 7-9, Abstract, S.4.2.

K0004 Kitonyi, G.W., T. Bowry, *et al.*, 1987, "AIDS Studies in Kenyan Haemophiliacs," III International Conference on AIDS, Washington, D.C., June 1-5, Abstract, p. 93.

K0002 Kreiss, Joan, Davy Keoch, Francis Plummer, *et al.*, 1986, "AIDS Virus Infection in Nairobi Prostitutes: Spread of the Epidemic to East Africa," *New England Journal of Medicine*, February 13, Vol. 314, No. 7, pp. 414-18.

K0010 Kreiss, J., M. Braddiek, F. A. Plummer, *et al.*, 1987, "Congential Transmission of HIV in Nairobi, Kenya," Second International Symposium on AIDS and Associated Cancers in Africa, Naples, Italy, October 7-9, Abstract, S.9.2.

M0017 Martin, Paul M.V., M. C. Georges-Courbot, and A. J. Georges, 1987, "Tentative Determination of AIDS Incidence and Risk Factors in the CAR," Second International Symposium on AIDS and Associated Cancers in Africa, Naples, Italy, October 7-9, Abstract, TH-26.

M0012 Mason, J. C., R. M. Bruce, B. S. Azadian, *et al.*, 1986, "HTLV-III Antibody in East Africa," *New England Journal of Medicine* July 24, Vol. 315, No. 4, pp. 259-60.

M0003 Melbye, Mads, E.K. Njelesani, Anne Bayley, *et al.*, 1986, "Evidence for Heterosexual Transmission and Clinical Manifestations of HIV Infection and Related Conditions in Lusaka, Zambia," *Lancet*, November 15, Vol. 11, No. 8516, pp. 1113-15.

M0014 Mhalu, Fred, E. Mbena, U. Bredberg-Raden, *et al.*, 1987, "Prevalence of HIV Antibodies in Healthy Subjects and Groups of Patients in Some Parts of Tanzania 1987," III International Conference on AIDS, Washington, D.C., June 1-5, Abstract, p. 76.

M0018   Mingle, Julis A. A., M. Hayami, M. Osei-Kwasi, *et al.*, 1987, "Reactivity of Ghanaian Sera to Human Immunodefiency Virus, and Simian T-Lymphotropic Virus III," III International Conference on AIDS, Washington, D.C., June 1-5, Abstract, p. 25.

N0008   Nsa, W., R. Ryder, and H. Francis, 1987, "Congenital HIV Transmission in a Large Urban Hospital in Kinshasa," Second International Symposium on AIDS and Associated Cancers in Africa, Naples, Italy, October 7-9, Abstract, F-1.

Q0002   Quinn, Thomas C., J. M. Mann, J. W. Curran, *et al.*, 1986, "AIDS in Africa: An Epidemiologic Paradigm," *Science*, Nov. 21, Vol. 234, pp. 955-62.

R0002   Ricard, D., S. M'Boup, A. N. N'Doye, *et al.*, 1987, "Prevalence of HIV-1 and HIV-2 HTLV-4 in the South of Senegal, in Casamance," Second International Symposium on AIDS and Associated Cancers in Africa, Naples, Italy, October 7-9, Abstract, TH-7.

S0012   Saracco, A., M. Galli, G. Zehender, *et al.*, 1987, "Low Prevalence of HIV Antibodies in a Remote Area of Kenya," Second International Symposium on AIDS and Associated Cancers in Africa, Naples, Italy, October 7-9, Abstract, TH-38.

S0007   Sow, L., S. Lu, E. Coll, *et al.*, 1987, "HIV-1 and HIV-2 Seroprevalence in a Hospital Worker Population, Dakar, Senegal," Second International Symposium on AIDS and Associated Cancers in Africa, Naples, Italy, October 7-9, Abstract, TH-6.

S0011   Surmont, I., and J. Desmyter, 1987, "Urban to Rural Spread of HIV Infection in Dungu, Zaire," Second International Symnosium on AIDS and Associated Cancers in Africa, Naples, Italy, October 7-9, Abstract, TH-33.

V0001   Van de Perre, P., J. B. Kanyamupira, M. Carael, *et al.*, 1985, "HTLV-III/LAV Infection in Central Africa," International Symposium on African AIDS, Brussels, Nov. 22-23, Abstract.

V0002   Verdier, M., A. Sangare, G. Leonard, *et al.*, 1987, "Co-Exposure to Three Human Retroviruses (HTLV-1, HIV-1, 2) in Prostitutes and Pregnant Women in Ivory Coast," Second International Symposium on AIDS and Associated Cancers in Africa, Naples, Italy, October 7-9, Abstract, Th-17.

Z0003   Zagury, D., K. Lurhuma, R. C. Gallo, *et al.*, 1987, "HTLV-III/LAV Infection in Central Africa," Second International Symposium on AIDS and Associated Cancers in Africa, Naples, Italy, October 7-9, Abstract, S.8.1.

PART II
Historic and
Ecological Implications

AIDS IN AFRICA: HISTORICAL ROOTS

Marc H. Dawson*

SUMMARY: AIDS is a new disease to central and eastern Africa, but it is not spreading in a social, political, and economic vacuum. Thus, the historical forces which have shaped the disease environment of twentieth century Africa are also important in the epidemiology of AIDS. These factors are explored in a comparative case study of the history of venereal syphilis in Kenya. This comparison reveals the importance and the need to examine more closely the role of labor migration, urbanization, and medical care in the dissemination of both diseases.

Introduction

The origins of the virus (HTLV-III) responsible for AIDS remain unresolved, but recent studies leave little doubt that this syndrome is not an old African disease suddenly spreading to the rest of the world.[1] Contrary to some initial reports from the continent in 1983-84, the disease only emerged as a problem in central Africa in the late 1970s and early 1980s. This new syndrome, however, did not spread in Africa in a social, political or economic vacuum. Consequently the same historical forces which shaped the disease patterns of twentieth century Africa are important in understanding the epidemiology of AIDS.

The current known risk factors for African AIDS are: living or working in an urban environment, having a large number of heterosexual partners, possibly injections with unsterilized syringes, and lastly the presence of genital ulcers possibly related to a sexually transmitted disease (STD). These factors resemble those which were responsible for the introduction and spread of venereal syphilis earlier in this century. If the analogy between the two diseases holds true, given the deadly results of AIDS, the situation in central and eastern Africa is truly disturbing.

---

* Marc H. Dawson is an Assistant Professor of History at Western New England College. He has published various articles on health and disease in colonial Kenya.

Some recent studies of AIDS in Africa have begun to ignore the wider picture of the disease's epidemiology by narrowly concentrating on individual risk factors. The many studies of prostitutes and their clients (certainly populations at increased risk) distract researchers from asking broader questions of possible epidemiological importance about both of these groups and other aspects of the society in which they live. Until these questions are investigated, a more complete understanding of the disease will not be achieved.

The major question Western health workers ask about African AIDS is why the disease in Africa is transmitted almost exclusively heterosexually, unlike in Europe and North America where it is transmitted mainly homosexually or through drug abuse. The question which followed for African AIDS was then what was different about Africans medically and sexually. The suggested answers to this question were that in Africa a large number of hetrosexual partners and possibly the presence of genital lesions (perhaps related to an STD) characterized the AIDS-infected population. These answers have not, however, generated a second set of broader questions including why in an African urban setting does this sexual behavior exist, and why is there a higher incidence of STD and genital lesions in Africa as compared to the much lower incidence in the West.

Part of the answers to these questions can only be found by examining the political and economic structure of modern African countries. These societies inherited those structures from their colonial past. In order to study the forces shaping the spread of AIDS, Kenya and its experience with venereal syphilis can stand as a valuable comparative case study.[2] The dominant economic pattern of colonial African societies, especially the countries where AIDS is a serious problem, was the presence of migrant labor systems.

Venereal Syphilis In Colonial Kenya

The colonial economy of Kenya was based on large estate agriculture and through time a small and growing industrial urban sector. Both parts of the economy relied on the availability of cheap, unskilled, and abundant African labor. To this end through taxes, land alienation, force, etc., colonial officials caused thousands of African males to become migrant laborers. Colonial authorities wanted African males to work as laborers in the European sector of the economy, but did not want them to lose their attachments to the newly created rural African reserves. This economic structure resulted in an unprecedented movement of people both in terms of numbers involved and in distances travelled. By 1920, tens of thousands of African males travelled to rural European estates for work as farm laborers, or to the new colonial cities to work as domestics or in shops or factories, or went to the city to sell agricultural produce. These men travelled back and forth from their rural homes to their work place.

During this same time period, the influx of new populations of Europeans, Asians, and Africans resulted in the growth of urban areas. These new cities and towns began to grow up around the administrative outposts of the colonial regime. For instance, Nairobi grew from a few Europeans living in tents and corrugated iron buildings in 1899 to a multiracial city of 20,000 by 1920. The number of Africans going to urban areas continued to accelerate especially after the 1940s. This movement was not only into the large cities, like Nairobi, Mombasa, and Kisumu, but also into smaller towns, like Fort Hall, Machakos, Naivasha, etc.

The influx of Africans was not, however, the movement of people from rural homes to set up new households in the city. It was the movement of men without their families to take up temporary (but lengthy) residence while working in the city. The African urban population had a very skewed sex ratio; as early as 1911 in Nairobi males out-numbered females six to one.[3] Given the need to keep up their farm in the Reserve and the lack of housing in the city, few African migrant laborers brought their wives to the city. The long absences (perhaps up to a year) from their wives or in the case of young men, no wives at all, led men to seek female companionship from prostitutes who began to practice their profession very early in Nairobi's history.

Women who came to urban areas had few employment opportunities open to them. Men took most of the jobs as cooks and domestic servants. Consequently, they could only earn a living preparing food for African men, brewing beer (forbidden by law in 1921), or becoming prostitutes.[4] The latter choice was the most lucrative. Many of these women also began to practice this profession in the smaller towns, railway stations, and administrative outposts to the consternation of colonial officials.

In this new environment venereal syphilis began to spread. The disease had been confined at the start of the century to coastal communities, but began to spread more widely in the 1910s and 1920s. The major risk factors for venereal syphilis infection for Africans were those of working in an urban environment, being a migrant laborer, and visiting prostitutes. The disease began to spread rapidly in some rural areas owing to infections carried home by returning labor migrants. Prostitutes, soldiers, and colonial employees, who lived in rural administrative and colonial towns were also important sources of introducing the disease into rural Kenya.

Venereal syphilis did not spread widely, however, among rural Kikuyu in the 1920s and 1930s, despite the fact that they formed a large part of Nairobi's urban population and were heavily involved in labor migration. The disease could not gain a foothold among these people because of the widespread presence of yaws. These two treponematoses offer a partial cross-immunity to infection with each other. In the late 1940s, however, a rapidly rising incidence of venereal syphilis in the rural Kikuyu reserves drew the attention of medical authorities. The sharp increase in the incidence was the result of removal of the former limited immunological protection offered by active yaws infections combined with the changes described above.

In the 1920s and 1930s colonial medical authorities had conducted extensive anti-yaws campaigns in rural Kenya, especially in the Kikuyu reserves.[5] Medical officials using a heavy-metal-based chemotherapy mistakenly thought they were curing cases of yaws. In reality they were only suppressing the patients' symptoms. Nevertheless, the symptom-suppressing therapy allowed a whole generation of Kikuyu children to grow up without having contracted yaws. This same generation also lacked that former immunological protection. The result was the rapid increase in cases of venereal syphilis in the 1940s, and the disease still remains a public health problem today.

Historical Roots Of The Epidemiology Of African AIDS

Thus this series of socio-economic changes of the colonial era related to colonial economic policies, labor migration, urbanization, the rise of prostitution, and colonial health efforts led to the widespread incidence of a new disease, venereal syphilis. This same set of factors also plays a role in the dissemination of AIDS in Africa. The risk factors for AIDS listed at the outset are not only similar to those of venereal syphilis but are also the result of the historical processes discussed above.

This statement does not suggest that there has not been any socio-economic change in the twenty-five years or so since independence for Kenya and most of sub-Saharan Africa, but that much of the change can only stem from roots set in colonial patterns. Since independence, there has been much more stability in most African labor forces. Men stay in wage employment for most of their lives usually only returning to rural areas for holidays or to retire. At the same time there is still some labor migration and a great deal of movement between the city and rural areas, as the week-end bus traffic from Nairobi, Harare, or Lusaka will attest. The social and economic ties of urban workers to rural areas remain strong.

Urbanization continues to occur at ever increasing rates, but the sex ratios in African cities have begun to balance out. The structure of urban populations, however, still bears some resemblances to the colonial city. For example, a 1971 survey of employed workers in Nairobi revealed the following pattern of family distribution: 45.9 percent of the wives of these men lived completely outside of Nairobi, 34.0 percent of these men's wives all lived in Nairobi, 6.9 percent of these men had wives both in Nairobi and in rural areas, and the remaining workers were unmarried, either single, widowed or divorced.[6] Thus, roughly 57 percent of the employed males in Nairobi were without spouses in the city. Similar figures can be found for towns in Zambia's Copperbelt and other central and eastern African cities. The consequence of this pattern is that many urban males seek female companionship and frequently from prostitutes.

Women in many African urban areas have more job opportunities than they did in the colonial era. These jobs, however, tend to be at the lowest level of the pay scale and the demand for such jobs is high. Women without jobs who are alone in the city, possibly because of family problems (divorce), are forced to find ways to live. Given the structure of the urban male population there is a high market demand for female companionship. In Nairobi for example, there are clearly two different markets: less well-to-do residents of Nairobi, and tourists, travelling businessmen, and the wealthy elite.

One study of AIDS in Nairobi recently revealed that the prostitutes working in these two markets have a significantly different rate of testing positive for AIDS and suffering from an STD.[7] The study found that 55 percent of the women working in an average African working-class area suffered from syphilis, and 45 percent suffered from gonorrhea. The respective percentages for the other group of women were 31 percent and 19 percent. Clearly, this latter group of women dealt with clients who were probably healthier, but they also, probably because of higher income, had better access to health care.

The more disturbing finding from this study was the different rates of seropositivity for the AIDS virus. Two thirds (66 percent) of the first set of women, who dealt mainly with average African clients, tested positive, whereas only 31 percent of the other group tested positive. Other data found in the survey made these figures more disturbing. The first set of women had an average of 963 contacts per year without using any barrier forms of birth control. The clients of these women would tend to be the groups of employed males who were without their spouses in the city. Even if female to male transmission of AIDS is not efficient, there would appear to be a significant opportunity for a substantial number of male infections.

In turn some of these infected men will return to their rural homes and their spouses. The disease will accompany these men who will infect their wives, who in turn will infect any subsequent children. This urban-rural pattern of disease dissemination was true not only for venereal syphilis, but for also a number of other infectious diseases, such as tuberculosis and gonorrhea. Consequently studies for AIDS must be carried out in rural areas from which labor migrants come to track fully the spread of this epidemic.

The pattern of dissemination of venereal syphilis into rural areas suggests that another area which should be studied is small towns. The movement of colonial employees, soldiers, and "followers" to rural administrative outposts (future small towns) was important in the spread of venereal syphilis. In Kenya both medical reports and oral testimony cited these groups as introducing syphilis.[8] This same pattern will possibly be true for AIDS, except the groups will include travelling businessmen, truck and bus drivers, government officials, as well as prostitutes. These small urban centers have become the focus of regional economic activity with many rural visitors to their market places.

This last group of labor migrants, prostitutes, are geographically mobile. Verhagen surveyed prostitutes in Mombasa and found that they travelled widely, some throughout East Africa.[9] Many of the women were foreigners (20 percent from Uganda), and 40 percent had lived in the city less than a year. Movement of these women between larger cities and smaller towns is probably not unusual. Thus the nature of their profession and their geographic mobility amply justify the attention given them by medical researchers. However, almost all of the published studies of this particular population have all been conducted in large urban centers, and disappointingly few have examined smaller rural towns. Lastly and perhaps not surprisingly, limited data have been collected concerning the clients of prostitutes.

Another mobile population involved in the transmission of both diseases is truck drivers. They were accused of helping to spread venereal syphilis in western colonial Kenya. As early as 1910, Kavirondo elders claimed that African and Asian truck drivers introduced syphilis to that area. The drivers picked up female hitchhikers and accepted payment in kind for the favor.[10] Recently, East African authorities have been concerned about the possible role of long-distance lorry drivers in the spread of AIDS. These men travel between large urban areas, Nairobi-Mombasa, Nairobi-Kampala, Mombasa-Kigale, etc., but also stop in small rural urban centers to make deliveries or rest for the night. They also visit local bars and hotels and have families with ties to rural areas.

The last major risk factor for AIDS is the presence of genital lesions possibly related to STD.[11] Venereal syphilis and chancroid are two frequently occurring STDs. The reasons for the continued widespread incidence are discussed above, but with perhaps two additional factors. Both conditions are readily curable with either antibiotics or chemotherapy. A high standard of personal hygiene can reduce the incidence of chancroid. Poverty, however, makes access to health care and maintenance of personal hygiene much more difficult. Consequently the higher rate of STD in Africa as compared to Western countries is probably most closely linked to the differences between access to and availability of their health care systems. The presence of genital lesions may also prove a more important explanatory factor than the number of sexual partners.

The role of injections in the transmission of AIDS in Africa is an issue which has received some attention. In Africa the popularity of injections in treating all types of afflictions stems from the successful campaigns to eradicate yaws in the 1920s and 1950s.[12] Thus, many Africans expect an injection as part of any treatment at a medical clinic. African medical systems have also incorporated the use of syringes for herbal medicines. Cost factors, however, have required that most African medical facilities continue to use non-disposable syringes which could pose hazards. Also one can easily find many "amateur injectionists" who use the same type of syringes but with only minimal, if any, precautions of sterilization.

The high incidence of AIDS among intravenous drug abusers sharing needles in the West would appear to indicate that injections play an important role in the dissemination of AIDS in Africa. The debate on this issue has been heated.[13] The evidence to date suggests that needles do not play a major role in the spread of the disease. The age distribution of African AIDS patients falls into two main groups: sexually active young adults and children under five.[14] If injections do play a major role in transmission, why are the five to fifteen age bracket and old men and women virtually unaffected? Since these groups also receive injections, heterosexual contact would appear to be the major means for the spread of African AIDS. As AIDS continues to spread and the number of seropositive individuals grows, the use of poorly sterilized or unsterilized syringes may become a more serious problem.

Conclusion

Clearly the movement of labor and the structure of the economy is an important determinant in disease patterns for both colonial and modern Africa. The spread of venereal syphilis and AIDS serve as ample proof. An understanding of the patterns of these movements can help predict regions which may require more careful screening for the appearance of AIDS. An awareness of the pressures faced by employed urban workers will also be valuable in designing educational campaigns to prevent the spread of AIDS. The behavior of these workers cannot be written off as simply promiscuous, as some past and present medical literature has suggested.

The most disquieting aspect of comparing the history of venereal syphilis and AIDS is the current extent and speed with which venereal syphilis spreads. In 1940 colonial medical officials surveyed the dispensaries in the rural Kikuyu reserves and found that around 6 percent of the cases were diagnosed as venereal syphilis, and signs of congenital, cardiovascular and neuro-syphilis were rare. By 1944 the incidence of venereal syphilis had changed dramatically. Investigations revealed that the case load had risen to 20 percent and that cases of congenital syphilis had begun to be observed.[15]

This dramatic spread can also be seen with AIDS from studies done both in Kenya and elsewhere in Africa. Two Kenyan studies have tracked groups of prostitutes and clients. The first study found seropositivity rates for prostitutes had gone from 4 percent in 1981 to 59 percent in 1985.[16] A similar study tracked another group of women from 1985 to 1987 and saw the seropositivity rate rise from 0 percent to 67 percent.[17] Some other African cities from limited samples show disturbing rates of seropositivity. If AIDS follows a pattern similar to venereal syphilis and given its eventually deadly results, the disease will spread into the rural countryside with possibly devastating demographic effects.

ENDNOTES

[1]An earlier version of this paper was given at the 30th annual meeting of the African Studies Association, 20 November 1987, Denver.

[2]I have chosen Kenya not because AIDS is more of a problem there than in other parts of the continent, but only because I am most familiar with the medical history of the country. For a more complete treatment of the history of venereal syphilis in Kenya, see, Marc H. Dawson, "Socio-economic and Epidemiological Change in Kenya:1880-1925," (Ph.D. thesis, University of Wisconsin-Madison, 1983), pp. 190-261.

[3]Janet M. Bujra, "Women 'Entrepreneurs' of Early Nairobi," *Canadian Journal of African Studies* 9 (1975):213-17.

[4]Interviews conducted by the author in Murang'a District with Macaaria Ndegwa, 28 September 1978; Elijah Gicheru Mugera, 12 January 1979; Adam Karanja Kiruri, 18 and 29 December 1978; and Bujra, pp. 217-20, and 222-23.

[5]Marc H. Dawson, "The 1920s Anti-Yaws Campaigns and Colonial Medical Policy in Kenya," *The International Journal of African Historical Studies* 20 (1987):417-35.

[6]Sharon Stichter, *Migrant Labor in Kenya: Capitalism and African Response 1895-1975*, Longman, 1979, p. 154 n. 87.

[7]Joan K. Kreiss, D. Koech, F.A. Plummer, *et al.*, "AIDS virus infection in Nairobi prostitutes: spread of the epidemic in East Africa," *New England Journal of Medicine* 314 (1986):414-18.

[8]See note #4.

[9]A.R.H.B. Verhagen, "Gonorrhoea," in *Health and Disease in Kenya*, edited by L.C. Vogel, A.S. Muller, *et al.*, East African Literature Bureau, 1974, p. 377.

[10]John A Carman, *A Medical History of the Colony and Protectorate of Kenya: A Personal Memoir*, 1976, p. 34; and P.A. Memon, "Some Geographical Aspects of the History of Urban Development in Kenya," *Hadith* 5 (1975):136-37.

[11]Francis A. Plummer paper given to 3rd International Conference on AIDS, Washington, D.C. as reported in *Chronicle of Higher Education*, 10 June 1987, p. 8.

[12]See discussion above, and for a fuller discussion, Dawson, 1987.

[13]For a review see, N. Clumeck, "Epidemiological Correlations Between African AIDS and AIDS in Europe," *Infection* 14 (1986):97-99.

[14]Robert J. Biggar, "The AIDS Problem in Africa," *The Lancet* 11 January 1986, p. 81.

[15]Dawson, 1983, pp. 190-262.

[16]N. Clumeck, "Heterosexual Transmission of AIDS: No Time for Complacency," *European Journal of Clinical Microbiology* 5(1986):610.

[17]See note # 10.

BIBLIOGRAPHY

Biggar, Robert J. "The AIDS Problem in Africa." *The Lancet* 11 January 1986, p. 81.

Bujra, Janet M. "Women 'Entrepreneurs' of Early Nairobi," *Canadian Journal of African Studies* 9(1975):213-34.

Carman, John A. *A Medical History of the Colony and Protectorate of Kenya: A Personal Memoir*. 1976.

Clumeck, N. "Epidemiological Correlations Between African AIDS and AIDS in Europe." *Infection* 14 (1986):97-99.

Clumeck, N. "Heterosexual Transmission of AIDS: No Time for Complacency." *European Journal of Clinical Microbiology* 5(1986):601-11.

Dawson, Marc H. "The 1920s Anti-Yaws Campaigns and Colonial Medical Policy in Kenya." *The International Journal of African Historical Studies* 20 (1987): 417-35.

Dawson, Marc H. "Socio-economic and Epidemiological Change in Kenya:1880-1925." Ph.D. Thesis. University of Wisconsin-Madison. 1983.

Kreiss, Joan K; Koech, D.; *et al*. "AIDS virus infection in Nairobi prostitutes: spread of the epidemic of East Africa." *New England Journal of Medicine* 314 (1986)414-18.

Memon, P.A. "Some Geographical Aspects of the History of Urban Development in Kenya." *Hadith* 5 (1975):128-53.

Stichter, Sharon. *Migrant Labor in Kenya: Capitalism and African Response 1895-1975*. Longman. 1979.

Verhagen, A.R.H.B. "Gonorrhoea." In *Health and Disease in Kenya*. Edited by L.C. Vogel, A.S. Muller, *et al*. East African Literature Bureau. 1974. pp. 375-80.

HISTORICAL AND ECOLOGICAL RAMIFICATIONS
FOR AIDS IN
EASTERN AND CENTRAL AFRICA

Rodger Yeager*

SUMMARY: As in other Third World areas, socioeconomic and political development in eastern and central Africa is closely associated with the ability of human societies to master their natural environments, and also with the tendency for this mastery to result in environmental overexploitation. One of these regions' greatest developmental constraints now involves rapidly growing and predominantly rural populations taxing the capacities of their increasingly endangered ecosystems. The possibility of a rural AIDS epidemic suggests a somewhat different scenario of ecological imbalance, and one with even graver consequences for political stability and sustainable development.

Introduction

We should not discount the real possibility that African AIDS is and will continue to be overestimated in its current magnitude. Rumors abound, many local areas are inaccessible to systematic data collection, diagnostic facilities are rare, and a host of deaths from other causes can be mistakenly attributed to AIDS.

On the other hand, it would be just as imprudent totally to discount the possibility of African AIDS triggering epidemics and destabilizations to rival those initiated by the Black Death, which in the fourteenth century helped depopulate Europe and its food-producing regions by one-third. I will argue that if AIDS spreads widely from African urban to rural areas, even lesser population reductions could produce equally disastrous consequences for the countries subjected to this epidemic. My present concern is not so much with the actual epidemiology of AIDS, but rather with a now totally hypothetical situation involving the possible impact of the

---

*Rodger Yeager, Ph.D., is Professor of Political Science and Adjunct Professor of History, West Virginia University.

disease if it were to reach epidemic proportions among African rural populations.

The eastern and central regions of Africa, and seven countries in particular, are particularly important in this regard because of their proximity to the apparent epicenter of the African AIDS outbreak, and because of their relatively high (although vastly understated) reported incidences of the disease. These countries include Burundi, Kenya, Rwanda, Tanzania, Uganda, Zaire, and Zambia. Their aggregate 1985 population was 100 million, of which 76 percent was rural and 24 percent urban.[1] The average annual population growth rate was 3.2 percent between 1980 and 1985, slightly above the African average. The average annual urbanization rate was 5.6 percent. Some of the potential implications of AIDS can be estimated for these countries along two vectors, urban and rural.

The Urban Vector

As we know, the most immediate effects of human immunodeficiency virus (HIV),[2] and consequently of AIDS, will be experienced in the urban areas of eastern and central Africa, because it is here where the greatest concentrations of infection appear to have become heterosexually established. To date, AIDS seems to have spread most rapidly among the several countries' limited pools of educated white-collar workers and professionals, including civil servants and public-sector technocrats. As such, AIDS threatens to "decapitate" already overstressed policy-making, administrative, and technical cadres by decimating their ranks at home and by denying overseas training opportunities to new generations. In the essentially statist social and economic environments of these countries, the resulting decline in policy performance alone portends increasing urban disorders. When they occur, these disturbances may be akin to recent anomic outbursts in some African cities, prompted by basic commodity shortages following policy-induced lapses in production and distribution, and also by reform-oriented consumer price increases and anti-inflationary currency adjustments.

Over the somewhat longer run, structural economic and political dislocations can be anticipated from sharp decreases in urban-centered foreign investment, and also in international tourism which likewise requires a strong urban infrastructure. This latter prospect is particularly ominous for Kenya, where tourism has become the second largest earner of hard currency.

In terms of checking the spread of AIDS along major trunk routes linking cities with each other and with the rural areas, no African country has been successful in preventing rural-to-urban migration through direct policy interventions. Even if such controls could be imposed, the disease seems already to be entrenched and is constantly reinforced by traders, prostitutes, and other itinerants. Added to this problem is the tendency for governments still to deny or downplay the seriousness of AIDS, which must limit the effectiveness of admittedly weak controls provided by blood screening, mass education, widespread distribution of condoms, and other countermeasures.

This reluctance to report AIDS cases results from African elites' unwillingness to have their countries viewed as cultural - and racial - pariahs of sexually communicated lethal disease. It also stems from a determination to protect foreign revenues, and from an equal fear of losing personal political legitimacy garnered through highly fragile patronage networks linking elites with each other and with their ethnic and sectional power bases.

Unfortunately, official denial also exercises a depressing influence over attempts by foreign aid agencies to help limit the scope of the disease.[3] Nor can private foreign initiatives presently be expected to receive unqualified political support. The Kenya government, for example, has created a cabinet-level committee to screen all AIDS-related information and expatriate research.[4]

A possible way out of the current dilemma could entail the quiet transfer of ameliorative research technology from industrial countries to Africa. This option faces three major obstacles in eastern and central Africa as in other parts of the continent; the rudimentary state of health-care delivery systems, the high cost of drugs likely to be effective in treating and/or preventing AIDS, and the length of time probably required to develop and test these drugs.

AIDS research performed *in* Africa has been primarily epidemiological, and suggests that infection rates are much lower in the rural areas than in the cities. At face value, this finding should be encouraging in terms of governments' ability to preserve some semblance of economic and political order, simply because most of the human population and its productive capacity continue to reside in the countryside. This conclusion must be balanced, however, against possible losses in rural productive capacity caused by decimations of urban technical cadres. It must also be weighed against other factors linking the fate of African urban centers with that of their rural hinterlands.

The Rural Vector

As is widely appreciated, the rural-urban relationship remains much closer throughout Africa than in the industrial world. In a few countries (e.g., Botswana) the majority of city dwellers divide their time seasonally or even more frequently between town and countryside. This nexus carries political significance in that policy-making and administrative elites maintain, enhance, and sometimes lose their preferred statuses through the highly personalized patronage relationships mentioned earlier, which unite them not only with peers and subordinates, but also with their rural bases of mutual assistance and support.

This close association of patronage interests (if not necessarily policy interests) means that a rapid and widespread increase in rural AIDS may bring forth an equally rapid and widespread epidemic of elite instability, as these leaders jockey for position and struggle to survive amid the ruins of their defunct patronage hierarchies. A spillover of AIDS into the countryside is favored by certain demographic and public-health realities in contemporary eastern and central Africa, in addition to the high levels of physical mobility and close social bonds just noted. The possible effects of rapidly occurring and widely felt rural depopulations[5] include not only short-term elite destabilizations, but also long-term ecological collapses causing more-or-less permanent political and developmental crises.

An obvious demographic factor must be that more than 40 percent of these predominantly rural populations occupies the sexually most active age group, the highest percentage in the modern world. The risk of a woman contracting AIDS is increased by term pregnancy, with an even chance of transmitting the disease to the child. This not only extends high risk to yet another large age cohort, but it also raises the possibility of a Malthusian population involution accelerating into the next century. This prospect is enhanced by the actively pronatalist quality of African rural society, and by the nutritional problems and lowered resistances to disease already present there.

If AIDS massively compounds these survival problems, population growth will slow and local depopulations may well appear. Until now, one of eastern and central Africa's greatest developmental constraints has involved rapidly growing and yet productively unassisted populations taxing the capacities of their countries' increasingly endangered natural resources and environments. From a human if not an environmental recovery standpoint, AIDS-related reductions in rural population growth and density will exacerbate rather than lessen these imbalances. Not only will the survivors be compelled to support larger numbers of younger and older dependents. Their ability to do so will be severely hampered by a loss of ecological control over the environment, creating what Kjekshus has described as "a frontier situation where the conquest of the ecosystem [has] to recommence."[6] This scenario may depict AIDS' most lasting threat to African political stability and development.

The Ecological Control-Loss Scenario
In trying to estimate the impact of events that could but have not yet happened, it is often useful to look for historical parallels to such occurrences. Clues to what may result from a rural AIDS epidemic can in fact be found in the late nineteenth and early twentieth-century experiences of Tanzania and parts of Uganda and Kenya. Before this time, rural dwellers provided confirmation to a thesis argued by Ester Boserup,[7] which rejected the neomalthusian hypothesis that population growth must always subject

subsistence societies to progressive environmental destruction and eventual food shortages.

Instead, Boserup contended that high human fertility and rising population densities prompt an intensification of land use and farm labor in arable environments, which leads to the adoption of technical innovations that maintain soil fertility, increase agricultural productivity, enable farm surpluses for trade, and facilitate a diversification of economic activity into nonagricultural pursuits. Conversely, less-arable ecosystems are typically inhabited by scattered pastoral and farming populations which employ land-extensive agricultural practices requiring fewer inputs of labor and technology, and also producing fewer if any agricultural surpluses. Owing to their intermittent land-use tendencies, however, such practices incur little environmental damage which is not self-correcting.

In its eastern African setting, this dual system of population and land use was mutually reinforcing. The fertile agricultural "center" was protected by the low-density "periphery," in that widely dispersed peripheral communities provided a human and livestock buffer separating larger population concentrations from the scourge of trypanosomiasis (sleeping sickness). This was achieved through a partial displacement of indigenous wildlife species, including those hosting trypanosomes and transmitting them through the tsetse-fly vector. In return, the agricultural centers contributed food surpluses and useful manufactures (e.g., textiles and metal products such as spear tips) which eased life at the periphery.

This balance resulted from specialized controls exerted by human societies over their different ecosystems. It was fundamentally disrupted during the final years of the last century and the first decade of this, by a series of natural and artificially created catastrophes. First, rinderpest swept over eastern Africa in the 1890s, destroying perhaps as much as 95 percent of the region's cattle population and breaking peripheral societies' accommodation with their savanna ecologies. This epidemic was swiftly followed by a recurrence, after many years' absence, of smallpox which combined with dysentery to decimate the rural periphery and the center as well. At about the same time, sand fleas spread into eastern Africa from

Brazil via Portuguese Angola, laying their eggs in human flesh and causing infection, mutilation, and still more death.

As these tragedies unfolded, indigenous societies' control over their ecosystems lapsed, leaving them most vulnerable to yet other, and this time policy-related, demographic calamities. The denouement of ecological collapse, famine and trypanosomiasis, resulted from the direct (famine) and indirect (widespread human sleeping sickness) effects of European colonization. German "pacification" campaigns included a scorched earth policy that lay waste to vast areas of what is now mainland Tanzania. European land acquisition and labor procurement displaced many communities from the agricultural centers of Tanzania and Kenya, and also separated these communities from their most productive workers. To such dislocations were added locust swarms from the north, followed by the ravages of world war, which pitted Germans against British in mainland Tanzania and finally drove the former from Africa. Widespread famine could not help but result from this combination of crises.

As eastern Africa entered the 1920s, the inevitable consequences of the previous two decades' ecological disruptions occurred - sleeping sickness rapidly spreading from the peripheries of human settlement to the once-protected centers. This epidemic led to further colonial policy interventions, from which some rural areas have not yet recovered.

What had changed were the geographical and intergroup relationships of five long-standing populations in eastern Africa: humans, domestic livestock, wild fauna, trypanosomes, and tsetse fly. Previously controlled by the first two, the latter three groups were confined to discrete areas so that they worked some, but not epidemic, hardship on local African societies and their livelihoods. With the initial depopulations of the 1890s and early 1900s, wildlife and tsetse expanded their territories, returning infested zones to bush and threatening the surviving people and their livestock.

In order to combat sleeping sickness and to protect now-endangered wildlife, the colonial authorities established concentrated settlements in what remained of the agricultural center. They also began creating a vast system of national parks and game reserves, under the distinctly European notion that the only way to preserve wild animals was by denying human access to them. These highly unpopular actions took yet more land out of managed use, again upset local economies, led to new outbreaks of trypanosomiasis, and further intensified human conflict with wildlife. The last two unintended consequences created an impetus for additional settlements and game preserves.

The Postindependence Political Factor: The Tanzanian Case

Sleeping-sickness settlements were most emphasized in mainland Tanzania, which had become a League of Nations territory mandated to British administration. The settlements were successful from the standpoints of political control and public health, bringing people together into governable units and preventing major epidemics of trypanosomiasis. From an ecological perspective, however, they set precedents for a series of policy errors which continue to confound Tanzanian socioeconomic and political development nearly 70 years later. These include the independent regime's nationalization of sisal production, and also its reconsolidation of once again-disbursed rural populations through the 1970s policy of *ujamaa vijijini* (socialism in the villages).

Following its commitment of Tanzania to populist socialism in 1967, the independent leadership decided to increase its own control by nationalizing the "commanding heights" of the economy. Included in this move were the country's commercial sisal estates, originally established as part of a colonial enclosure movement, which had once served as Tanzania's most important earners of foreign exchange. Unfortunately, nationalization was not matched by adequate capitalization and management capacity, and was accomplished during an historically low slump in the international sisal market. Located in boundary areas separating the agricultural periphery from its arable center, and often bordering on national parks and game reserves, the estates quickly fell to incursions of bush, tsetse flies, and trypanosomes. This process continues today, although the current regime is now attempting to attract foreign investment on behalf of reprivatizing the estates.

The *ujamaa vijijini* policy offers further insights into the ecological effects of rural depopulation. In the decades following Tanzania's sleeping-sickness crisis, rural dwellers reestablished their widely scattered homesteads in the agriculturally peripheral areas. The colonial government failed to follow its public-health initiatives with effective measures to raise agricultural productivity and food sufficiency on these lands. Following independence in 1961, African policy makers announced their determination to reorder local governance and to reverse the production losses and environmental deterioration that were presumably exacerbated by a lack of developmental inputs. Agreeing with President Julius Nyerere's preference, they reasoned that if these goals were to be reached, large numbers of peasants would have again to be moved from scattered homesteads and isolated hamlets into consolidated and easily accessible village communities.

The ultimate product of this decision was the compulsory villagization of the Tanzanian rural society, so that by 1977 over 90 percent of the peasantry were reportedly assigned to more than 7,000 villages at an average occupancy of over 1,000 people per nucleated settlement. This huge exercise in directed migration was not applied equally in all parts of the country, and today about 60 percent of the resettled population lives in areas of low rainfall prone to density-related ecological problems.

Like their colonial predecessors, Tanzanian elites proved far more successful in resettling rural dwellers than in providing for their basic economic needs. In fact, the now all-encompassing public sector not only failed to deliver the essentials for sustainably intensive agriculture, it also prevented them from being obtained from private sources. By 1980-1982, per capita food output had fallen to about 88 percent of its 1969-1971 level.

The villagization program was centered on peripheral food-producing areas, in part to avoid disrupting production in the already densely settled export-crop regions. Ecologically, the speed and scope of *ujamaa vijijini* meant that villages were hastily and often poorly sited, so they lacked access to basic amenities such as water and fuelwood. Given the available agricultural technologies, moreover, many were far too large for the carrying capacity of the land. The noted French agronomist René Dumont visited the rural areas in 1979. He discovered extensive soil exhaustion and erosion barely two years after the completion of villagization.

Writing two years earlier, Kjekshus described the perils then facing Tanzanian agricultural systems and environment.

> Nucleated settlement will mean overcrowding of restricted areas with people and domestic animals and the accompanying soil erosion, gully formation and dust-bowls which are all common features in situations where the human initiative has suddenly overtaxed the carrying capacity of the land without compensatory inputs to increase the quality of cultivation. Centralized settlements will mean time wasted in long walks between the new dwellings and the productive fields and will result in the almost certain falling into disuse of the peripheral shambas [farming plots] and their gradual takeover by bush and vermin.[8]

Kjekshus' predictions have since materialized in large parts of Tanzania. Under these circumstances, it is difficult to imagine coherent economic and political survival, let alone development, if AIDS intervenes on the side of a new wave of trypanosomiasis and other diseases - to effect yet another round of rural depopulations extending into the twenty-first century.

Conclusion

These same outcomes can be imagined for other African countries possibly facing rural AIDS outbreaks - for example, Uganda where years of political violence have severely damaged a once thriving rural economy; Kenya where 80 percent of the world's fastest growing population is compressed into less than 20 percent of the available space with the remaining people and land developmentally neglected; Zaire where bureaucratic inefficiency and corruption both arise from and feed on ethnic and sectional instability; Rwanda where rural overcrowding and natural resource degradation may already be approaching a terminal state; and Zambia where a collapse of copper revenues and near bankruptcy prevent economic recovery and developmental investment in the long-deprived agricultural sector.

Predicting the future is always a hazardous business. Yet it can be argued that if African AIDS were to spread massively from the urban to the rural areas, the resulting human-ecological collapses would bring devastation in every other respect. And even if the two vectors do not merge and reinforce each other, the political and economic chaos created by a growing urban AIDS epidemic may well wreak its own havoc on already weakened rural societies throughout eastern and central Africa.

ENDNOTES

[1]All standard demographic, nutritional, and health statistics are taken from World Bank, *World Development Report, 1987* (New York: Oxford University Press, 1987), pp. 202, 212, 254, 256, 258, 259, 260, and 266.

[2]In some eastern and central African countries (e.g., Uganda and Zaire), between 6 and 10 percent of the total population is thought to be infected with HIV, making its incidence more than 100 times greater than in the United States. Moreover, men and women are infected in about equal numbers, suggesting that HIV may correlate with other venereal diseases that go untreated.

[3]Official intransigence may finally be lessening as African governments come more fully to appreciate the collective dangers presented by AIDS.

[4]One should not become too self-righteous in criticizing African governments' reluctance to acknowledge their AIDS epidemics. Denial of this sort is commonly expressed in low-incidence areas of industrial countries including the United States. According to Harry Hull, New Mexico state epidemiologist, "everywhere in the country we're seeing denial. I hope [New Mexico, with less than 4 percent the incidence rate reported in New York City] can learn the bitter lessons vicariously" (*Science News*, August 22, 1987).

[5]If AIDS contraction rates encountered in the United States also prevail in Africa, decimations of local populations seem possible. According to one estimate (which may soon be revised upward for both incubation period and final ratio of HIV to AIDS cases), HIV incubates in five to six years. About 20 percent of the HIV-seropositive population contracts AIDS, with half dead in two and one-half years and the other half in five years. Robert J. Biggar, "AIDS and HIV Infection: Estimates of the Magnitude of the Problem Worldwide in 1985/1986," *Clinical Immunology and Immunopathology*, 45 (1987): 299.

[6]Helge G. Kjekshus, *Ecology Control and Economic Development in East African History* (Berkeley: University of California Press, 1977), p. 184.

[7]Ester Boserup, *The Conditions of Agricultural Growth* (Chicago: Aldine Publishing Co., 1965).

[8]Helge G. Kjekshus, "The Tanzanian Villagization Policy: Implementational Lessons and Ecological Dimensions," *Canadian Journal of African Studies*, 11 (1977): 282.

PART III
Issues of Management, Policy and Politics

MANAGEMENT OF AIDS PATIENTS:
Case Report From Uganda

Cynthia Haq*

SUMMARY: AIDS, now endemic in many areas of Uganda, has complex interactions with the management and treatment of other infectious tropical diseases. The impacts on primary health care in a rural area and on child survival are described, with some consideration of psychological and economic effects. Two case reports exemplify some of the clinical dilemmas of treating AIDS when limited diagnostic and therapeutic resources are available. Educational and preventive programs now underway in Uganda are briefly described.

Introduction

The epidemic of AIDS, now spreading extensively through Central and East Africa, has added complexities to the management of basic health care services in communities which already had tremendous needs and limited resources. The following observations were made while working in Kasangati, Uganda, a rural community village north of Kampala, in child survival and community-based primary care projects.

The appearance of "Slim's Disease," or AIDS, in Uganda was first noted in 1982 and in some areas is still unrecognized among the people. The number of reported cases of AIDS has grown from 17 in 1983 to over 2,000 in 1987. Estimates of the prevalence of the infection are based on small, possibly unrepresentative samples and range from less than 1% in adults and in some rural areas to over 80% in high-risk groups such as urban prostitutes.

The problem of AIDS in Uganda, though devastating and critical, has had relatively minor impact when compared to other health problems. In 1986 less than 20% of the population had ready access to clean water, 25% of children surveyed were malnourished, and less than 10% of the nation's children were immunized against preventible diseases. Less than half the

---
* Cynthia Haq, MD, an Assistant Professor of Community and Family Medicine at Dartmouth Medical School worked in rural Uganda as a physician dealing with HIV and AIDS.

population has access to local health care, and most women receive no prenatal care.[1] The incidence of malaria, tuberculosis and other respiratory infections is high, as well as that of diarrheal diseases and dehydration. Each year an estimated 600,000 children die of preventible diseases; this is compared to 300 reported deaths to date from AIDS.[2]

The epidemiology of AIDS in Uganda is similar to that throughout Africa. The majority of patients are between 20 and 40 years of age with very few cases in the 5 to 14 and over 60 year age group. An increasing number of infants and young children under 5, however, are now being affected. Heterosexual transmission is the primary means of spread, and risk increases rapidly with a larger number of sexual partners. The disease is present primarily in urban areas but is spreading into the southern regions of Lake Victoria and along the Trans-African highway to the east and west. In 1987 surveys showed 13% HIV seropositivity among pregnant women in Kampala, 33% seropositivity among long distance truck drivers, and 85% seropositivity among prostitutes in the Rakai district.[3]

The health impact of AIDS in Ugandan communities is tremendous and complex. Morbidity from infectious diseases is increased in patients with AIDS, and infections are more likely to be transmitted from them to patients without AIDS. The high incidence of sexually transmitted diseases enhances susceptibility to AIDS, and once AIDS has developed, the impact of these infections is worsened. Respiratory infections, including pneumonia and tuberculosis, are common in AIDS patients and may be spread extensively through communities where crowded conditions exist. When access to clean water and effective human waste disposal systems are limited, as in much of rural Africa, exposure to viral, bacterial and amoebic gastrointestinal infections is common in AIDS patients. Once these infections are contracted they readily spread to other persons in the community with or without AIDS. The interactions of AIDS with other common infectious tropical diseases is not completely understood, but one would expect all infectious diseases to be worsened in settings where individuals have experienced damage to the immune systems.

The effect of AIDS on mortality rates among adults is also beginning to be felt in most areas where AIDS is endemic. For example, up to one-quarter of the adult population in some communities in southern Uganda has reportedly died from AIDS. The effects of the death of adults in their most productive years results in significant loss of economic productivity. The elderly will be left without adult children to provide economic support; children will be orphaned or dependent on the ill and dying. These economic and social effects are intensified by the high rate of infection of the educated elite in many communities.

Public Health Dilemmas

Child survival will also be affected by AIDS in many ways. Since maternal rates of infection are nearly 25% in some areas, transmission of HIV to newborn infants will be significant, resulting in the infection of over 10% of infants born. The effects of endemic malnutrition, diarrhea, illnesses, and respiratory infections will probably speed the death of these children, the majority of whom will die in early childhood.

Children in areas of endemic AIDS who are not yet infected with HIV face significant risks. Massive national immunization programs are now being mounted to counter the low level of immunizations for diphtheria, tetanus, pertussis and measles among most children in Uganda. Due to limited needles, syringes, fuel for sterilization, and antiseptic agents, immunizations can risk transmission of HIV. Although no cases of HIV infection following immunization have been documented to date, parental fear of HIV transmission through immunizations could result in much lower immunization rates and consequent increases in deaths due to entirely preventable diseases. In areas with a high prevalence of parasitic infections and sickle cell disease, in which severe anemia is common, transfusions of unscreened donor blood also carry significant risk of HIV transmission.

The psychological effect of AIDS on communities, families and those infected can be devastating. Communities confronted by this new, fatal illness, which is incompletely understood and carries significant social stigma, frequently develop widespread fear and depression. Since neurologic impairment and depression is frequent in patients with AIDS, mental health needs will increase in areas where AIDS is endemic. AIDS reverses the natural order of death; the loss of young adults creates a war time atmosphere. As Uganda is still recovering from a long series of civil wars, the impact of AIDS is even more acute.

AIDS has significant impact on the economics of health care in Uganda as in all developing African nations. In 1987 Uganda spent less than $2 on health care per citizen. Providing treatment for one AIDS patient, comparable to that delivered in the United States, would exceed the entire annual budget of a rural health center in Uganda. Government health officials must make difficult decisions of allocating scarce health care resources. Choices must be made between providing clean water, sanitary facilities, immunizations, or controlling the spread of AIDS. Neither resources nor manpower are available to undertake the needed public health measures and to simultaneously launch AIDS control programs.

Case Studies: Mother and Child

The following medical case histories illustrate the complexities of dealing with AIDS in a rural Ugandan community.

CASE 1: *A.S. is a 20 year old single mother of two who came to the physician with diarrhea of nine months duration, 10 kg weight loss and fatigue. For several weeks she had been vomiting frequently after meals and had become anorexic. She had become gradually more withdrawn and spent much of her time in bed.*

The patient was the second youngest in a family of five children who was raised in a semirural area, 20 miles from Kampala, a large urban center. At age 16 she left home to live in the city, where she worked at various odd jobs, including prostitution. She delivered two children within three years; the second child was born three months prior to her illness. After becoming ill and unable to care for herself and the children, the patient returned to her rural home to live with her parents and extended family. Because of her illness and fatigue, the patient discontinued breastfeeding her second child at five months. This child was experiencing failure to thrive with slow weight gain and frequent episodes of diarrhea.

Examination revealed an alert, oriented, thin young woman, who appeared depressed. The skin was dry, warm and had multiple darkly pigmented lesions, especially prominent over the lower extremities. Her mouth showed dry mucous membranes and extensive white patches extending into the throat. No involvement of the lymph system was noted. Lungs were clear. Her abdomen was thin and soft with hyperactive bowel sounds and diffuse mild tenderness. Laboratory studies revealed anemia and gastrointestinal infection.

The patient and her family were informed of the diagnosis of possible Slim's Disease (AIDS). Education was provided about the nature of the illness, its mode of transmission, and the lack of curative therapy. Arrangements for obtaining confirmatory HIV testing were offered, but due to the expense (Uganda shillings 6,000; U.S. $1.20) and lack of transportation, the patient declined. She was given oral electrolyte solutions, oral washes for treatment of her mouth infection, and repeated antibiotics for her intestinal infection, but this was never eradicated. Daily care was provided in the home by extended family members. The patient died within four months of the initial treatments. A follow-up examination of her children revealed persistent failure to thrive and diarrhea in her youngest child, but HIV infection was not verified.

CASE 2: E.K. is a 3 year old female who had a three week history of fatigue, shortness of breath and swelling of the extremities. The mother had noted a decreased appetite and decline in activity as well as intermittent fever and apparent joint pains.

Physical examination revealed a pale lethargic child in mild respiratory distress. Her skin showed no pigmented lesions. Her heart rate was high, and she had fluid in both lungs. The liver was enlarged. Laboratory studies revealed severe anemia. The patient was diagnosed as having sickle cell anemia. She was referred to the nearest hospital for a blood transfusion. The parents were informed of the risks and benefit of transfusion and elected to have the transfusion performed. Despite a reported prevalence of 30% of donor blood contaminated with HIV, no blood screening was performed due to lack of resources. The child improved significantly following blood transfusion and continued to do well two months later at a follow-up visit.

These cases illustrate some of the common dilemmas of dealing with HIV in a rural African setting. CASE 1 describes a typical patient who probably contracted AIDS sexually in an urban area. Her youngest child was probably also infected. Confirmatory diagnostic testing was not practically available, and therapy was primarily supportive and palliative. Education of the patient and her family was of primary importance. When the patient died, her children were taken over and supported by the grandparents.

CASE 2 highlights the dilemma of performing blood transfusions for patients in HIV endemic areas where screening of donor blood is not performed. The child had severe congestive heart failure secondary to profound anemia and sickle cell disease, but did not yet have AIDS. Transfusion therapy, though immediately life-saving, conferred significant risk of transmission of HIV.

For a health worker in an area of endemic AIDS there are multiple concerns. First, the fear of contracting the illness through provision of health care services is real. Exposure to blood is frequent; surgical gloves are scarce, usually unavailable, and are re-used many times. Antiseptics and fuel for sterilization are in short supply. Second, the extent of preclinical AIDS in rural communities, being unknown to health care workers, makes determination of priorities in providing basic health care services and educational programs difficult. Third, the ability to care for patients with obvious AIDS is limited by the lack of drugs and trained health workers. Fourth, diagnostic testing for HIV seropositivity and infectious diseases is generally unavailable. Fifth, profound ethical questions are raised when the treatment required to save a life may be dangerous. Preventive and curative medical services which confer a significant risk of transmission of HIV violate the basic medical ethic of "first do no harm."

Management: The Ugandan Response

During a relatively short period of time in Uganda, dramatic progress toward curbing the spread of HIV infection has been made. The government has formed a National Committee for the Prevention of AIDS (NCPA), which includes health workers, educators, administrators, and political and church leaders to develop priorities and set national policies. An AIDS Control Program has been independently established to avoid diversion of funds from other crucial health programs. A primary health care infrastructure already exists which serves as a vehicle for dissemination of information and policy.

The main purpose of the AIDS Control Program is prevention of the spread of AIDS through health education. Education of health care workers is now widespread with a focus on prevention of transmission, clinical diagnosis, and supportive therapy. The risks of transmission of HIV through blood transfusions, injections, and surgery are now recognized, and measures are being implemented to reduce these risks. In 1986 only very limited blood screening for HIV was available in Kampala, but by May 1987, 13 ELISA screening centers were established in Uganda, primarily in HIV endemic areas. Serious limitations are the costs and lack of availability of blood screening procedures in many areas, the shortage of needles, syringes, and gloves necessitating their re-use, and shortage of fuel and disinfectants to permit effective sterilization of medical instruments.

Research efforts to investigate various aspects of AIDS are being conducted in many areas. Longitudinal epidemiologic studies are being coordinated to improve surveillance. Sociological research is being conducted on cultural factors in the risk of transmission and to investigate the acceptability of condom use. Virological research and laboratory test quality control studies are being conducted at the Uganda Virus Institute.

Large scale public education campaigns are also underway. These programs are being facilitated by WHO, UNICEF, and other volunteer programs. Educational literature has been developed and disseminated in urban areas and through the school systems, focusing on curbing the transmission of the HIV. Radio Uganda carries frequent messages with "Love Carefully" as a catchphrase, describing the transmission of AIDS by sexual intercourse and the importance of condoms and reducing the number of sexual partners. Church and political leaders are encouraging villagers to maintain "zero grazing," the concept of having only one sexual partner, to reduce HIV transmission. Condoms are now available in many areas, provided free by the Ministry of Health.[2] Community health workers have been trained to deliver the information in many areas. Local political "resistance committees" and church groups are also spreading information.

Serious limitations in these efforts are the current high level of illiteracy in Uganda, and a shortage of health workers to convey information to the people, especially in rural areas.

Funding for an effective AIDS control program at the local level is a major limiting factor according to Ugandan sources. The costs are staggering on the scale of Uganda's economy. An ELISA testing center costs almost U.S $10,000 to set up. One ELISA test costs U.S. $1, while average per capita spending on health care in Africa is U.S. $1.70.3 The WHO has committed $7 million to be spent in Uganda over the next 5 years. In May, 1987 an additional $6 million was pledged by 15 countries and nine international agencies to support the first year of Uganda's National AIDS program, but assistance is still needed for expansion and development of control measures and management techniques.

It is too early to judge the effectiveness of Uganda control and education campaigns dealing with AIDS. As in most African nations there are complications with other tropical infectious diseases, with a shortage of health care workers, and with a lack of funding. The hopeful sign in Uganda is that serious, collaborative, international efforts are underway to meet the challenge of AIDS.

ENDNOTES

[1] World Health Organization, Annual Statistics, 1986.

[2] Combating AIDs in Uganda, (Editorial) *Lampada*, 1987 Spring (11):16-7.

[3] Okware, Samuel: Towards a National AIDS Control Program in Uganda, *Western Journal of Medicine*, 147(6)726-29, December, 1987.

TRADITIONAL HEALERS AND AIDS MANAGEMENT

Charles Good*

SUMMARY: Traditional healers (THs) are urgently needed as co-workers in public health strategies designed to 1) contain the spread of HIV and AIDs and 2) care for AIDS/ARC victims. Incorporating THs is a socially sound and pragmatic policy. They are key opinion leaders in health matters as well as therapists in and beyond their own rural and urban communities. THs are geographically and functionally well-situated to perform positive interventions. They are at risk of exposure to HIV and potential co-factors of AIDs through their patients, and vice versa. Consequently, many are already informally engaged in AIDS "management." Involvement of THs in the (integrated) urban and rural sectors of national AIDS control programs will build upon the informal interaction that already exists among the traditional, biomedical, and "popular" elements of African ethnomedical systems.

Introduction

The true incidence, prevalence and geographical extent of HIV (Human immunodeficiency virus) infections and AIDS/ARC (AIDS-related complex) cases in African populations are unknown. AIDS is a disease that progresses after antibodies that should provide immunity to the HIV have formed. It includes a number of clinical conditions that are produced or intensified by profound suppression of the immune system (Biggar, 1987).[1] One million HIV infections and 10,000 new AIDS cases per year is a present minimum estimate for Africa; however, no world region has a greater problem with HIV than Africa in terms of the estimated proportion of the population currently HIV seropositive and estimated AIDS cases (Mann, 1987). Heterosexual transmission and, overall, an almost equal male:female ratio of infection characterize the epidemiology of HIV seropositivity and AIDS in Africa as it is known at this time. Young adults in the 18-40 age

*Charles M. Good, Ph.D., is Professor of Geography at Virginia Polytechnic Institute and State University, Blacksburg, Virginia, 24061.

group and children under two (vertically transmitted congenital or perinatal infections) appear to be at greatest risk (Biggar, 1987). However, a recent study of HIV seropositive persons in Kinshasha revealed a female:male ratio 6:1 in the age category of 15-30 years, while in the over 30 years group the ratio showed a dramatic drop to 0.64:1 (Ryder, *et al.*, 1987) and Green (this volume). In contrast to North America and Europe, homosexuality as a lifestyle, intravenous drug abuse, and hemophilia are not significant risk factors for AIDS in Africa (Barker and Turshen, 1986). While AIDS is certainly not the most common or widespread disease affecting the population of Africa south of the Sahara *at this time*, if left unchecked it may soon reach a hyperepidemic scale in many regions. Such a tragedy could precipitate the breakdown of social systems and reverse previous gains in levels of health.

Populations with HIV seropositivity have been officially reported from 36 African countries and are known to be present in many others. Highest levels of confirmed cases of AIDS are reported from an epidemic "belt" in central and east Africa that includes Uganda, Tanzania, Rwanda, Burundi, Kenya, Zambia, Congo, Central African Republic, Zaire, Zimbabwe and Malawi (Mann, 1987; Family Health International, 1987). However, it must be emphasized that HIV and AIDS are *not* uniformly distributed, or of equal incidence and prevalence levels throughout the cities, towns and countryside in the present AIDS belt. Case reporting is improving but remains grossly incomplete and sporadic. In Uganda, for example, it is estimated that only 1 in 50 AIDS cases is currently being seen and/or reported by health authorities (Ankrah, 1988). As Biggar observes elsewhere in this volume, most of the available evidence about the spatial distribution of HIV and AIDS depends on extrapolations from small, selected risk groups (hospital-based studies, prostitute surveys, etc.). Careful random sampling of urban and rural populations is necessary in order to develop more comprehensive and reliable estimates of the regional distribution and structure of HIV prevalence and at-risk populations.[2] At this time the geographical epidemiology of AIDS is one of the least known aspects of the disease.

Within Africa the early pattern of clinically recognizable AIDS and ARC cases suggested rapid spread (or emergence) of HIV and co-factors, or perhaps other triggering mechanisms (Leishman, 1987 and *Daily Nation* [Nairobi], 1987), from an elite network "downward" into urban non-elite classes and then into rural zones (Klondahl, 1985; Tinker and Sabatier, 1987). However, the pattern of AIDS in rural southern Uganda (e.g., Rakai) and the Kagera-Buhaya region of northwest Tanzania (see, e.g. *Daily Nation* [Nairobi], 1987a, *The Weekly Review* [Nairobi], 1987, and Hooper, 1987) where it is locally known as "Slim disease", suggests that the elite network hypothesis model characterizes just one of several transmission processes. The Uganda evidence indicates that AIDS is spreading *from* villages as well as outward from the towns and along transportation corridors (Ankrah, 1988). In reality, the pattern of AIDS in many localities is interconnected with the synergisms of income uncertainty, malnutrition and infection in poor households (cf. Barker and Turshen, 1986) -- and a high degree of local, regional, and transnational population mobility.

This paper highlights a critical need to involve *bona fide* traditional healers (THs), including traditional birth attendants (TBAs), as co-workers in public health strategies designed to accomplish two basic goals: to 1) contain the spread of HIV and AIDS and 2) care for AIDS/ARC victims. The argument--essentially a hypothesis that must be evaluated through sound fieldwork--is summarized as follows. Traditional healers are key health opinion leaders as well as therapists in and beyond their own rural and urban communities (Green, 1986; Last and Chavunduka; and Good, 1987). They are at risk of exposure to HIV and potential co-factors of AIDS through various forms of contact with their patients, and vice versa. Consequently they are *already* informally engaged in AIDS "management".[3] Involving THs in the (integrated) urban and rural sectors of national AIDS control programs will build upon the informal interaction that already exists among the traditional, biomedical, and "popular" (lay) elements of African ethnomedical systems (Chavunduka, 1978; Good, 1987; and Last, 1986).

Overview Of Traditional Medicine

Before proceeding further it will be useful to briefly note the essential character of African traditional medicine in the late 1980's. The main features of the changing traditional systems have been examined empirically and in theoretical discussions at considerable depth, particularly during the last decade (e.g. Janzen, 1978; Chavunduka, 1978; Sargent, 1982; Feierman, 1985; Githagui, 1985; Last and Chavunduka, 1986; Stock, 1987; and Good, 1987). Many of the strengths and weaknesses of traditional medical practices have been identified (Good, 1987a). Social and behavioral profiles of THs and their clientele are now available for a small but instructive range of societies. More is known about when, how, and why THs are consulted. It is now well-established that the search for health care, and referral practices by THs, often result in patients consulting practitioners in two or more therapy systems. Self-treatment, visits to THs, and resort to biomedical services may occur serially or concurrently during episodes of the same illness. This full complement of therapy options available to a particular population is what forms the basis of an African (or any other) "ethnomedical system" (Good, 1980; 1987). Similarly, another observer has defined "African medicine" as "medicine of whatever kind available to the patient...including not only all the varieties of 'traditional medicine' but all the varieties of non-traditional medicine, too, whether Islamic, homeopathic or 'Western'" (Last, 1986:5).

African health ministries may choose to initiate cooperative endeavors with THs, or pay lip service to their roles and continue to ignore them. In either case, THs will continue to comprise large, diverse, and more or less organized cadres that are increasingly influenced by contact with local forms of biomedicine and modern pharmaceuticals. As such THs are both subjects and agents of change: they participate in an on-going, essentially unsystematic process in which they variously "borrow," reinterpret, and apply selected biomedical ideas and practices--including the use of mass-produced drugs--in everyday contacts with patients. While different forms of intentional cooperation between biomedical workers and THs have long been advocated (W.H.O., 1985) and policy options are well-known (Pillsbury, 1982; Stepan, 1985; and MacCormack, 1986), traditional medicine and THs continue to occupy an ambiguous position in national health policies.

Meanwhile, their influence in society and in health remain strong and there are mounting pressures for increased professionalization of their membership and activities (Last and Chavunduka, 1986).

Unfortunately, *bona fide* THs are sometimes stereotyped together in the public mind with charlatans and other unqualified "fringe" practitioners-- including "bush doctors" and "backstreet doctors"--whose goals seem limited to cash accumulation obtained through fraud and preying on the innocent and needy. Such abuses appear to be growing in volume and lead to blurred distinctions between credible and disreputable practitioners. This growing trend of real and perceived charlatanism and "medical entrepreneurship" is exacerbated by the inequities in biomedical services and the failure of health ministries to adopt sound policy initiatives in respect of both *bona fide* THs and various kinds of practitioners in the "popular" health care arena such as faith healers, astrologers, and injectionists.

As used here, bona fide THs are individuals who are formally or informally "accredited" by their own communities and clientele to practice various health-oriented services. They charge reasonable fees and often do not expect full compensation until the patient is satisfied with the outcome of therapy. In much of rural Africa and in many urban neighborhoods, THs are the most frequented source of health care after self-treatment. At their best, THs offer an authentic application of their culture's experience with the healing arts--modified and adapted according to their own experience in a rapidly changing society. Their functions include diagnosis, prevention, and elimination of imbalances in physical, mental, social well-being. THs provide *traditionally-based* therapy in the sense that indigenous beliefs and practices about health and disease-- such as the dichotomy between etiologies of natural and human agency and the ritualization of herbs--are typically their central point of reference.

Generally speaking, most rural areas have at least one TH (typically part-time) for every 200-300 people. In towns the crude ratios range from 1:400-800, and many practitioners are full-time. THs continue to serve in various specific roles, including those of religious-medical specialist, counselor, psychotherapist, herbalist, birth attendant, and surgeon as well as different combinations of these specialities.

A large proportion of THs concentrate on a few diseases or syndromes. They are consulted for acute ailments such as diarrhea, convulsions, fever, and burns, as well as chronic disorders involving the human reproductive systems, the abdominal tract, and a wide range of stress-induced illness. In general, there is considerable diversity among THs from the same or related ethnic groups concerning the kinds of diseases they are best qualified to treat, their empiric or spiritual orientation, skill proficiency, reputation, and spatial mobility. Such factors must be carefully weighed in proposals that call for cooperative activities involving THs and the biomedical sector (Stock, 1983).

Rationale For Linking Traditional Healers To AIDS Management

Incorporating THs into a formal strategy for combatting AIDS is a socially sound and pragmatic policy. THs are situated spatially and functionally--to perform positive interventions. As the morbid consequences of AIDS unfold in the months and years ahead THs will be visited by growing numbers of people who carry the virus but are still apparently healthy, and others with early symptoms and signs of AIDS/ARC. They will also increasingly encounter triage--the problem of caring for those in the later stages of AIDS. Indeed, in many cases the triage decision will be made *for* THs by others because hospitals generally cannot provide long-term support for the terminally diseased and will discharge such patients to provide spaces for patients who can survive (*World Press Review*, Sept. 1987:53; and Murtagh, Feb. 4, 1987). When this happens THs will often be the patients' only real alternative. Moreover, if the epidemic consequences approach predicted case levels (Mann, 1987; Tinker & Sabatier, 1987; *World Press Review*, 9/87; Kitchen, 1987), many symptomatic individuals may not even gain admission to a hospital. Responsibility will thus fall heavily upon families of the sick who will in turn look to THs for support.

Geographically, much of the care for AIDS/ARC victims will occur in rural villages, with added risk for THs and other care-givers. Unless intense fear of AIDS transmission (among victims' social relations and THs alike) alters customary social behavior, a growing volume of adults and children who have been living in towns will return to their home villages to die amidst family members and the graves of their ancestors (Konotey-Ahulu, 1987, Murtagh, Feb. 5. 1987). Such behavior is already commonplace in Uganda and northwest Tanzania and is placing enormous pressures on family support systems (Ankrah, 1988, and Rutayuga, 1988). Villages are serving as "hospices" in which THs are perceived as the only hope for AIDS victims.[4] Similarly, urban-based THs, many of whom also have a substantial rural clientele, will be called upon to assist a growing volume of patients at various stages of progression to AIDS/ARC. THs and their non-infected (and HIV infected?) clientele are thus *both* at risk. Consequently, THs must be included in health education strategies that will lead to substantial reduction of high-risk behaviors, decreased AIDS incidence, and safe, humane care of the sick and orphaned. In short, failure to involve THs in AIDS management is likely to further endanger public health and social stability throughout Africa's AIDS belt.

A Conceptual Model of HIV Transmission Among Traditional Healers And Their Patients

THs risk personal exposure to the HIV from their patients, who may be asymptomatic carriers, have ARC, or present clinical AIDS. Similarly, THs with HIV infection can transmit the virus to healthy patients and also to other THs. Potential transmission pathways are shown in Figure 1, together with person-person contacts which probably do not result in HIV transmission.[5] It is reportedly unknown scientifically whether high-risk behavior between THc and Pc/Pt, resulting in repeated infection of already-infected individuals, magnifies or intensifies HIV pathogenicity and or virulence.[6]

Risk Factors For Traditional Healers And Their Patients

Given the pathways in Figure 1, what kinds of behavior involving TH->P, P->TH, and TH->TH risk HIV transmission? *Population mobility,*

Figure 1

Transmission of the Human Immunodeficiency Virus Among Traditional Healers and their Patients

Reservoir
Population

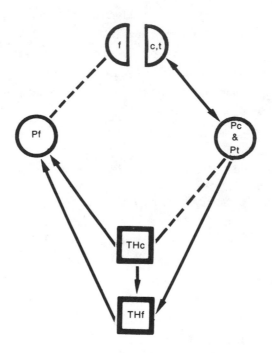

TH Traditional Healer (includes midwives)

P Patient of Traditional Healer

c HIV Carrier (clinical/subclinical)

f Free of HIV

t HIV "triage" case

————— Potential HIV Transmission Route
(includes mechanical infection)

— — — Social/Intimate Contact
(no transmission ?)

including rural-urban, urban-rural, rural-rural, and urban-urban movements of varying distance and permanence, is a major, neglected epidemiological factor (Prothero, 1977) that helps to generate and maintain a substantial volume of potentially high-risk contacts. Any AIDS strategy which ignores mobility cannot succeed. The documented movements of THs and their patients provide confirming evidence that "rural" and "urban" are part of a unified system rather than functionally separate spaces. For example, in a study of the origins of patients consulting THs based in Nairobi, I found a strong inward flow of patients from the rural areas (Good, 1987:235). Indeed, the search for healing can become an extended, costly endeavor that brings the patient into contact with geographically dispersed biomedical, traditional medical, and popular therapies *and* uninvited pathogens. Such interactions exemplify the epidemiological importance of Parkin's (1975:3) observation that East and Central Africa's rural and urban areas form "part of single field of relations made up of a vast criss-crossing of peoples, ideas, and resources." In addition to interactions of THs and their patients, long-distance truck and bus routes, local bars and commercial sex, market-place systems and seasonal labor movements are just a few examples of other established circulatory systems and socioeconomic institutions that have real or potential significance in the epidemiology of AIDS.

Blood, saliva, diarrheal fluids, semen, and other bodily discharges[7] are primary *media* in which HIV and its co-factors spread from TH->P, P->TH, or TH->TH. The blood of domestic animals (chicken, goat) is commonly used in sacrificial rituals throughout the AIDS "belt" and is potentially a source of infection. Wild monkeys, such as the vervet (green) are also extensively trapped, sold, and eaten by peoples who inhabit the vast forest--savanna transition regions of equatorial Africa (Harden, 1987 and Owen, 1981). Such factors emphasize the need for a veterinary component in AIDS research.[8]

Table 1 identifies possible HIV transmission modes and specific risk factors together with the pathways that link THs and patients (Fig. 1).[9] Such information is essential to developing appropriate targets and methods of health education for THs and their biomedical co-workers. As in the general population, heterosexual relations probably explain much of the actual

Table 1

HIV Transmission Modes & Risk Factors

Potential/Actual Modes of Transmission & Risk Factors	Human Pathways
A. *Mechanical.* Use of contaminated cutting/piercing instruments:	
1. *knives & razors* (circumcision of M & F[1],	THc → Pf
uvulectomy, cord-cutting, scarification[2],	THc → THf
blood-brotherhood)	THf → Pf
2. *needles* (injections, ear piercing)	—same—
B. *Oral/Recal-Oral:*	
1. Foreign saliva ingestion; ritual spitting on infants	THc → Pf
2. Ingestion of animal blood in sacrificial elements	THf & THc
of therapy/ceremony	Pf & Pc
3. Contact with diarrheal fluids (water & blood) of	THf & THc
children and adults	
C. *Contact Between External Lesions of Two or More Persons or Species*	
1. *Intentional:*	
—blood-brotherhood ceremonies	THc → THf
2. *Unintentional:*	
—TBA during deliveries (contact with infected birth	Pc THf
canal and/or newborn)[3]	THc → Pf
—first-aid (trauma) & dentistry	THc → Pf
—Interspecies transfer (e.g. simian → human via	Pc → THf
inoculation or bite)	Pf & Pc
D. *Sexual* (infection via contact with internal lesions	Pc → (HIV-
and/or semen)	free kin)
1. E.g., ritual intercourse with widows of male	THc → Pf
AIDS victims	THc → THf
2. Intercourse (conjugal/other partners)	Pc → THf

[1]Female genital surgery may result in bleeding during intercourse. Bacterial infection of circumcision wounds may enhance spread of AIDS via open lesions (Kitchen, 1987).

[2]A case-control study of hospitalized children 2-14 years old in Zaire indicated that "a history of scarification in the previous year was significantly more common" among 40 seropositive children compared with 92 seronegative children (Quinn *et al.*, 1986: 959 citing J. Mann, in press).

[3]Contact with blood during delivery places TBAs "at special risk" (Morley and Ibrahim, 1986: 147 and Tinker and Sabatier, 1987: 25).

transmission of HIV that may occur between THs and their patients. However, mechanical, fecaloral, and other means of contacting or spreading infected blood or other bodily fluids are potentially significant epidemiologically and must be taken into account. A less crude typology awaits biological and behavioral research that will illuminate the natural history of AIDS and the associated environmental factors and behaviors that expose people to the disease.

Approaches To Collaboration

Collaboration between biomedical workers and THs is feasible and can contribute to better AIDS management. One such effort was begun in 1986 at the South African Institute of Medical Research, where it was hoped that THs would provide "an early warning system" when AIDS symptoms appear (Thurow, 1986). The general case for intersectoral cooperation is outlined in a recent analysis of policies and strategies for involving THs in African Primary health care (PHC) programs (Good, 1987a). The Primary Health Training for Indigenous Healers (PRHETIH) Program, for example, is a model which has already been adapted with good results by several local PHC programs in Ghana (Warren, *et al.*1982; Dormaa, 1986; Good, 1987a). PRHETIH incorporates a training syllabus developed and taught cooperatively with THs, adult education methods, evaluation and follow-up, and linkage to a base of support such as a hospital or District PHC program. In Swaziland, Ministry of Health workshops for THs, nurses, and allied health workers have also demonstrated imaginative use of existing resources to develop culturally acceptable means of upgrading and applying the new practical knowledge and skills available to "healers" in both medical traditions (Green and Makhubu, 1984; Hoff and Shapiro, 1986; Hoff and Maseko, 1986; Good, 1987a). Such schemes build upon what the participants already know and upon the existing linkage of the traditional and biomedical systems established informally through patient behavior and referrals by THs. Current evidence thus indicates that it is irrational and unscientific to assume that THs *cannot* learn to recognize the major signs and symptoms of

AIDS (and co-factors such as TB) and provide improved care of the sick and dying who are brought to them.

An appeal to the increasingly visible THs associations in urban areas and some rural localities can be an effective means of enlisting the participation of individual THs in a multi-pronged AIDS action strategy (Last and Chavunduka, 1986, and Good, 1987: 210-213). A dialogue with *bona fide* THs can also help to check the emerging practice by some unethical individuals who advertise bogus cures for AIDS (*Daily Nation* [Nairobi], 1986). In rural areas large gatherings of THs are possible--for purposes of communicating and gathering information--when such meetings are called by a respected local chief or other official.

African traditional healers form a large and varied body of practitioners who will continue to provide many health-related services to the general population in the decades ahead. THs are still underrated and neglected by the biomedical sector, and I have recently argued that they are a "missing link" in African PHC (Good, 1987a). If THs are to be equipped to reduce their own and their patients' risk of exposure to AIDS and its co-factors, and to provide appropriate care to patients with AIDS, their anti-AIDS training should be an integral part of a concerted effort to engage them in the broader disease prevention and family health goals of PHC. Such an approach will be less sensational and alarmist--and hence more acceptable and productive--than could be obtained by introducing a separate AIDS curriculum.

ENDNOTES

[1] The WHO's provisional approach to clinical case definitions of adult and pediatric AIDS is designed for locations "where diagnostic resources are limited." It relies on combinations of major and minor signs that are manifest in the absence of known causes of immunosuppression, including cancer or severe malnutrition. See Quinn (1986:961).

[2] The emergence of HIV-2 infections in West Africa, in a zone extending from Cape Verde to Niger, (Kitchen, 1987; and Colburn, 1987) expands and complicates the challenge to comprehend the natural history of AIDS and to provide preventive education, disease control, and care of the sick. HIV-2 is now reported to be spreading also within and from Kinshasha, Zaire (Piot, 1988).

[3] An AIDS study in Kinshasha, Zaire indicated that 29% of patients utilized traditional medical practitioners, although lack of a control group disallowed direct assessment of associated risk. Quinn, et al. (1987), 957.

[4] The case of an urban TH who provided a hospice-type environment for a terminal cancer patient is described in Good, 1987: 286-289.

[5] Figure 1 is an open system since subsets P and TH also have contact with a variety of individuals who are not patients, including the patients' therapy managers and many others in non-therapy settings. The model assumes that HIV is the non-vectored agent of AIDS.

[6] Personal communication, Peter Drotman, M.D., Medical Epidemiologist, AIDS Program, Center for Infectious Disease, CDC, Atlanta, GA., October 7, 1987.

[7] HIV is not known to be transmitted by casual contact. However, contact with body fluids must be presumed to create the potential for transmission. "The concentration of virus in body fluids is proportional to the number of white cells in the fluid. Therefore, HIV concentrations are highest in blood and semen, somewhat lower in vaginal secretions, and significantly lower in saliva and tears" (FDA, 1987:16). Only blood, semen, vaginal secretions and "possibly breast milk" have been implicated in HIV transmission (*Virginia Epidemiology Bulletin*, 1987).

[8] A report by an African anthropologist that the Idjwi people of Lake Kivu inoculated monkey blood into the thighs, pubes, and back of men and women to heighten sexual response also has possibly important epidemiological implications (*The Economist*, July 25, 1987, citing *The Lancet*.) Ingestion of animal blood (most often from chickens) in summoning spirits during voodoo ceremonies has been hypothesized as one link in a possible Haitian origin of AIDS (Moore and LeBaron, 1986.)

[9] An alternative classification might be based on the theoretical efficiency of a given transmission mode (e.g., intercourse vs. contact with diarrheal fluids) or on a hierarchy of risk based on the proportional concentration of HIV in a specific body fluid (e.g., blood vs. breastmilk). See footnote 7.

BIBLIOGRAPHY

Ankrah, M. "The Social Context of Multiple Sexual Partners" (and discussion). National Institute of Allergy and Infectious Diseases/USAID Workshop, *Anthropological Perspectives on AIDS in Africa: Priorities for Intervention and Research*. Department of State, Washington, D.C., Jan. 7-8, 1988.

Barker, C. and Tershen, M. "AIDS in Africa." *Review of African Political Economy* (*The Health Issue*), 36 (September, 1986), 51-54.

Biggar, R.J. "AIDS and HIV Infection: Estimates of the Magnitude of the Problem Worldwide in 1985/1986." *Clinical Immunology and Pathology*, 45 (1987), 297-309.

Chavunduka, G. *Traditional Healers and the Shona Patient*. Gwelo, Rhodesia: Mambo Press, 1978.

Colburn, D. "Tracking the Other AIDS Virus." *Washington Post/Health*, October 27, 1987, 14-21.

Daily Nation [Nairobi], July 28, 1986 and November 8, 1986.

Daily Nation [Nairobi], "AIDS Blamed on Fight Against Smallpox," May 14, 1987; "Uganda Fights AIDS with Education," July 17, 1987.

Dormaa Presbyterian PHC Programme. Mimeographed report. Sunyani District. Brong Ahafo Region, Ghana. 1986.

Family Health International. Research Triangle Park, North Carolina 27709. USA. *AIDS Case Reported to WHO by Countries and Territories in Africa by 6-month Period* (21 October, 1987).

FDA Drug Bulletin, 17,2 (September, 1987).

Feierman, S. "Struggles for Control: The Social Roots of Health and Healing in Modern Africa." *African Studies Review*, 28 (1985), 73-147.

Githagui, N. *Traditional Healing Practices in Kenya--A Study of Four Kenyan Communities*. Nairobi: African Medical and Research Foundation, September, 1985.

Good, C.M. "Ethnomedical Systems in Africa and the Third World: Key Issues for the Medical Geographer." In *Conceptual and Methodological Issues in Medical Geography*. M. Meade (ed.). Department of Geography Studies in Geography No. 15. University of North Carolina, Chapel Hill, N.C., 1980. Pp. 93-116.

Good, C.M. *Ethnomedical Systems in Africa. Patterns of Traditional Medicine in Rural and Urban Kenya*. New York: Guilford Press, 1987.

Good, C.M. "The Community in African Primary Health Care: Problems of Strengthening Participation and a Proposed Complementary Strategy." Takemi Program in International Health, Harvard School of Public Health, June, 1987a.

Green, E.C. Personal communication, June 25, 1986.

Green, E.C. and Makhubu, L. "Traditional Healers in Swaziland: Toward Improved Cooperation Between the Traditional and Modern Health Sectors." *Social Science and Medicine*, 18 (1984), 1071-1079.

Harden, B. "Down the Zaire: An African Mainstream." *Washington Post*, November 8, 1987.

Hoff, W. and Maseko, D.N. "Nurses and Traditional Healers Join Hands." *World Health Forum*, 7 (1986), 412-416.

Hoff, W. and Shapiro, G. "Traditional Healers in Swaziland." *Parasitology Today*, 2,12 (1986), 360-361.

Hooper, E. "AIDS in Uganda." *African Affairs*, 86,345 (October, 1987), 469-477.

Janzen, J. *The Quest for Therapy in Lower Zaire*. Berkeley: University of California Press, 1978.

Kitchen L.W. "AIDS in Africa: Knowns and Unknowns." *CSIS Africa Notes*, No. 74, July 17, 1987, 104.

Klovdahl, A.S. "Social Networks and the Spread of Infectious Disease: The AIDS Example." *Social Science and Medicine*, 21, 11 (1985), 1203-1216.

Last, M. Introduction. "The Professionalisation of African Medicine: Ambiguities and Definitions." In Last and Chavunduka (eds.), *The Professionalisation of African Medicine*. Manchester: Manchester University Press, 1986. Pp. 1-19.

Last, M. and Chavunduka, G.L. (eds.). *The Professionalisation of African Medicine*. Manchester: Manchester University Press and International African Institute, 1986.

Leishman, K. "AIDS and Insects." *The Atlantic Monthly*, September, 1987, 56-72.

MacCormack, C. "The Articulation of Western and Traditional Systems of Health Care." In M. Last and G.L. Chavunduka (eds.), *The Professionalisation of African Medicine*. Manchester University Press, 1986. Pp. 151-162.

Mann, J.M. "The Global AIDS Situation." *World Health Statistics Quarterly*, 40 (1987), 185-192.

Moore, A. and LeBaron, R.D. "The Case for a Haitian Origin of the AIDS Epidemic." In D.A. Feldman and T.M. Johnson (eds.), *Social Dimensions of AIDS, Methods and Theory*. New York: Praeger, 1986. Pp. 77-93.

Morley, D.C. and Ebrahim, G.J. "AIDS: Third World Beware?" *Journal of Tropical Pediatrics*, 33 (August, 1986), 146-147.

Murtagh, P. *The Guardian* (U.K.), February 4, 1987.

Owen, D. *Grasslands of Africa*. New York: National Audubon Society, 1981.

Parkin, D. *Town and Country in Central and Eastern Africa*. London: International African Institute, 1975.

Piot, P. "Epidemiological Overview." National Institute of Allergy and Infectious Diseases/USAID Workshop, *Anthropological Perspectives on AIDS in Africa: Priorities for Intervention and Research*. Department of State, Washington, D.C., January 7-8, 1988.

Pillsbury, B.L.K. "Policy and Evaluation Perspectives on Traditional Health Care Practitioners in National Health Care Systems." *Social Science and Medicine*, 16 (1982), 1825-1834.

Prothero, R.M. "Disease and Mobility: A Neglected Factor in Epidemiology." *International Journal of Epidemiology*, 6, 3, (1977) 259-267.

Quinn, T.C., Mann, J.M., Curran, J.W. & Piot, P. "AIDS in Africa: An Epidemiologic Paradigm." *Science*, 234, 21 November, 1986, 955-963.

Rutayuga, John. Personal communication, January 8, 1988.

Ryder, R. *et al.*, "Community Surveillance for HIV Infection in Zaire." Paper presented to the Third International Conference on AIDS. Washington, D.C., June 1-5, 1987.

Sargent, C.F. *The Cultural Context of Therapeutic Choice*. Dordrecht, Holland: D. Reidel, 1982.

Stepan, J. "Traditional and Alternative Systems of Medicine: A Comparative Review of Legislation." *International Digest of Health Legislation*, 36, 2 (1985), 283-341.

Stock, R. "On the Diversity of Healers: The Hausa Example" Unpublished paper presented at Annual International Health Conference of the National Council for International Health, Washington, D.C., June 13-15, 1983.

Stock, R. "Understanding Health Care Behavior: A Model, Together With Evidence from Nigeria." In R. Akhtar (ed.), *Health and Disease in Tropical Africa--Geographical and Medical Viewpoints*. Chur, Switzerland: Harwood Academic Publishers, 1987. Pp. 279-292.

The Economist, "The Monkey's Blood." July 25, 1987.

The Weekly Review [Nairobi], "Strong Anti-AIDS Programme," August 28, 1987, p. 34.

Thurow, R. "Physicians Enlisting 100 Witch Doctors In War On AIDS." *Wall Street Journal*, December 16, 1986.

Tinker, J. and Sabatier, R. "AIDS The Hidden Enemy." *Development International*, January/February, 1987, 22-27.

Virginia Epidemiology Bulletin. Vol. 87, 11 (1987), 1.

Warren, D.M. *et al*. "Ghanaian National Policy Toward Traditional Healers: The Case of the Primary Health Training for Indigenous Healers (PRHETIH) Program." *Social Science and Medicine*, 18 (1984), 375-385.

World Press Review, September, 1987.

World Health Organization. *Report of the Consulation on Approaches for Policy Development for Traditional Health Practitioners, Including Traditional Birth Attendants*. NUR/TRM/85.1. Geneva: WHO, 1985.

THE HIV/AIDS PANDEMIC IN AFRICA: ISSUES OF DONOR STRATEGY

Gary Merritt

William Lyerly

Jack Thomas*

SUMMARY: The pandemic of human immunodeficiency virus (HIV) infection and acquired immunodeficiency syndrome (AIDS) in central and southern Africa poses a new challenge to international donor assistance strategies. Some influential observers predict that demographic and socio-political impacts of the disease might become catastrophic -- insofar as HIV prevalence estimates in some urban areas can be extrapolated to general populations. However, time trend data and statistical models are still inadequate for confident projections. Many activities have begun to improve understanding of the epidemiology of HIV/AIDS, but definitive results may be several years hence. Meanwhile, policy makers and technical officers in donor agencies must frame issues, allocate funds and take action based on what is known now. This paper reviews some key donor strategy issues.

Demographic Background

Current international donor responses to the pandemic of human immunodeficiency virus (HIV) in sub-Saharan Africa must be seen in a recent historical context. Fears of catastrophic demographic and socio-political consequences of HIV may be exaggerated, however understandable. It is important that current support for other areas of public health not be undermined since, for example, child survival and family planning (contraceptive delivery systems) represent powerful counter balances to HIV mortality. Based on available information about HIV epidemiology, understanding of institutional absorptive capacities, and the momentum now underway in programs that seemingly must compete for relatively fixed

---

* Gary Merritt, Ph.D., is a medical sociologist; William Lyerly, an immunologist, and epidemiologist; and Jack Thomas, a program officer, all in the Bureau for Africa, U.S. Agency for International Development, Washington, D.C. The views expressed herein are entirely those of the authors and do not necessarily represent those of the Agency for International Development. The authors wish to acknowledge helpful suggestions on an early draft from Mr. Bradshaw Langmaid and Dr. Jeffrey Harris.

health resources, there is insufficient reason as yet to significantly alter donor strategies for health, family planning and human resource development.

Africa's remarkable demographic changes over the past four decades provide a critical frame of reference for understanding how international donor responses to the HIV/AIDS pandemic are likely to be organized over the next few years. From the late 1940's through the late 1970's high death rates fell markedly over most of the continent. These declines, combined with historically high fertility rates (which actually increased in most groups during this period), led to the highest population growth rates ever recorded at national and regional levels by the "1980 round" of censuses. Doubling times between 17 and 30 years produced extremely youthful populations and high dependency ratios across the continent.

Mortality declined during this time, mostly due to basic improvements in diet, sanitation and water supplies linked, in turn, to rising educational standards and economic development. However, death rates remained high by international standards, especially among infants and children. By the late 1970's, it seemed clear to most public policy advisors that further major improvements in mortality and morbidity required more deliberate mass efforts in vaccination and control or management of infectious and other diseases.

High fertility had become the main factor in extraordinary population growth and also was closely correlated with infant and child mortality. Rapid socio-economic development had become virtually hostage to the demographic imperatives of rapid growth and high dependency burdens. By 1980 a growing number of public policy advisors in Africa, both indigenous and expatriate, were urging deliberate efforts to induce rapid fertility decline.

Africa became an arena for policy efforts to directly effect public health and demographic changes. "Western" government and voluntary agency donors vigorously joined this effort. The United Nations' (A.I.D, several European development agencies and the U.S. Agency for International Development (USAID) in recent years have helped stimulate intensive child survival efforts. Likewise, the United Nations Fund for Population Activities (UNFPA), The World Bank and A.I.D. have vigorously assisted efforts in most of sub-Saharan Africa to publicly promote small family concepts and wide public access to modern techniques of contraception.

Now in the late 1980's donor assisted public and private sector programs are showing great promise of reducing infant and child mortality. Likewise, studies show that family size aspirations are declining and that levels of use of modern contraception are rising rapidly wherever quality services are made accessible. Despite many justifiable criticisms of donor programs, most people who follow these issues would agree that donor resources are contributing significantly to important and highly desirable demographic changes.

To whatever extent there is renewed momentum in Africa towards improved public health, and donor efforts are effective in this, the pandemic of HIV represents a serious challenge. Cost of dealing with HIV morbidity and mortality obviously could be quite high, but opportunity costs may be greater. These involve less obvious trade-offs of budget, scarce skills and organizational capacities of both African countries and external donors, diminishing alternative priority efforts.

Perhaps the foremost questions for most policy makers and their technical advisors are these: (1) How extensive is the pandemic and its demographic impact likely to become; (2) what is the probable socio-economic and political impact; (3) are existing funding levels adequate to meet needs for prevention; and, (4) given relatively fixed donor resources for public health, how much should existing donor health and family planning programs be diminished in order to support HIV prevention activities? This public policy context leads us to highlight aspects of the problem that may differ in tone, substance and conclusion from those of most commentators. We hope these issues will be further spelled out and debated by others.

Demographic Impact

The World Health Organization (WHO) estimated in mid-1987 that perhaps ten million people worldwide were infected with HIV. About one half were estimated to be in sub-Saharan Africa. To date these appear to be concentrated in some eleven countries across Central and Southern Africa where infection levels among "high risk behavior" urban groups, both male and female, appear especially high by international comparison (WHO:1987). No one knows to what extent HIV infection has spread among Africa's mostly rural peoples; the few studies available suggest low but detectable levels of HIV sero-positivity in several of the affected countries.

Estimates of infection levels vary greatly. Predictions of HIV prevalence levels and eventual demographic impact therefore involve much guesswork. Crucial information from rural areas, where 80% of the population lives is quite limited in extent and quality. Experts on the African data do not agree on best guesses about key factors for projections. The WHO estimate of current prevalence put the number of persons in sub-Saharan Africa with HIV infection in 1986 at between two and one half to five million (WHO:1987), while a leading N.I.H. epidemiologist estimates the number to have been no more than one million in 1985 and well under two million in late 1987 (Biggar:1987). This variation should not be surprising: in the U.S.A., where epidemiologic surveillance presumably is much better, the U.S. Public Health Service in December, 1987 estimated that the number of infected persons ranged between about 500,000 and 1.4 million.)

Aside from the near certainty of eventual death from infection, at least two aspects of the disease in Africa are especially troubling: (1) the apparent predominance of *heterosexual* modes of transmission, (perhaps 80% of cases) rather than the pattern of intravenous drug use and homosexual anal intercourse found in relatively small portions of the population in North America and Europe; and (2) an apparent very rapid "doubling time" in estimates of prevalence of the disease based on urban data during roughly the period 1983-86. These aspects of the disease lead some to predict that the disease will spread widely, and insidiously, since the average latency may be longer than nine years and the period of infectiousness perhaps almost as long. To most epidemiologists, a significant rise in death rates in affected countries seems sure to follow (WHO:1987).

Neither "period of infectiousness" nor "incubation period" is adequately defined at this time. Epidemiologists differ widely, with estimates of the former ranging between five and fifteen years (Anderson: 1987), though the preferred figure appears to be nine (Bongaarts:1987). Projections also depend on estimates of the rate of spread. Did HIV begin its spread in the 1960's? Or much earlier? Estimates of "doubling time" in projections depend heavily on these assumptions.

It is possible that HIV in fact could be spreading very slowly among rural people and that earlier underlying assumptions about transmissibility, susceptibility and "promiscuous" sexual behavior based on selected urban sites do not apply well to most rural peoples. Very wide variation in the design of models and their calculations result from lack of data and differences in assumptions.

This year A.I.D., through the U.S. Bureau of Census and the National Academy of Sciences, is sponsoring development of statistical models that incorporate factors known to be involved in the spread of HIV. These will permit better projections of the scale of overall demographic effects. As part of the same effort the U.S. Bureau of Census has designed a computer database system for organizing all published and unpublished data, worldwide, as it pertains to epidemiologic findings on HIV/AIDS in developing countries.

In October, 1987 a conference of international experts from various disciplines reviewed HIV epidemiology. Ten initial efforts to model the spread of the disease were presented. Many assumptions built into the models were based on U.S. and/or European data since findings from Africa are quite limited. Results of this conference were predictably vague about demographic effects of the disease in Africa, with large differences between the implied results of these efforts.

Preliminary results of the leading model from the Population Council suggest that under *worst-case* AIDS assumptions, net population growth rates in affected countries might decline as much as one percentage point, (e.g., 3.5% to 2.5%) sometime after the turn of the century. Population growth will remain high because almost 50% of Africans are under age 15 and not yet sexually active (the "age pyramid" effect). This model assumed constant marital fertility and constant mortality from other causes (Bongaarts: 1987). Subsequent efforts with this model will test more realistic assumptions. Mortality has been declining rapidly over the past two decades and shows every sign of continuing to decline with further socio-economic development and expansion of improved infant and child mortality programs. Also, fertility almost certainly will show some decline in the next two decades in response to the rising levels of prevalence of use of contraceptive methods in several of the countries, including the rapid rise in use of condoms in several countries in response to the HIV threat.

With more realistic assumptions about changing mortality and fertility, the independent effects of HIV may contribute to a worst-case decline of as little as 0.5 percentage point in the growth rate between 1980 and 2010 (i.e., from 3.5% to 3.0%) in those eleven or so most affected countries. Although this means many tragic early deaths, the long-term demographic effects may not be great, certainly nothing like the "negative" growth rates informally suggested by some concerned observers.

Perhaps the key issue is whether the pandemic will remain mostly concentrated among "high risk behavior" people in urban areas or spread easily across groups. The size and degree of sexual endogamy of African sub-populations is undocumented, making it impossible to estimate levels of "saturation" and potential spread across groups. Although the cumulative number of HIV/AIDS cases continues to grow in the U.S., the incidence in the population at large does not appear to be growing. Rather it now seems to be concentrated in "high risk behavior" groups, with only a limited "leakage" into the broader heterosexual population. If comparable transitional processes hold in African populations, HIV may not have the broad impact that many fear is almost inevitable.

Socio-Political Impact

Some commentators believe that the worst effect of HIV will be not in absolute levels of mortality, but in potentially devastating levels among economically active adults upon whom young and old depend and upon whom acceleration of economic development is most dependent. HIV/AIDS is concentrated among adults in urban areas. It is well documented that the disease has claimed the lives of African elites, including members of presidential families, cabinet minister, some bankers, a neuro-surgeon and several high ranking military officers. These observations, combined with an underlying assumption that Africans typically have a large number of heterosexual partners, suggest that HIV could undermine much of the urban, more highly trained occupational structure (Tinker:1987).

However, fears of social, political and/or economic collapse or upheaval in Africa resulting from the HIV/AIDS pandemic probably have been exaggerated, though well intentioned. There is little evidence to suggest that urban elites will be devastated. We do know that the case gender ratios are about 1:1; that females are younger (20's) and males older (30's). One study showed more cases with reported higher education (to 12 years, at least) and several reports show that many military personnel in at least two countries are infected. HIV/AIDS in fact so far appears to be concentrated among the least fortunate people in urban areas (especially so for females). HIV/AIDS is most likely to show virtually the same social pattern as other sexually transmitted diseases.

No HIV/AIDS studies as yet have revealed anything about the average productivity or leadership qualities of men (or women) with HIV/AIDS compared to those not infected. We cannot yet infer that parts of Africa are about to lose their most productive intelligentsia. We can only guess about most victims' sexual preferences (e.g., some involvement with "prostitution"), and should *not* assume, as worst-case scenarios seem to, that African leaders and males in general are widely promiscuous with high risk behavior females.

African societies are probably much more robust than recognized. Even given some level of elite mortality to HIV, the potential for sizable upward social mobility (occupational replacement) should not be underestimated. Kenya, for example, has high unemployment and underemployment among the educated and may not differ qualitatively from most other countries. Though many of these people are comparatively inexperienced, societal loss of leadership to HIV/AIDS would never be instant; there will be time for occupational induction. In most countries there is some inherent capacity to replace skilled people lost to HIV/AIDS. Indeed, pervasive unemployment and underemployment in contexts of rising aspirations may carry far greater potential for revolutions and massive disruptions than selective mortality from HIV/AIDS.

The point is not that we should be less concerned, but rather that we still lack critical information to judge whether parts of Africa are facing catastrophes, as some suggest. Entire societies probably are not. However tragic HIV/AIDS will be for some countries and for hundreds of thousands or even millions of people in the next few years, the overall demographic and socio-political effects of HIV/AIDS probably will be far less than some people have feared.

Finding Issues Of HIV/AIDS Control

Coping with the pandemic may severely tax affected African countries. Hospitals and clinics lack capacity to care for a rising number of HIV victims while trying to meet existing needs. If African nations make policy decisions to care for HIV victims, there will be displacement effect, i.e., consumption of limited drugs and hospital beds otherwise needed for non-HIV patients.

If many victims are among the more affluent there will be especially strong pressure on already limited care facilities since most health care delivery systems usually respond most to demands of the affluent. Even if severely affected countries adopt a pattern of simply sending victims home to die (e.g., as in Uganda today), costs of preventive measures alone introduce new burdens on budgets for health, inevitably reducing investment in other preventive and curative problems.

Equipment and reagents for testing, training of personnel and screening blood supplies are costly but must be undertaken as a high priority. So are intensive national and targeted educational campaigns, including those that focus on abstinence and monogamy ("zero grazing," in the words of a Kenyan Minister of Health). Condoms, by far the best available HIV prophylaxis for the sexually active, cost about $6 for one year's supply per average (male) user at base procurement prices.

The most marketable spermicides (foaming vaginal tablets with nonoxymy 1-9) are also probably quite effective as an HIV prophylaxis and have the great advantage of being largely under the control of women. They cost about twice as much per unit as the condom. Education, distribution and promotion (i.e., "marketing") of these methods on a large scale probably adds about 70% more to the commodity costs.

If we assume provisionally that about 100 million people live in the areas of highest HIV prevalence and another 100 million live in areas adjacent, and that about 15% are those in the age of highest risk (15 to 40), then about 30 million couples represent the immediate priority for control of HIV transmission. If one-third were to use the above prophylaxes (ratio of 4:1 -- condoms:tablets) procurement costs would be on the order of US $75 million. Marketing and distribution costs would likely raise the total cost to about $135 million per year. Per capita costs would run about $0.75 per day for these two methods alone and only in the highest priority areas of Africa.

Of course, there is little likelihood of this demand in the near future, but it is helpful to simulate the budgetary context. Annual health budgets of most African countries now run between $1 to $6 per capita, much of which already is supported by external donors. These countries confront excruciating budgetary decisions. They will have to allocate more funds to confront HIV and donors will have to raise their contributions. Delays in initiation of preventive measures may have large adverse effects in the future. What should the scale of the budgetary response be?

International Funding

During the past two years virtually all international donors have volunteered commitments of funds through the World Health Organization (WHO) and directly to African countries through bilateral programs. To date, limited A.I.D. funding, *per se*, seems not to be a main constraint on HIV prevention programs in Africa.

A.I.D. overseas assistance for HIV/AIDS prevention began with $2 million in FY86, more than one-half of which went to Africa. In FY87 roughly $17 million went as follows: W.H.O. ($5 million); extra condom procurement ($3 million); U.S. contractors for technical assistance ($4.2 million); and the remainder went for direct bilateral support of which total slightly more than one-half supported activities in Africa that are now getting underway.

Of the total FY88 $30 million for HIV prevention $15 million will be granted directly to W.H.O., of which W.H.O. estimates perhaps 50% will go to Africa. A.I.D., through its Science and Technology Bureau, expects to spend $3 million extra for condoms and $7 million for contractor and grantee work, of which about 50% will go for Africa. Finally, about $5 million will be allocated for direct bilateral activities, of which perhaps $3 million will go to Africa. Therefore, of the total $30 million in FY88, about one-half will go to programs in Africa.

HIV/AIDS has arisen at an inopportune juncture in the history of U.S. efforts in foreign assistance. Constraints include the steadily declining overall federal budgetary appropriation levels for foreign aid compounded by the diminishing value of the U.S. dollar. Nevertheless, the limited budget increase planned for HIV activity in FY89 over FY88 by A.I.D. in Africa, and possibly level requirements thereafter, takes into consideration the following:

—large contributions will be available from donors, other than the A.I.D.;

—in many affected countries there is a limited capacity to absorb additional funds;

—most African countries are currently making only limited expenditures on HIV/AIDS control;

—there has been limited offical U.S. government domestic policies and commitment, (or budgetary experience in U.S. Programs);

—The U.S. has considerable and unique U.S. domestic technical expertise on HIV and AIDS;

—earlier funds from the U.S. Government and other donors have not yet been fully absorbed;

—the private sector in African nations is largely untapped; Significant increases in funding requirements could occur if:

—estimates of the spread of HIV to rural areas increase;

—other donors withdraw or significantly reduce commitments;

—African governments increase their commitments *and* turn more to the U.S. for help;

--contraceptive use increases greatly *and* the U.S. Government is asked to supply needs.

Most African countries themselves have not yet budgeted HIV/AIDS control adequately in their formal national budgets. This context constrains program development far more than most well-meaning outsiders are usually able to recognize. Official national budgets guide the allocation of civil service effort far more than "off budget" resources. Experiences in many other areas of health and family planning over the past twenty years show that actual commitment and long term sustainability of initiatives depends heavily on overt budgetary commitment. As African countries budget more for HIV/AIDS prevention, expanded donor funding for personnel and country infrastructures can be absorbed more usefully. A.I.D.'s planning levels for HIV assistance should be pitched according to the levels of commitment in Africa.

Issues Of Strategy

Mindful that resources available for assistance in health are quite limited and already focused on priority infant and child survival programs that are gaining momentum in Africa, efforts to combat the spread of HIV/AIDS must be focused. The Bureau for Africa's strategy is built around the following key elements:

1. A *Region-Wide* approach -- control of the pandemic cannot otherwise be achieved. However, the scale and type of A.I.D. assistance by country are most influenced by:

–the estimated current prevalence of HIV;

–the probable potential for transmission of the disease, estimated by:

-prevalence of other known sexually transmitted diseases;

-the size and proportion of the population that is urban;

–government (or other indigenous) commitment and capacities;

–A.I.D. Mission capacity to design and monitor a program.

2. Concentrates almost exclusively on applying current knowledge to *preventive measures*. Basic research and/or treatment activities will not be funded.

3. Consolidates *surveillance* so that spread of the disease and evaluation of impact of interventions can be monitored, working closely with the U.S. Bureau of Census and the U.S. Public Health Service (Centers for Disease Control and the National Institutes of Health).

4. Fully supports W.H.O.'s *leadership role* in the Global Programme on AIDS, with its main emphasis on African countries and its strong focus on health education, serologic screening and improvements in blood supply.

5. Concentrates on implementation of two large new agreements ($15 & 28 million for five years each) with U.S.-based firms for worldwide *assistance in communications and technical services*, respectively; about half of these resources are planned for Africa.

6. Provides *condoms*, and funds and technical assistance for programs to *encourage sexual abstinance by adolescents and marital monogamy*, and discourages "*high risk behavior.*"

7. Places emphasis on *African leadership* in defining the scale of the pandemic and the most appropriate measures; host government commitments are indexed by official budgetary levels (either or both attribution to host government and donor) for HIV/AIDS prevention.

8. Seeks to *mobilize private and voluntary sector institutions* across the range of potential interventions.

Conclusion

HIV control depends directly on how African governments view the scale of the problem, how best to intervene, and identification of priority actions. Donor organizations have special responsibilities to assist and have been eager to help. However, representatives of donor countries have sometimes spoken out too quickly on the HIV subject in Africa, sometimes stating conclusions for which there has been insubstantial evidence. African leaders and scientists sometimes have not been adequately consulted. Deep irritations and suspicions have been aroused needlessly.

Based on available information there is no reason yet to significantly alter overall USG strategies for health and human resource development. Without effective vaccines and/or chemotherapeutics, control of the disease is possible only by rapid behavioral changes. Such changes involve having few sexual partners, at least among people with high risk behaviors.

We must have confidence that prevention programs prompted by the epidemic will change behavior and improve health care standards. These changes could save the lives of many millions of young Africans who have yet to become sexually active. The fact that AIDS may be concentrated in urban areas and among the literate actually suggests that it should be easier to control: these people may respond more readily to education campaigns and modify their behavior.

Concerns for elites should be balanced by sustained commitment to children as the central focus of public health. In fact, one of the more tragic consequences of the HIV pandemic will be that many children will be left without parents. The extended family, an integral and durable part of African social life, has the capacity to absorb most of these victims. The death threat is very serious indeed, but it is important to note that HIV/AIDS mortality is and probably will remain less than mortality caused by malaria, respiratory and diarrheal diseases -- mostly among infants and children. The impact of donor assistance on children should remain the central ethical issue in setting current priorities.

This analysis concludes with the argument that international donors steer a steady course in Africa, continuing a balance of sectoral efforts given what we now know about HIV/AIDS. Not only is this not the time to diminish family planning efforts, but instead such efforts could be redoubled at this time due to the need to:

(a) more rapidly improve reproductive health (e.g., reduce sexually transmitted diseases);

(b) improve access to and more effective use of barrier techniques (condoms, spermicides) in sexual relations;

(c) support those who encourage more widespread adoption of controlled sexuality: abstinence among adolescents; and monogamous or minimally changing sexual relations; and

(d) address increasing dependency ratios due to increased mortality expected among the economically productive and sexually active adult populations.

These efforts will have a profound effect on controlling the disease. Likewise, the focused international assistance by UNICEF and A.I.D. for child survival is having a real impact on saving young lives, perhaps more than will be dying of AIDS. These efforts are all the more important because of the new burden of mortality from AIDS. Likewise, we should emphasize human resource development: mortality among comparatively more urban and possibly skilled people should heighten needs for education and training.

BIBLIOGRAPHY

Anderson, Roy (1987) "The Epidemiology of HIV Infection: Variable Incubation Plus Infectious Periods and Heterogeniety in Sexual Activity." Presented at the Workshop on Modeling the Spread of Infection with Human Immunodeficiency Virus and the Demographic Impact of Acquired Immune Deficiency.   National Academy of Sciences. Washington, D.C. October 15-17, 1987.

Bongaarts, Jon (1987) "A Model of the Spread of HIV Infection and the Demographic Impact of AIDS." (Preliminary Draft) Paper presented at the Workshop of Modeling Impact of AIDS (see Anderson, above). National Academy of Sciences. Washington, D.C. (October 15-17)

Biggar, Robert (1987) "Africa and AIDS: An Epidemiological Perspective." African Studies Association Meetings. Denver, (November 20-22)

Colgate, S.A., Hyman, J.M., Stanley, E.A. (1987) "A Risk-Based Model Explaining the Cubic Growth In AIDS Cases." Presented at the Conference on Modeling the Impact of AIDS (see Anderson), National Academy of Sciences, Washington, D.C. (October 15-17)

Tinker, John (1987) "AIDS: A Gathering Death-March for the World's Poor." Paper of The Panos Institute. (October)

U.S. Bureau of Census (1987) Personal communication with Dr. Peter Way. (November 12)

World Health Organization (1987) Speech by Dr. Jonathan Mann at the Second International AIDS Conference. Washington, D.C. (June 6) The countries are: Burundi, Central African Republic, Congo, Kenya, Malawi, Rwanda, Tanzania, Uganda, Zaire, Zambia, Zimbabwe.

THE ROLE OF NON-GOVERNMENTAL ORGANIZATIONS IN AIDS PREVENTION: PARALLELS TO AFRICAN FAMILY PLANNING ACTIVITY

Edward H. Greeley[*]

SUMMARY: NGO's operating in Africa offer a wide range of community-based support that could be harnessed in prevention campaigns concerning HIV/AIDS. Specifically, family planning efforts that have focused upon contraceptive techniques may be well-suited as prevention strategies.

Introduction

Non-governmental Organizations (NGOs) show significant promise for addressing all aspects of the AIDS problem in Africa.[1] Because of their close association with local communities, virtually all NGOs may be able to serve in some way as vehicles for information concerning AIDS and its prevention. (See resource guides to NGOs concerned with AIDS in Africa found elsewhere in this book.)

One group of NGOs, those involved in ongoing family planning and health service delivery programs, appears to offer exceptional potential for addressing the AIDS problem. The purpose of this paper is to explore this potential by first briefly reviewing existing information on the extent of community-based NGO programs, and second by analyzing illustrative examples of ongoing NGO activity, particularly church-based health and family planning programs which suggest the scope of such activity for dealing with AIDS. The major propositions of the chapter are three-fold:

The role of NGOs in providing sustainable health and family planning services throughout urban and especially rural Africa is significantly underrated. This leads to a tendency of

*Edward Greeley, Ph.D., an anthropologist, is Chief, Policy Planning and Evaluation, Bureau for Africa, USAID, Washington, DC. Views are those of the author and do not necessarily represent those of the Agency for International Development.

policy planners to overlook its potential in preventing HIV transmission.

Given their knowledge of the local community and ability to handle culturally sensitive issues, NGOs may be especially well suited to intervene in slowing the spread of HIV/AIDS. Such programs could deal with the types of difficult behavior modification necessary in combatting AIDS, *e.g.*, changes in culturally-rooted sexual roles and behavior, relations between husband and wife, and adoption of contraceptive practices.

Of the various types of NGOs involved in family planning service delivery, church-based medical systems offer the highest promise in combatting AIDS.

Much of the NGOs promise in this arena lies in developing -- through interaction with the community -- a rapid and constructive learning process. It might include not only introduction of new technologies for screening blood and diagnosing patients with seropositivity, but also culturally appropriate guidelines for counseling AIDS patients and their families. Solutions systematically developed and tested in such a setting should provide useful direction to governments and donors on the wide range of problems associated with AIDS.

This chapter is organized in three sections. The first focuses on the extent of the role of NGOs in providing health and family planning services throughout Africa. The second, using illustrations from Kenya, explores the unique fit between what family planning services NGOs are currently providing and what they could do to deal with HIV/AIDS and its impact. The third section concludes the paper by suggesting key strategies for action.

Scope Of NGO Activities In Health And Family Planning

NGOs are active throughout Africa, and many build on long traditions of service established during the colonial period. Missionary health services, for example, formed the backbone of medical services in countries currently affected by AIDS and once controlled by England (Kenya, Uganda,

Tanzania, Zambia), and Belgium (Rwanda, Burundi, Zaire). Church-based health care still accounts for a significant portion of overall health services and is increasingly instrumental in providing family planning services throughout Africa.

Despite broad involvement in the health sector, relatively little of a systematic nature is known of NGO activities. This data gap is explainable in part due to the diffuse nature of the organizations involved, the difficulty in defining and delimiting what is being delivered, and also the difficulty in distinguishing NGO activity from government activity.

In many cases government and NGOs work in partnership. A local health institution, for example, receives significant resources from government health systems. Some institutions operate under direct supervision of governments. Such partnerships make it very difficult to quantify the relative contributions of government and NGO. It is also very difficult to document to what extent resources are provided for curative, as opposed to preventive, services. In fact, this is an important distinction in assessing the contribution of the NGOs to provision of primary health care and family planning as well as HIV/AIDS prevention services.

In order to analyze how NGOs might help reduce AIDS prevalence, an assessment of how such organizations have performed in a parallel endeavor is illustrative. Table 1 includes an estimate of the extent to which delivery of contraceptive methods is shared by government and NGOs in a number of countries most affected by AIDS. Note that "for profit" organizations such as plantations, mining and manufacturing corporations in AIDS prevention programs are also included in this comparison under "commercial." Like NGOs, these private sector organizations may run clinics or even hospitals for workers and families of workers, thereby offering an alternative to or replacement for over-burdened government services.[2]

An important implication of the table involves the variability of NGO involvement across countries. In Senegal, a predominantly Islamic country, there has been relatively little Christian Church health delivery. In Zaire there is in fact *vast* scope of NGO delivery, because church-based activities play a *dominant* role in the government health service.[3]

Table 1

Contraceptive Methods by Source
Among Current Users from Selected African Countries

(Taken from Maureen Lewis and Genevieve Kenney, *The Private Sector in Developing Countries: Its Role, Achievement and Potential*, Urban Institute, Washington D.C. May 1987, p. 44.)

Country (year)	Contraceptive Prevalence Nationwide	Government (percent)	Commercial[a] (percent)	NGO (percent)	Other[b] (percent)
Kenya (1984)	17	58.3	8.4	32.2	1.1
Liberia (1986)	6	31.1	18.3	48.2	2.3
Senegal (1986)	12	45.0	50.0	— —	5.0
Zaire (1984)		64.1	28.7	3.6	3.5
Zimbabwe (1984)	38	42.8	9.2	46.2	2.0

SOURCE:
Contraceptive Health Survey; Demographic Health Survey; Bogue et. al. (1987); U.N. (1987).

[a]Includes private physicians, hospitals, pharmacies, and any other private, non-NGO.

[b]Unspecified source, may encompass NGOs when private, nonprofits are not a category, and may include commercial where it is not a separate category.

Although there is a variation in the patterns of health and family planning services in the countries affected by AIDS, reference to the pattern in Kenya, where some systematic estimates have been drawn, may be useful. Church-related medical systems account for about 30% of hospital beds in Kenya, and for about the same percent of rural health facilities. In the early 1980s, there were 374 rural health facilities that were being operated by non-governmental organizations, and virtually all were church-sponsored. Of these, 28 were health centers, 7 health subcenters, and 339 were dispensaries.[4] Kenya has been one of the leading countries in Africa to provide such family planning services. Currently the contraceptive usage is estimated at 17% (See Table 1), with a third of the services provided from sources outside the government system. In fact, it is in the family planning area that a model for AIDS prevention may be found.

Family Planning As A Model For Preventing AIDS

NGOs involved in health and family planning programs offer unique potential in combatting HIV transmission. Perhaps most important is the potential for a NGO with strong roots in a community to provide the means not only to educate people and change attitudes, but also to modify patterns of behavior. The goal of such a program would be the reduction of behaviors that significantly increase the risk of exposure to HIV/AIDS and the concomitant increase in behaviors which which minimize the risk. Examples of such behavior include the use of barrier contraceptive techniques (spermacides and condoms), early treatment of sexually transmitted diseases, sexual fidelity, and avoidance of promiscuity and prostitutes.

There are also a range of other reasons why NGOs can be important in campaigns to prevent AIDS. NGOs are often in the position to provide family planning information and services, often as a complement to overburdened government health systems. They have credibility in the community, may be led by some of the most important opinion leaders, and are well placed to mobilize public opinion to support a particular activity.

Examples of NGOs' potential role in modifying behavior can be illustrated with reference to three successful approaches to the introduction of family planning information, education, and communication, and community based services in Kenya. The case examples each illustrate a number of important points. First, the potential scope of NGOs in providing information and contraceptive methods of use in preventing HIV transmission. Second, the effectiveness of church-based medical programs in promoting use of contraceptive practices, and finally, the wide range of problems posed by HIV/AIDS which can be effectively addressed by the institutions that provide health and family planning services -- particularly the church-based hospital system.

- *Maendeleo Ya Wanawake* (MYWO) is the national women's organization of Kenya. There are over 10,000 women's groups registered nationwide by MHWO, the average size of which is about 30 women. The organization obviously has high potential for communicating ideas to rural women. An example is a recent newsletter in Kiswahili sent to groups that carried a message from UNICEF on the benefits of breast feeding. MYWO is also involved in a pilot community-based family planning program in several locations. In these areas some 75 volunteers work with 150 families each to provide information on family planning and sell selected contraceptives, including condoms and spermacides. Assuming such an undertaking can be established on a cost-effective basis, the wide scope of the organization offers high potential for introduction of a program to prevent HIV transmission. The program would include provision of contraceptive techniques.

- *The Christian Organizations Research Advisory Trust* (CORAT) is an organization designed to provide management assistance to Christian churches. Among other organizations, it provides support to the Protestant Church Medical Association (PCMA). One of CORAT's current programs is management assistance to five church dioceses in Kenya implementing a project on child survival, family planning, and other primary health care services at the community level. This program has a broad reach, with plans for training of 835 new community health workers, retraining of 2240 existing community health workers, and improving services for some 696,000 beneficiaries. In one of the five dioceses, 47% of the costs will be covered locally; in the other four, local contributions will amount to 33% of the overall project costs.

The five-diocese project follows an earlier pilot program with one of the five dioceses. This operations research project (carried out in conjunction with Johns Hopkins University and funded by USAID) demonstrated that a church organization can substantially increase family planning use through outreach efforts. In this project, community health workers visited households to offer family planning information and sell supplies. Consequently,contraceptive prevalence rates increased from 21% to 34% over a period of two and a half years, and reported contraceptive prevalence rates for illiterate women visited in the program went from 19% to 38%.

CORAT also worked with Johns Hopkins University researchers and the Kenya Catholic Secretariat in Nyeri diocese on a pilot project introducing natural family planning methods (ovulation) to couples in rural Kenya. In a three-year interval, contraceptive prevalence of all methods increased from 14% to 21% and use of natural family planning methods increased from zero to 7%. Among contraceptors, use increased from zero to 32%, with accidental pregnancy rates at twelve months recorded at 18%.[5]

A further factor suggesting the attractiveness of church-related programs, particularly when compared to the free health care provided at government services, is the system the NGOs have for cost recovery. It is estimated, for example, that church-related medical institutions (which charge fees for drugs and services) offset more than 50% of all recurrent costs for their medical facilities (excluding costs of medical staff, many of whom serve in a voluntary capacity.)[6] A possible next step would be for CORAT to work with other church dioceses within the PCMA and the Kenya Catholic Secretariat on an expansion of community-based programs. A program for prevention of HIV transmission associated with Christian teachings could reinforce avoidance of promiscuous behavior and, where appropriate, use of barrier contraceptive techniques.

- *The Chogoria Program.* In Meru District, Kenya is located an exemplary church and hospital-based family planning and health care system. Run under the auspices of the Presbyterian Church of East Africa, the system comprises a hospital, 28 village health clinics and a grassroots cadre including 42 full-time field health educators and 500 volunteer family health workers who serve 350,000 on the slopes of Mt. Kenya. Although the dominant program, the Chogoria system is also complemented by government clinics.

Chogoria is one of several rural hospitals established by the Church of Scotland now associated with the Presbyterian Church in Kenya. Established by medical missionaries in 1922, Chogoria's prominent and wide-reaching role in the community suggests how church hospital systems throughout Africa can complement and extend government and donor resources in coming up with new community- based solutions to the full agenda of new problems posed by HIV/AIDS. Chogoria's support for a successful family planning program demonstrates this prominence and potential.

A World Bank publication singles out the Chogoria area as having one of the highest contraceptive prevalence rates for couples in rural Africa, some 27%. More recent reports include an estimate of 43% of all couples.[7]

Some of the reasons for relatively easy adoption of modern contraceptive techniques are related to the indigenous culture of the Meru people of the area. Other reasons, however, relate to the powerful impact the Church of Scotland Mission, and its successor, the Presbyterian Church, have had on family life since getting established in Meru in the 1920's.

Among the key influences were the introduction of a monogamous model of the family (encouraged by Scottish missionaries), marital fidelity in sexual relations, abstinence from liquor, and an openness to new technologies and behaviors such as those promoting good health and sanitation, and since the 1960s, family planning. Other changes illustrating the power of the church system included proscribing traditional female circumcision for church members and promoting construction and use of latrines in direct opposition to indigenous mores regulating toilet practices.

The effects of these influences for a program in preventing HIV transmission are obvious, as they promote monogamous behaviors which reduce the risk of exposure to HIV. Promoting abstinence from alcohol is also significant because it greatly reduces the likelihood of men frequenting bars. In a rural area such as Meru, drinking of alcohol in bars is closely associated with prostitution. Many bar girls, who work as prostitutes, represent the highest risk of exposure to HIV of any group in Kenya.

Church-based medical systems not only offer great potential for assisting in finding solutions; they can also pose formidable barriers if they are not taken into account. An early experience in Chogoria illustrates this point. Prominent Meru medical staff at Chogoria Hospital played an instrumental role in successfully challenging and terminating a pilot program to introduce the sale of condoms on a commercial basis in Meru District in the early 1970s. The church medical staff's reason for their (effective) objections was that condoms were being promoted openly in a manner not compatible with Meru and Christian morality, and so were objectionable.[8]

NGO Activities: The Broader Possibilities.

In addition to playing a very important role in supporting behavioral changes which decrease the risk of HIV/AIDS, a church hospital-based system like Chogoria, or the CORAT and MWYO programs, can also serve as key local institutions in dealing with a wide range of problems posed by AIDS. Proposed solutions include the following:

Introduce Interventions. Systematically introduce and field test newly developed interventions to prevent the spread of HIV/AIDS -- such as screened blood supply, drug therapy, vaccines, spermacides, educational and counseling programs. Church hospitals in rural areas offer a unique capability in being staffed by professional medical personnel that can sustain implementation of such programs while taking into account local ethics and values.
Community Participation. Develop community-based guidelines governing medical laboratory, diagnostic, and surveillance capability through existing hospital and clinic networks.

Counseling. Identify, counsel and care for persons tested positive for AIDS. Related to this are questions concerning the financial burden that treatment of AIDS patients places on hospital services.

Social Solutions and Support. Develop locally appropriate solutions to deal with the clinical and social manifestations of HIV/AIDS, such as care of parentless children, prevention of destructive social behavior, and social and economic support, for AIDS patients and their families.

Manage Donor Resources. Serve as a community-based catalyst (often under the guidance of the church hospital medical board), broker, or mediator to utilize resources provided by donors and government.

Training. Provide educational training and support to medical personnel and community based workers and support a program in which the pilot-testing of innovative approaches can be conducted.

Outreach and Dissemination. Ensure *spread* of successful, cost-effective approaches (as has been done with successes in family planning service delivery), to other systems operating within the region, Kenya, and/or other countries.

Action For Immediate Action

What activities can NGOs undertake today to address the urgent problems posed by AIDS? How can they incorporate state-of-the-art technologies and mobilize community and family resources? It is essential that all NGO activities be carried out only under the auspices of the government, particularly since these NGO activities touch on the delicate and sensitive nature of interventions to deal with HIV/AIDS. At least three direct activities can be delineated.

First, the development of a church-based AIDS prevention program focused on couples about to enter matrimony. Such a program would include education and counseling on AIDS, and on a trial basis, testing for sexually transmitted diseases including HIV/AIDS. The purpose of the program would be to enable couples to commit themselves to marriage knowing they and their spouses were free of infection. Additionally, they would be initiated into a program of periodic counseling (including provision of appropriate contraceptives) sustained within the framework of the church community, thereby increasing protection for the community as well as for the couple.

In many cases counseling and testing should be provided on a fee basis, the proceeds to be used to maintain a revolving fund to support a broader AIDS prevention program. A challenge of the program would be working on procedures acceptable to the community for identification and counseling of persons who are tested seropositive. The church leadership, within the framework of the government medical system, would take the lead in defining locally appropriate guidelines for addressing these and related issues, such as use of hospital resources for clinical care and support for affected families.

A second intervention particularly appropriate for community-based NGOs would be partnership between an international NGO and church hospital which might jointly assess the resources required in an affected community to deal with the social and economic costs of AIDS. A likely outcome of such a program would be to increase the recognition of the local hospital staff concerning the costs and benefits of an active AIDS prevention campaign. This would also highlight the resources needed to cope with the needs of those affected, such as the care of parentless children, prevention of destructive social behavior, counseling of AIDS patients, and management of hospital patient workload.

A partnership between NGO and Church Hospital might also serve as a means to generate international contributions for HIV prevention and related programs in family planning, nutrition, and health. As the AIDS problem interacts with other problems on the agenda of hardpressed government health ministries, support provided directly to nongovernmental activities can reduce the burden on the government. This, in turn, could increase the overall absorptive capacity for assistance within the health sector.

Third, NGOs could also support an array of operational research problems similar in vein to the approach described above with Maendeleo Ya Wanawake or CORAT (working on family planning information and service delivery) in Kenya. Key questions especially appropriate for NGOs to address might be tests on the cost-effectiveness and efficiency of various interventions, studies of the dynamics of behavior modification of risk behavior for HIV/AIDS, and promiscuity and other behavior related to travel of rural job seekers, etc., in and out of urban areas [rural and urban migration patterns].

Looking Ahead:
Barriers To And Possibilities For NGO Activities

Some NGOs may be slow in responding to the AIDS crisis, much as they have been slow in responding to the need to provide family planning information and/or services. Issues of morality permeate the topic of AIDS, and a portion of NGOs, especially those with a conservative religious orientation, cannot be expected to address the problem in a systematic manner, at least in the near term.

These organizations, however, deserve the attention of development planners and analysts as they may well present *barriers* to effectively dealing with AIDS, just as some have put road blocks in front of provision of family planning information and services. In short, it is important that the full spectrum of NGOs receive attention in strategy that addresses the AIDS problem at the community level.

Other NGOs are anxious to respond to the AIDs crisis, as the resource articles in this volume attest. In addition to community-based NGOs which are well-suited to combat AIDS, there are NGOs with medical expertise which also have the potential for leadership in this area. Many have experience in implementing activities in several countries and are well placed to work with governments as well as donors. Others can speed the collection of information and analysis to be gained through AIDS-related pilot activities. Such information will be invaluable in identifying what is *essential* to a successful program that attempts to control AIDS. Such information will also give African policymakers an understanding of what kind of interventions will effectively *modify* behavior that puts their peoples at risk in the HIV/AIDS pandemic.[9]

ENDNOTES

[1]I am grateful for helpful comments provided by Dr. Gerald van der Vlugt, Dr. Norman Miller,Dr. Maureen Lewis, Jack Thomas and Indirwa Biswas. The views expressed herein are those of the author.

[2]For a description of a successful (USAID-funded) project which works through private channels including companies, plantations, factories, private health clinics, parastatals and NGOs in Kenya, see "New Paths to Family Planning," written and produced by the IMPACT project of the Population Reference Bureau, Washington, D.C., November, 1987.

[3]Experience in Ghana also underlines the long-established role of the Church in family planning in Africa. The Church Council of Ghana (CCG) has actively supported family planning activities since 1960. The CCG Committee on Christian Marriage and Family Life started the first marriage counseling clinics to provide family planning information and advice in 1961, and even during the unsupportive regime of Dr. Nkrumah worked quietly and earned the credit for creating an initial awareness about family planning in Ghana.

[4]See Patrick Fleuret and Edward Greeley, *The Kenya Social and Institutional Profile*, Washington, DC: U.S. AID/Kenya, 1982, p. 214.

[5]See the paper, "Teaching and Practicing the Ovulation Method in Rural Kenya," Research Division Office, Population Agency for International Development, September, 1987. See also Mark L. Jacobson, Marian H. Labbok, Anne Murage, "Community Health Workers in Kenya: A Comparison" in the *Journal of Health Administration Education*, 5:1 Winter, 1987, p. 83-94.

[6]Fleuret, p. 14.

[7]For a discussion of the background to Chogoria's success in providing support for a relatively high level of contraceptive use, see Edward H. Greeley, "Planning for Population Change in Kenya: An Anthropological Perspective," (forthcoming in D. Brokensha and P. Little, *The Anthropology of Development and Change in East Africa*, Westview Press). See also "Making Community Distribution Work," a booklet about Chogoria written and produced by the IMPACT project of the Population Reference Bureau, Washington, D.C., November, 1987.

[8]See Edward H. Greeley "Men and Fertility Regulation in Southern Meru: A Case Study from the Kenya Highlands," Catholic University of America, 1977:111-16 (Ph.D. Dissertation).

[9]There is a substantial literature on the role of the Christian church as well as health in Eastern Africa. For further reading see: Beck, Ann. *A History of the British Medical Administration of East Africa 1900-1950*. Cambridge, MA: Harvard University Press, 1970; Bond, George, Walter Johnson, and Sheila Walker, eds. *African Christianity: Patterns of Religious Continuity*. New York: Academic Press, Inc., 1979; Hyden, Goren. "Religion, Politics and the Crisis in Africa," Universities Field Staff International Reports, No. 18, 1986; Long, Norman. *Social Change and the Individual: A Study of the Social and Religious*

144

Responses to Innovation. Manchester, U.K.: Manchester University Press, 1968 (Zambia); Mbiti, John. *Love and Marriage in Africa*. London, Longman Group Ltd., 1973; Oliver, Roland. *The Missionary Factor in East Africa*. London: Oxford University Press, 1970; Reining, Priscilla, *et al*., eds. "Impact on Family Life: Kenya," in *Village Women: Their Changing Lives and Fertility*. Studies in Kenya, Mexico and the Philippines. Washington, DC: American Association for the Advancement of Science, 1977.

THE POLITICS OF DISEASE: THE AIDS VIRUS AND AFRICA

Gloria Waite*

SUMMARY: This essay surveys several political issues that have arisen with respect to AIDS in Africa. It utilizes African and American press reports, journals and other studies on the political economy of health care in Central and East Africa. The primary themes investigated are the responses of African governments to the epidemic, the political and economic constraints involved in meeting the threat posed by AIDS, and the role of racism in the global response to AIDS in Africa.

Introduction

Within five years of the first AIDS case being diagnosed in Africa, responses to the disease have become highly political. This is true for several reasons. Large numbers of people are affected and state authorities are responsible for providing the resources for the public health response. National governments have numerous roles in the epidemic. They are responsible for mobilizing resources, coordinating national education programs, instituting whatever precautionary measures are necessary, appealing for international funding, and supplying materials such as self-destruct syringes to reduce the spread of AIDS through intravenous means. Choices have to be made regarding the distribution of resources. AIDS has also become a political issue because persons other than public health officials are concerned about the disease. These other interest groups have been seeking to protect or advance their interests vis-â-vis the health officials or those with the disease. Internationally, political issues have arisen, partly concerning African students and other travelers who encountered discrimination in immigration procedures.

This paper explores these issues in three parts. The first reviews the responses of government and industrial interest groups to AIDS in Africa. A second section focuses on health care budgets and financial priorities and

*Gloria Waite, Ph.D., is Assistant Professor of African and Afro-American Studies at Brandeis University. She spent part of her childhood in Liberia and did dissertation research in Zambia and Tanzania.

considers the politics of AIDS from an economic standpoint. The third section concerns the manner in which racist perceptions and stereotypes have influenced the discussion of African AIDS, and the consequences of these perceptions of Africans.

Government Responses To AIDS

AIDS cases were first identified in Rwanda, Uganda, and Zaire between 1982 and early 1984. Government-sponsored education programs began in Rwanda and Uganda in 1985. Although there was a time lag between the diagnosing of these first cases and the beginning of the campaign to stop the spread of AIDS, this lag may have been due more to the lack of resources, communication facilities and an inadequate understanding of the threat than to indifference on the part of the governments.

The Rwandan and Ugandan programs were considered in 1987 to be the best-coordinated ones in the Third World.[1] The Rwandan program includes radio broadcasts of a ten-part series to raise people's consciousness about the disease and how it is transmitted. It also involves the distribution of leaflets in clinics, libraries, government offices and schools, and will eventually include the integration of AIDS information into the general school curriculum. Because women have unequal access to printed information, different means of reaching them are being attempted. Uganda, despite its material shortages and numerous local languages, has established a similar program of national education in many of these languages. A half a million leaflets and numerous posters have been distributed. Information is being spread by word of mouth, by theatre groups, singers, and by local political workers.[2]

Zairean officials at first only distributed educational materials in hospitals in Kinshasa.[3] It was not until the end of 1986 that a national education program began with a six-part series on SIDA (French initials for AIDS) in *Elmina*, one of the national newspapers.[4] On the other hand, Zaire moved faster than any other African country to open its doors to research on AIDS, including the testing of vaccines on its citizens.

In other East and Central African countries responses to AIDS cases moved more slowly. Tanzania's first case of AIDS was identified in 1983. But it was not until 1985 that an education program was launched.[5] Kenya's first case was identified in 1985. It was not until July 1986 that the Kenyan Red Cross began to distribute leaflets, posters, and booklets in English and Swahili.[6] The Central African Republic (CAR) began an education campaign in late 1986.[7] Zambia[8] and Zimbabwe[9] began their programs in the spring and summer of 1987, and West African countries initiated programs in 1987 as the spread of the epidemic became irrefutable.[10]

Almost everywhere plans are afoot for expanding educational programs and in some cases for evaluating the relative success of these programs, and redesigning them as necessary to reach the greatest number of people. Consortiums of international donors in 1987 began to fund 5-year programs in Uganda[11] and Rwanda[12] that are designed to gradually expand the target populations, make follow-up studies on responses, and create information packages that serve the various population groups, taking into account cultural, educational, and social differences.

There are other measures besides public education that are essential to checking the spread of AIDS. These include the screening of blood to eliminate HIV-positive donations that could accidently be used in transfusions, and national distribution of non-reusable syringes for use in inoculation programs.

It would not have been possible to screen blood any earlier than 1985 because no reliable test was available until then. After 1985 the ELISA and other tests were developed for detecting antibodies to the AIDS virus in blood serum. During this period, however, the World Health Organization (WHO) cautioned that allocating what limited monies are available to preventive work on blood screening can deprive other areas that may be of more pressing concern.[13] Nevertheless, a recently published study indicates that transfusions for malaria-related anemia have been an important source of AIDS infection for children.[14]

Donated blood is presently being screened in a few African countries. The first African country to do so was Rwanda, which in the spring of 1985 began to screen blood for HIV-positive supplies.[15] Limited screening in

Kinshasa was initiated in 1986.[16]   Kenya began the process in Nairobi in January and in Mombasa in March of 1987.[17]

In spite of the caution about spending for blood screening, in the latter part of 1985 the World Health Organization sought $30 million from industrial countries for support staff and equipment needed to detect seropositive blood supplies in Africa.[18]   The response was less than enthusiastic, for a year later, in October 1986, the Commonwealth African health ministers were still appealing for massive financial assistance to buy the laboratory and medical equipment needed for screening blood supplies and to purchase disposable syringes.   These materials are needed because large numbers of Africans have diseases such as malaria and measles that require transfusions and inoculation respectively.[19]

Besides public health officials, other government officials and lay persons are also concerned with the epidemiology of AIDS.   There are sometimes conflicts between these parties.[20]   Persons in charge of ameliorating or controlling the problem may be pitted against those who suffer from or are at risk for the disease.   Conflicts may arise between one or both of these parties and others whose profit or prestige may be affected.

Specifically, African ministers in charge of tourism are concerned about the loss of national incomes that may result from the fear attached to AIDS.   Ministers of health are concerned, naturally enough, with containing the epidemic but must also weigh this particular disease against others that affect the lives of even greater numbers of people.   In addition, the health ministers must be concerned about the degree to which panic is created in their countries through irresponsible news reporting.

A case in point is Kenya, whose first AIDS case was identified in May 1985.[21]   The local press called for the government to make public the number of known cases and to begin informing the public about AIDS transmission.[22]

While these calls went out, the government was reacting angrily to reports that surfaced in Sweden and London about AIDS cases in Kenya.[23]   The Swedish television company wrongly reported that twenty percent of Kenyans had AIDS in 1985.   Although the company never named its sources, it went on to warn potential tourists to Kenya.[24]   At the time there were about 15 known AIDS cases in the country.[25] Another report appeared at the same time in Boston, Massachusetts, stating that between ten and fifteen percent of the blood donor population in Kenya had AIDS.[26] However, the blood samples from the Kenya Medical Research Institute indicated only one percent exposure, and the doctors at the institute had pointed this out to the reporter, as well as the fact that the ELISA test used to detect antibodies gives false positives to the AIDS virus because of the test's sensitivity to the antibodies of other, more common diseases in Africa.[27] Nevertheless, the writer reported the 15 percent assertion without qualifying the data.

The Kenyan government reacted to these reports by confiscating copies of the *International Herald Tribune* that carried a story from the *New York Times* on AIDS in Kenya.[28] Despite this hostility to the western press, Kenya became the first country in East and Central Africa to report AIDS cases to the World Health Organization when it reported eight cases in November 1985.[29] At that time, however, Kenyan government officials, including the director of medical services, insisted that they were not sure if AIDS warranted national priority, given the other more pressing health problems affecting larger numbers of people.[30]

Why had the Kenyan Government responded this way? One possible explanation is that it was concerned with the economic consequences of a sensational overseas reporting of its AIDS problem. Antibody tests did show high rates of exposure to the AIDS virus among prostitutes in the two major cities--Mombasa and Nairobi--but nationally there were still few other cases.

Undoubtedly, the minister in charge of tourism was concerned that unsubstantiated or exaggerated stories about AIDS would deprive Kenya of its second biggest source of foreign revenue after coffee.[31] Official confusion also compounded the problem. One official stated categorically that no AIDS cases were to be found in the country, despite statements from the ministry of health to the contrary.[32] During this time the British Royal Navy and the U.S. Navy were also already warning their sailors to avoid prostitutes in Mombasa, an important port of call.[33]

Even today, it is not clear how much the tourist trade has been affected by the western reports of AIDS in Kenya. One source claimed in February 1987 that tourism was being hard hit,[34] while another publication reported at the same time that the trade went up ten percent in 1986 because of the attraction to Kenya created by the film, *Out of Africa*.[35]

In another sphere, the politics of disease in Africa also involves the private interests of mine owners and other foreign companies that have either historically been unwilling to pay the cost of treatment for their workers, or else believe they will face bankruptcy if their profits are reduced because of rising health bills and death benefits. One indicator of these concerns surfaced when the Panos Institute in London was approached by representatives of several multinational corporations and asked to make a cost analysis of health care for their African employees. These corporate officials wanted to know how many African employees with AIDS they could afford to have before having to shut down their operations.[36] Other expressions of concern have been heard from companies in Zaire's mining and financial sectors that have expressed doubt about their ability to give sickness benefits if the rate of increase in AIDS cases continued to soar.[37]

In the bedrock of South Africa's economy--the migrant labor system in the mines--mine owner officials have discussed repatriating workers found to have AIDS.[38] Such a policy would shift the cost of treatment to migrants' families and their own countries (or "homelands" if within South Africa) and thereby deny the miners' compensation for the termination of their services. Throughout the history of South Africa's mining industry, black workers have borne a disproportionately large share of the cost of their own social security and social welfare.[39] AIDS thus becomes another excuse for shifting responsibility for health care onto the workers and preserving the profits of their labor for the mine owners and the white population in that country. The major mine workers' union vowed to resist forced repatriation.[40]

Health Care Budgets And Priorities

There are a number of economic issues involved in the politics of AIDS. Indeed, one reason why African countries have been in dire need of international assistance for this epidemic, and why the nature of reports on AIDS in Africa in the international media becomes of great consequence, is that most African countries were becoming increasingly impoverished even prior to the advent of the AIDS epidemic. It is no coincidence that AIDS and poverty are found together.

Despite the occurrence of AIDS among the elites of Central African nations, AIDS is closely linked to the poor. Among the first people to contract AIDS were women prostitutes in Central Africa, and male and female prostitutes in the U.S. and Haiti. A large number of homosexuals with AIDS in the U.S. are poor, as are the majority of drug addicts.

While analysts have been quick to point to the economic consequences of the AIDS epidemic on Africa's future,[41] some socioeconomic factors such as poverty that have contributed to the spread of the epidemic are rarely mentioned. An analysis of socioeconomic factors would point to the role of multinational corporations and foreign governments, in conjunction with their African collaborators, in the impoverishment of the African people. Perpetual underdevelopment gives rise to spiraling poverty and limited health services. The problem is not, as one writer calls it, "low health standards in Africa,"[42] but rather inadequate health-care resources. It is not aberrant cultural traits of Africans that must be searched for in the quest for the spread of AIDS in Africa, but rather the aberrant nature of the African economies--which are still dependent on external forces or, in the case of South Africa, bound by apartheid constraints.

A key issue turns on financial resources. Medical equipment, research facilities, supplies and staff salaries are all failing to expand or improve because of a continuing decrease in national incomes. For example, Zambia's per capita income has decreased by forty-five percent since the 1970s and its health spending has declined by twenty percent. Uganda, ravaged by civil war for over a decade, presently has a per capita annual income of $230.[43] Obviously, there is not much available to spend on health. In fact, only about $2 per capita is available in Uganda for all health expenditures.[44] If these funds are siphoned off for AIDS, there would be nothing left to deal with diseases that currently kill more people, namely measles, malaria and tuberculosis. As it is, the proportion of the national budget spent on health care has dropped from a high of ten percent between 1935 and the mid 1970s, to less than three and a half percent in the early

1980s.[45] In the Central African Republic the health expenditure is even less than Uganda's: $1.67 per annum per capita.[46]

These figures do not reflect skewed national budgets, but rather poor economies. Uganda has only a small percentage of its national budget going to its health ministry because agriculture, industrial development, transport, minerals, energy, and other parts of the social infrastructure have been given higher priorities in order to reverse the negative growth rate the country has been experiencing.[47]

On the other hand, health care in Kenya ranges from modern, extensive services in urban centers to inadequate services in remote rural areas. In some, infant mortality and malnutrition remain a problem.[48] Zaire's situation is even more skewed. In 1985 the *Financial Times* of London reported for Zaire that "the social infrastructure of schools and clinics has deteriorated to a degree where an entire generation has grown up with only the most rudimentary education and health care."[49] Commenting on the situation, a Zairean authority, Nzongola-Ntalaja noted the following:

> The absolute decline in [the ordinary Zairean citizens'] standard of living as well as the corresponding deterioration of all social and economic services has made them highly vulnerable[50] to malnutrition, cholera, AIDS...and other epidemics.

The contrast between Zaire and Uganda is illustrative in other fields related to health. While Uganda earmarked twenty-seven percent of its national budget to agriculture in 1985,[51] Zaire's was less than one percent in 1985, despite the regime's slogan that agriculture was "the priority of priorities."[52]

Racism And AIDS

Racism has risen as another political by-product of AIDS. Stereotyping of Africans has led to screening and immigration changes, suggestions of bizarre sexual behavior and other denigrating allegations. Issues of prejudice have of course also arisen outside the African AIDS arena, particularly in the stigmatizing of homosexuals and drug addicts in the United States and Europe.[53] In both western and African cases of prejudice, the problem is more one of sexuality than of disease. Moral questions are raised about behavior. Race and other characteristics of those with the disease permit heterosexual and white people who do not have the disease to blame the values and behaviors of those that do. Irrational fears result; information about the disease, its origin, its spread, its numbers, its "risk groups" are misconstrued and racial sterotyping increases.

Nor are the issues unique to AIDS. Syphilis, the other important sexually-transmitted disease of the twentieth century, brought about very similar fears, prejudices, inequalities and inequities in treatment.[54] When syphilis surfaced in the late nineteenth century, ideas abounded about "corrupt sexuality," which was in turn based on the "dirt-causes-disease" paradigm.[55] These ideas surfaced again with AIDS, in part because the AIDS epidemic emerged first among the homosexual male community whose sexual behavior was widely regarded as deviant and excessive. AIDS was initially thought to arise from perversion. The leap to the stereotyping of Africans was not difficult. There were already well-established myths about African sexuality, going back to the era of New World slavery when black women were used by white planters and black men were regarded as a threat to white womanhood. The views had political and economic context as well as sexual underpinnings; in some respects it was more a political issue than a sexual one. Thus, when Europeans went into Africa in the nineteenth and early twentieth centures as colonists, they had already formed distorted ideas about black people. Missionaries denounced polygamy, puberty rites were regarded as evil, and African dress was often considered immoral.

Most of the stereotypes were based on myths. Unlike the bathhouses in San Francisco, there was nothing inherent in African practices to support the notion that sexual excesses were widespread. Nor did these ideas end with colonial rule. Today, or at least until AIDS became an issue, prostitution thrived in major African cities, particularly for western military visitors. African prostitution has been encouraged by western beliefs about the sensuousness of African women, foreigners seeking exotic experiences, and by disparities in money and power.

Further problems have arisen because some journalists, scientists, and even homosexual groups have assigned responsibility for the AIDS epidemic to Africa. This is based on the suggestion that the virus may have originated in Africa. Especially in 1984 and 1985, such distinguished scientific journals as *The Lancet*, the *British Medical Journal, Science*, and *Scientific American* carried material suggesting a relationship between the AIDS virus and other viruses of supposed African origin, in effect locating the origins of the AIDS virus in Central Africa and speculating on its diffusion from Africa to Europe and America. The suggestion has also been made that the virus mutated from an animal virus. Many of these assertions have been proven erroneous and unfounded.[56] Nevertheless, such ideas about AIDS and Africa became established, as though set in concrete. The assumption was made, and continues to exist today, that AIDS spread from Africa to Europe. In Africa the view is just the opposite, but seems just as permanently cast.[57] Another problem lies in allegations that African governments are hiding the facts, that in fact there are far more AIDS cases than these officials are willing to admit.

Still another issue lies in the reports of social scientists who have also contributed their share of distortions surrounding the AIDS in Africa picture. Female circumcision (clitoridectomy), for example, is said to be "widespread in central and east Africa,"[58] "hidden homosexuality"[59] is alleged, and ideas of exotic practices in African sexual behavior are reported.

Many of these views have historic underpinnings. Modern western racism first flourished in the context of rationalizing southern slavery in the United States and the Caribbean after 1820. Such attitudes became a part of western European colonial expansion into Africa and Asia in the last third of the nineteenth century. There are views built upon physiological, cultural, political and economic differences, all reinforced by institutional inequalities.[60]

One important political result of stereotyping has been both screening programs, or discussion of screening programs that strike directly at Africans. The main targets are the large numbers of immigrants, migrant workers and students. For example, a government report in Britain that was ordered by the Foreign Secretary called for the compulsory screening of students from Tanzania, Uganda and Zambia.[61] The media added its share to this particular problem. The *Times* of London said that Africa "represents a huge reservoir of infection to which other populations, such as in Europe and the

United States, are at increasing risk beca~

Sunday Telegraph concluded that the "bi~

Furthermore, it editorialized that the~

duty to discriminate in the matter of AID~

blaming the government for the mass immigration~

and 1960s.[63] In other countries screening measures ~

Although China at first dropped its plan to screen after widesp~

by African students there,[64] a year later it enacted the plan.[65] India~

testing African students in early 1987.[66] Belgium initiated a testing program~

for Central African students in early 1987.[67] And Bavaria in West Germany

likewise launched a screening program.[68] Elsewhere, "foreign workers and

visitors suspected of having AIDS or being HIV-positive" were to be

restricted, deported, or refused entry.[69]

Screening measures may be well-intentioned, insofar as the general

welfare of a host nation's citizenry is concerned, but they are hardly

appropriate, because they reflect racist and other scapegoating views.[70]

There is no medical evidence in support of these measures. Once AIDS

emerges in a community (as it had already done in all countries prior to the

implementation of screening measures) it is best dealt with through internal

education that reduces multiple and casual sexual activity, through the

improvement of living and health services, and through safe blood supplies,

rather than through erecting barriers and limiting movements of people. As

the World Health Organization has pointed out, screening measures are

expensive and detract from the main need of controlling the epidemic

through education.[71] In San Francisco, where the epidemic of AIDS first

emerged, the rate of increase in new cases had diminished by mid 1987

because of the education homosexuals initiated within their own community,

not through the initiation of barriers, and probably not even through the

closing of bathhouses where gay males gathered for anonymous sexual

contacts.

Finally, the sensationalistic reporting about AIDS in Africa by

journalists and scientists has created an enormous amount of conflicting

information[72] concerning the numbers that have contracted AIDS, the

numbers that are carriers, the rural and urban dimensions, the role of co-promoting the onset of AIDS, the number of viruses that are ⌐, the earliest evidence of AIDS in Africa, the kind of evidence that ⌐ts an African origin, and what social significance such a connection ⌐ have. Confusing and contradictory information has done a great ⌐sservice to our knowledge about the disease in Africa.

Conclusion

African governments have responded as well as can be expected to a disease about which little is known, and under circumstances that would challenge any country, including the resource-rich nations of the West. The politics of a public disease such as AIDS, however, are not limited to government services. There are other conflicting interest groups involved, including political parties, women's organizations, bi-lateral funding agencies, multilateral organizations such as UN offices, and probably most important for the future, the Private Volunteer Organizations (PVOs) or Non-Governmental Organizations (NGOs). As discussed elsewhere in this volume, PVO/NGO activity will play important parts in the campaign against AIDS in the immediate years ahead. Conflicts can also be expected as these organizations attempt to push their own mandates, and to do so in tandem with the changing policies of central governments.

Of great significance in the attempts of African nations to check the spread of AIDS is the fact that they have dependent economies that are easily subject to outside disruption. African economies are fragile because a combination of outside interests and internal self-interests have left them in this state. This situation, compounded by poverty seriously compromises the ability of even well-intentioned governments to meet the public threat posed by the spread of AIDS.

Underlying the current situation is the legacy of racism that permeates many of the African AIDS issues. Racism merges with ideas about "corrupt sexuality" and "contagious disease" to make Africans pariahs in several parts of the world. Within five years after the AIDS epidemic emerged, a campaign was discernible, sometimes very strident in tone, to check the immigration of African workers and students into Asia and Europe.[73] The overall consequence was to suggest that Africans should not only be banished from international travel, but in fact condemned to work out their problems in isolation. AIDS in this context had come full circle as a political issue.

ENDNOTES

[1]Panos Institute, *AIDS and the Third World*, pp. 29-31; *New York Times,* 1 November 1985, p. 25.

[2]Ed Hooper, "AIDS in Uganda," *African Affairs* 86 (Oct. 1987):476.

[3]*New York Times*, 22 December 1985, p. 29.

[4]*New York Times*, 4 Jan. 1987, p. 1.

[5]*Weekly Review*, 3 Jan. 1986, p. 15.

[6]*Weekly Review*, 25 July 1986, p. 13; *New York Times*, 24 Feb. 1987, p. B4.

[7]*New York Times*, 4 Jan. 1987.

[8]*AfricAsia*, May 1987, p. 54.

[9]*Herald* (Harare), 11 Sept. 1987, p. 7.

[10]*New York Times*, 15 April 1987, p. A12.

[11]*New York Times*, 26 May 1987, p. C1.

[12]*New York Times*, 29 May 1987, p. A2.

[13]*New York Times*, 3 June 1987, p. A1.

[14]Alan E. Greenberg, *et al.*, "The Association Between Malaria, Blood Transfusions, and HIV Seropositivity in a Pediatric Population in Kinshasa, Zaire." Some contaminated blood also was introduced into some Central African countries from the United States prior to 1985.

[15]*New African*, Jan. 1987, p. 13.

[16]*New York Times*, 22 Jan. 1988, p. A6.

[17]*New York Times*, 24 Feb. 1987, p. B4.

[18]*New York Times*, 22 Dec. 1985, p. 29.

[19]*Africa Now*, Nov. 1986, p. 34.

[20]And this is true of public health in general. See Paul Starr, *The Transformation of American Medicine*, for a discussion of such conflicts in a modern society. Gloria Waite, "Public Health in Pre-Colonial East-Central Africa" demonstrates how such conflicting interest groups were also found in pre-modern societies.

[21]*Weekly Review*, 13 Sept. 1985, p. 4.

[21]*Weekly Review*, 29 Nov. 1985, p. 9.

[23]*Africa Now*, Feb. 1987, pp. 11-12.

[24]*Weekly Review*, 29 Nov. 1985, p. 11.

[25]See *Weekly Review*, 14 Feb. 1986, p. 4, where 14 cases were confirmed by February 1986.

[26]*Boston Globe*, 14 Nov. 1985, p. 22.

[27]*Weekly Review*, 29 Nov. 1985, pp. 11-12.

[28]Alfred J. Fortin, "The Politics of AIDS in Kenya."

[29]*New York Times*, 22 Dec. 1985, p. 29.

[30]*Weekly Review*, 14 Feb. 1986, p. 4.

[31]*Africa Now*, Feb. 1987, p. 11.

[32]Ibid.

[33]Ibid., *New York Times*, 24 Feb. 1987, p. B4.

[34]*Africa Now*, Feb. 1987, p. 11.

[35]*New York Times*, 24 Feb. 1987, p. B4.

[36]*West Africa*, 22 June 1987, p. 1201.

[37]*New African*, Jan. 1987, p. 12.

[38]*Weekly Mail* (Johannesburg), 4-10 Sept. 1987, p. 2.

[39]See Shula Marks and Richard Rathbone, eds., *Industrialisation and Social Change in South Africa*. In the spring of 1987 black mine workers undertook a historically unprecedented strike in an attempt to get a living wage. They failed to reach their objective and thus continue to provide most of their own welfare and security.

[40]*Weekly Mail*, 4-10 Sept. 1987, p. 2.

[41]See for example, *Washington Post*, 31 May 1987, p. A1; *Boston Globe*, 9 October 1987, p. 1.

[42]Graham Hancock and Enver Carim, *AIDS: The Deadly Epidemic*, p. 119.

[43]Panos Institute, p. 35.

[44]*Africa Now*, Nov. 1986, p. 36.

[45]Cole P. Dodge, "Uganda--Rehabilitation, or Redefinition of Health Services?"

[46]*New York Times*, 4 Jan. 1987, p. 1.

[47]Ibid.

[48]Wilfred M. Mwangi and Germano M. Mwabu, "Economics of Health and Nutrition in Kenya."

[49]Quoted in Nzongola-Ntalaja, "Crisis and Change in Zaire, 1960-1985," p. 3.

[50]Ibid., p. 4.

[51]Dodge, p. 755.

[52]Ngongola-Ntalaja, p. 9.

[53]Nancy Krieger and Rose Appleman, *The Politics of AIDS*; Cindy Patton, *Sex and Germs*; Randy Shilts, *And the Band Played On*; and Richard Goldstein, "The Hidden Epidemic: AIDS and Race."

[54]Allan M. Brandt, *No Magic Bullet*. See also James H. Jones, *Bad Blood* on how the conjunction of syphilis, race, poverty, and greed in Tuskegee, Alabama was the basis for an experiment on black men with syphilis that continued long after effective treatments for the disease had been discovered. Such conditions exist in African nations today, and the role of AIDS research there is a very important issue that deserves a study in its own right.

[55]Brandt, *No Magic Bullet*.

[56]See Richard C. and Rosalind J. Chirimuuta, *AIDS, Africa and Racism* for a full discussion and critique of these writings.

[57]*Weekly Review*, 29 Nov. 1985, pp. 11-13; *Africa Events*, Jan. 1986, pp. 58-60; *New African*, Jan. 1987, p. 25; *West Africa*, 13 July 1987, pp. 1350-52; *New York Times*, 19 Nov. 1987, p. B13.

[58]*New York Times*, 22 November 1985, letters to the editor. This practice of clitoridectomy, by the way, is simply not practiced in the areas where the earliest cases of AIDS were concentrated and therefore could not have been a factor in the spread of AIDS.

[59]Ibid.

[60]Pierre L. Van den Berghe, *Race and Racism*, explains some of the basis for modern racism.

[61]*Times* (London), 22 Sept. 1986, p. 3

[62]*Times,* 22 Sept. 1986, p. 3.

[63]*Sunday Telegraph*, 21 Sept. 1986, p. 1.

[64]*Boston Globe*, 21 Dec. 1986, p. 19.

[65]*New York Times*, 22 Dec. 1987, p. A1.

[66]Reuter report from New Delhi in February 1987.

[67]*Salongo* (Kinshasa), 25 March 1987, p. 1.

[68]Panos Institute, *AIDS and the Third World*, p. 77.

[69]Ibid.

[70]For example, screening of all persons applying for permanent resident status in the U.S. and of prisoners, who are also powerless, in U.S. federal detention.

[71]*New York Times*, 3 June 1987, p. A1.

[72]See for example, Lynn W. Kitchen, "AIDS in Africa: Knowns and Unknowns."

[73]At the International AIDS Conference in London in January 1988, African health ministers spoke with great concern about this development.

BIBLIOGRAPHY

Brandt, Alan M. *No Magic Bullet: A Social History of Venereal Disease in the United States since 1880*. New York and Oxford: Oxford University Press, 1985.

Chirimuuta, Richard C., and Chirimuuta, Rosalind J. *AIDS, Africa and Racism*, London: Richard Chirimuuta, 1987. [Address: Bretby House, Stanhope, Bretby, Nr Burton-on-Trent, Derbyshire, DE15 OPT, U.K.]

Dodge, Cole P. "Uganda--Rehabilitation, or Redefinition of Health Services?" *Social Science and Medicine* 22 (1986):755-61.

Fortin, Alfred J. "The Politics of AIDS in Kenya," *Third World Quarterly* 9 (July 1987):906-19.

Goldstein, Richard. "The Hidden Epidemic: AIDS and Race." *Village Voice* 10 (March 1987):23-30.

Greenberg, Alan E.; Nguyen-Dinh, Phuc; Mann, Jonathan M.; Kabote, Ndoko; Colebunders, Robert L.; Francis, Henry; Quinn, Thomas C.; Baudoux, Paola; Lyamba, Bongo; Davachi, Farzin; Roberts, Jacquelin M.; Kabeya, Ngandu; Curran, James W., and Campbell, Carlos C. "The Association Between Malaria, Blood Transfusions, and HIV Seropositivity in a Pediatric Population in Kinshasa, Zaire." *Journal of the American Medical Association* 259, #4 (22/29 Jan. 1988):545-49.

Hancock, Graham, and Carim, Enver. *AIDS: The Deadly Epidemic*. London: Victor Gollancz, Ltd., 1986.

Holness, K., Wong, K., and Gazi, D. *AIDS--An African Perspective: A Report*. London: Black Health Workers and Patients Group, 1987.

Hooper, Ed. "AIDS in Uganda." *African Affairs* 86 (Oct. 1987):469-77.

Jones, James H. *Bad Blood: The Tuskegee Syphilis Experiment--a Tragedy of Race and Medicine*. New York and London: The Free Press, 1981.

Kitchen, Lynn W. "AIDS in Africa: Knowns and Unknowns," *Center for Strategic and International Studies* (CSIS) *Africa Notes* No. 74 (17 July 1987).

Krieger, Nancy, and Appleman, Rose. *The Politics of AIDS*. Oakland, CA: Frontline Pamphlets, 1986.

Marks, Shula, and Rathbone, Richard. Eds. *Industrialisation and Social Change in South Africa*. London and New York: Longman, 1982.

Mwangi, Winfred M., and Mwabu, Germano M. "Economics of Health and Nutrition in Kenya," *Social Science and Medicine* 22 (1986):775-80.

164

Nzongola-Ntalaja. "Crisis and Change in Zaire, 1960-1985" *In The Crisis in Zaire: Myths and Realities*, pp. 3-25. Edited by Nzongola-Ntalaja. Trenton, N.J.: Africa World Press, 1986.

Panos Institute. *AIDS and the Third World*. Revised and Updated Edition. London: Panos Institute, 1987.

Panos Institute. "The Talloires Conclusions on AIDS and Development." Talloires, Annecy, France: The Panos Institute, March 1987.

Patton, Cindy. *Sex and Germs: The Politics of AIDS*. Boston: South End Press, 1985.

Shilts, Randy. *And the Band Played On: Politics, and the AIDS Epidemic*. New York: St. Martin's Press, 1987.

Starr, Paul. *The Social Transformation of American Medicine*. New York: Basic Books, 1982.

Van den Berghe, Pierre L. *Race and Racism: A Comparative Perspective*. New York, London, and Sydney: John Wiley & Sons, 1967.

Waite, Gloria "Public Health in Pre-Colonial East-Central Africa." *Social Science and Medicine* 24 (1987):197-208.

PART IV
Issues
of Society and Education

OVERVIEW:
SOCIAL FACTORS in the TRANSMISSION
and
CONTROL OF AFRICAN AIDS:

David Brokensha[*]

SUMMARY: The overview discusses sexual relations and marriage, prostitution, social-sexual practices, movements of people, coping with illness, and technical issues of disease transmission.

Introduction

This brief essay focuses on social and behavioral factors of relevance to the transmission of HIV/AIDS in Africa and indicates some of the contributions social anthropologists and other social scientists might make. The questions are numerous. What specific information would assist epidemiologists and clinical researchers studying AIDS in Africa? How can this information be retrieved and communicated most efficiently? How can we and African social scientists present our detailed ethnographic knowledge of African societies in a usable form to the health and medical professions?

In order to provide an overview to the concerns of social analysts, six broad topics that illustrate social issues have been selected for brief delineation.

Sexual Relations And Marriage

Despite popular opinion that suggests otherwise, anthropologists have devoted relatively little attention to the systematic study of sexual behavior. There are many studies of marriage and divorce, of the social, economic and

* David Brokensha, Ph.D., is a Director, Institute for Development Anthropology, Binghamton, N.Y., and Professor of Anthropology, and Chairman of Environmental Studies, University of California, Santa Barbara. Kathleen MacQueen, MA. and Lewis Stess of IDA also contributed to the essay.

ritual roles of women, of changes in male-female relationships, and in other institutionalized forms of gender behavior. Where sexual practices are mentioned, however, they are often of a generalized nature.

To pursue greater understanding of sexual relations and marriage, more depth information on marital stability and divorce is needed. Admittedly some of the classics, such as Isaac Schapera's *Married Life in an African Tribe* (1940), are generally helpful, but these studies often refer to conditions that are generations out of date and cannot be expected to be an accurate presentation of contemporary life. Research on current sexual practices that surround migrant labor (for example from Botswana to the South African mines) may bear important insights. In this case, one obvious concern is the practice of absent husbands and stay-at-home wives taking lovers. Another issue concerns divorce. Divorced women, for example, are in many societies more likely than married women to enter into casual sexual unions.

To pursue this topic it is important to compile information on age at marriage for males and females, sexual permissiveness for males and females, and sexual permissiveness for unmarried and married males and females. Other issues include polygyny, particularly concerning the sexual relations of the parties. Another issue surrounds prohibitions relating to marital and sexual partners, particularly concerning such information as who may marry, at what age, under what conditions, and at what cost, and who may have sexual relations. Finally, data on post-partum sexual prohibitions are reported historically for many parts of Africa, but it is important to investigate to what extent these practices are followed today.

Prostitution

What happens to the children of prostitutes, given the high rate of mother-infant HIV transmission? What are the implications of ethnic specialization in prostitution? What are the causes of prostitution? Are there high rates of divorce, economic need, alcoholism or other factors behind prostitution, and what are the consequences of prostitution for the rural society? Some women become prostitutes in the classic western sense, but we must stress that this term is often used loosely, and inaccurately, by westerners in Africa.

Unquestionably, each large city, and many small towns (even some villages) has a group of "professional" prostitutes who earn their income in this way. But many other women "exchange sexual services" to augment their income, or to meet special needs. Sometimes women are steady partners of one man, referred to as "spares" (Zimbabwe), "meanwhilers" (Ghana) or "town wives" (West Africa). Variations of such relationships include forms of courtesanship in northern Nigeria among Hausa women who are generally uneducated, with few marketable skills, and hence few employment opportunities. There are also new "independent" women among various ethnic migrant groups in Uganda, who are economically independent with well-defined positions. In Uganda rural social structure, for example, women have the right to choose their lovers there as well as in urban settings.

Clearly the issue of prostitution in the transmission of AIDS is a complex and sensitive one, overlapping as it does with sexual mores, the economic dependency of women, and male-female power relations. Western cultural stereotypes and moral judgments can also present a problem in analysis. When we think of the term "prostitute" we think of a women who is aggressively marketing her sexuality. When we apply this label to single women who are economically dependent on a succession of lovers, the stereotype of the street hooker is often carried along with the term. That stereotype could prove detrimental not only to analysis, but also to counselling and education efforts where women are particularly sensitive to such negative interpretations of their behavior.

There is no doubt, judging from the high incidence of AIDS among prostitutes, that having multiple sex partners increases the risk of infection. Hard social data on this are nevertheless very scarce. Understandably, many Africans have protested at being labeled "promiscuous" on the basis of their rates of HIV incidence, and most social analysts would avoid the term because it implies a moral quagmire. A more fruitful tack would be to examine the range of tolerated sexual behavior found in different societies and to assess which individuals, and which groups, are more likely to have multiple sex partners and thereby run a greater risk of infection.

Social-Sexual Relations

Looking at social-sexual relationships more broadly, at least three important areas of inquiry may be set out. In school settings relations between male school teachers and female students are recurring areas of sexual activity. The situation often involves relatively few teachers in any one area, but many coerced student partners. Schools are important also in encouraging new ideas about sexual behavior.

A by-product of the problem involves teenage or pre-marital pregnancy. Parents are understandably upset when their daughters are impregnated at school because it reduces their attraction as potential wives and thus diminishes the bridewealth that is still expected in many African societies. Also, an interruption of education often occurs at a crucial time, just before examinations, either causing the girl to lose a year's schooling, or, more usually, to drop out of school.

Second, homosexuality, while clearly occurring on a minor scale in comparison to the West, is found in several circumstances and cannot be dismissed as a factor in HIV/AIDS. Wherever there are large numbers of white males present, there are usually some homosexuals, and there will almost certainly be a coterie of young African men who become, at least temporarily, homosexual. Second, in all-male compounds such as prisons or in the South African mines, homosexuality is reported to occur. And third, several African societies accepted in the past, and may continue to accept (though this is not clear) the assumption of female roles by certain individual men. In this third example, the relevance of homosexuality for the transmission of AIDS would depend on the number of sexual partners these men had.

A third factor concerns impotence and virility. There is a widespread fear of impotence which is, apparently, quite common. Several reports mention instances where older men ask younger men to impregnate a wife. The Gwembe Tonga of Zambia use euphemistic invitation in these circumstances - "go and cut wood for me, my friend" (T. Scudder, personal communication). The significance is both as a possible additional way in which AIDS might be spread and also as an illuminating factor on perception of sexuality and the importance of begetting children. On the other side of the picture, many men like to display and boast about their virility, as is indicated in novels, in ethnographies and in contemporary life.

Movement Of People

Population movement is one of the most significant themes in the study of AIDS, as it is through this means that HIV is carried from one region to another. Several questions are important: Who migrates? Why? When? For how long? Is migration correlated with an increase in extra-marital sexual acts or in sexual activity generally? What other types of population movement, such as tourism or military emplacements, are possible factors?

Topics that are important for analysis focus upon at least four groups. First, migrant labor groups, including rural-to-urban, rural-to-rural, to mines, industries, farms and plantations, are undoubtedly significant. Historically, migrant laborers were single men who circulated between their home villages and places of employment. With the transition from colonial rule to independence throughout Africa, this pattern is being replaced by one of permanent rural-urban migration of men, often with wives and children. There has also been an increase in the number of independent women migrants in recent years.

Second, truck drivers have been reported to be important contributors to the spread of AIDS, especially from Uganda to Kenya and Tanzania. The correlation between commonly used trucking routes and areas of high AIDS incidence are cited as evidence. Systematic studies, such as HIV testing of truck drivers, need to be carried out before conclusive statements can be made.

Third, elites are important to analyze. Many articles have commented on the apparent high incidence of AIDS among the leaders and educated elites. This has implications both for the political future of African nations, if they face a severe loss of leaders, and also for the families and others whom the elites have contacted sexually. Again, we have relatively little hard data on this topic.

Finally, other groups who move from their home areas include members of armed forces (soldiers and policemen), government officials, traders (and smugglers), university and high school students, pastoralists, fishermen, hunters and residents of the new "boomtowns". A group related to the above are those who are moved involuntarily, such as prisoners, refugees, and resettlers (e.g., from large dams). All of these may, in different ways, be at risk.

Coping With Illness

There is a substantial body of literature that attests to the resilience and adaptability of African societies in coping with major disasters. Many detailed studies have been made of the "adaptive strategies" and the social networks that have helped Africans to cope. To date, however, this factor has been underplayed in the literature about AIDS in Africa. A fruitful line of inquiry would analyze the ways of coping historically, seen as a positive contribution that Africans can make.

What are other related questions? One surrounds how local societies will cope with AIDS following traumatic changes such as on-going warfare and rebellion as seen in Uganda or the southern Sudan. A further issue surrounds how individuals cope with AIDS vis-à-vis traditional healers. As indicated by Charles Good elsewhere in this volume, traditional healers may be exceptionally important in helping fellow Africans become aware of AIDS. It should be noted that such healers are relevant to national efforts to contain the disease through their close community lines and roles as advisors and educators. Alternatively, traditional healers may become part of the problem as they interact closely with patients and thus risk infection themselves, thereafter spreading it to others.

Technical Issues Of Disease Transmission

Medical and technical issues concerning transmission of AIDS are also the legitimate realm of social investigators, particularly when behavioral issues are involved. For example, it is desirable to examine and document all cases where direct contact with blood may be a factor in HIV transmission, and to seek correlations with the incidence of AIDS. It is also true that these links are not well established, and caution is in order when extrapolating from cultural or medical practices to actual routes of infection. The major points of concern include: blood transfusions, injections, hospitals, or traditional surgical techniques, and such ritual practices as clitoridectomy, circumcision, scarification, tooth removal, incisions for healing, and incisions for protection.

The essays that follow in this section address other issues and other questions that portray the wide spectrum of topics in need of social analysis. The challenge will be to bring the insights and experience social scientists have built up in recent decades into the broad arena that the AIDS epidemic has created.

AIDS IN AFRICA: AN AGENDA FOR BEHAVIORAL SCIENTISTS

Edward C. Green[*]

SUMMARY: Behavioral scientists with experience in research and social analysis in Africa could play a vitally important role in developing and implementing programs to contain the spread of AIDS. First there is a need to establish an information base regarding beliefs and behaviors relevant to the cycle of AIDS transmission. Behavioral scientists are also needed to interpret and advocate the policy and programmatic implications of behavioral research findings, as well as to provide social analysis and forecasting to prepare African governments and donor organizations for the consequences of, and responses to, high morbidity and mortality from AIDS among the most productive segments of African societies.

Introduction

Acquired Immunodeficiency Syndrome (AIDS) is a fatal disease of pandemic proportion. Cases have been reported in over 120 countries, with highest current prevalence believed to be in sub-Saharan Africa. Prevalence levels for exposure to the virus are 25-30% among young adults in some parts of Africa, and among certain high risk groups such as prostitutes, truck drivers and soldiers, may be as high as 85-90% (Mann 1987:7; Potts 1987:3). The only means of stopping or slowing the spread of AIDS is for individuals to change behavior which promotes the transmission of the virus. In order to direct behavior change, an AIDS knowledge base is needed which will be comparable to--but will probably have to exceed in detail and complexity-- the knowledge bases that exist for family planning and child diarrheal diseases. To undertake directed behavior change prior to establishing an AIDS knowledge base could result not only in wasted resources but in a backlash against the U.S. or donor organizations involved in AIDS containment.

---
* Edward C. Green, Ph.D., administers programs in family planning and primary health care in Africa and the Caribbean for John Short and Associates, Columbia, Maryland, USA. He previously served as Social Science Advisor to the Swaziland Ministry of Health.

176

Changes in behavior which promote the spread of AIDS will go against social and cultural norms and values in Africa, and against deeply ingrained behavioral patterns. Any effective program of directed behavior change must be based on adequate behavioral and sociocultural information relating to the transmission of the HIV virus. A recent report from the National Academy of Sciences concludes:

> HIV infection is spread through particular types of behavior, and presently the best hope for stopping the epidemic spread of the virus is through changes in types of behavior responsible for its continued transmission. Yet the forces that shape human behavior, and the best approaches to influencing behavior to protect health, are among the most complex and poorly understood aspects of society's response to the AIDS epidemic...(the biological bases of AIDS are relatively well understood)...In contrast, the knowledge base in the behavioral and the social sciences needed to design approaches to encouraging behavioral change is more rudimentary... (NAS 1986: 230-1. Paren. mine)

There is an urgent need for behavioral scientists to shed light on those poorly-understood behaviors which are integral to the cycle of AIDS transmission, including patterned sexual behavior and traditional health and healing beliefs and practices. Anthropologists are in a unique position to conduct or direct the social and behavioral research needed to establish the requisite information base for AIDS in Africa, not to mention the interpretation of such research findings and the advocacy of policies or programs implied by research. Behavioral scientists associated with international development agencies have also developed skills in social forecasting, skills now of critical importance in planning for the social, economic, institutional, political and other consequences of high morbidity and mortality associated with AIDS. This chapter will discuss the role of behavioral scientists in containing the spread of AIDS in Africa. Emphasis will be given to the role anthropologists, sociologists and others could play in connection with the U.S. Agency for International Development (AID), since this organization will be the major implementing organization coordinating U.S. assistance in AIDS containment in Africa and other parts of the developing world (NAS 1986).

Establishing The Information Base

Information needs to be gathered relating to the categories of Africans at highest risk for AIDS, the specific types of behavior that promote the spread of AIDS, the attitudes that both infected and uninfected people hold about the disease and its carriers, what is understood about its transmission and prevention, and any beliefs and practices relating to treatment of what we know as AIDS and ARC symptoms.

Since HIV infection in Africa appears to be largely heterosexually transmitted, emphasis should be placed on understanding patterns of heterosexual behavior in their sociocultural context. Behavior promoting the transmission of the virus includes at least the following:

(1)   Having numerous sexual partners, which increases the risk of encountering an HIV-carrier;

(2)   Having intercourse unprotected by condom when one or both partners has a sexually transmitted disease, especially one characterized by open genital lesions;

(3)   Having intercourse with partners at special risk, that is, who tend to have many sexual partners and thus are more likely to be HIV carriers or to have an untreated STD.

(4)   Failure to use condoms, especially with partners likely to be carriers. According to the most recent Contraceptive Prevalence and Demographic and Health Surveys, prevalence rates for condom use are 1% or less in the AIDS-infected countries of Africa.

(5)   Male homosexuality and anal intercourse practices, whether homosexual or heterosexual.

Sexually Transmitted Disease (STD)

A most significant epidemiologic finding relating to heterosexually-transmitted AIDS in Africa is the apparent facilitating role of other sexually transmitted diseases (STDs):

In studies among Nairobi prostitutes, HIV seropositivity was significantly associated with current sexually transmitted diseases such as gonorrhea, genital ulcers, and syphilis....In another study in Zambia, seropositivity in men was also correlated with the presence of genital ulcers. These observations suggest that disruption of genital epithelial integrity caused by sexually transmitted diseases that are common in Africa may facilitate transmission of HIV during vaginal intercourse. (Quinn *et al*.1986:234-5)

It is important to note that STDs may not be recognized as such by many uneducated Africans, and in any case STDs often go untreated by trained medical personnel. Instead, they are commonly treated by traditional healers with ineffective therapies, in fact therapies that may involve use of needles and razor blades that may facilitate the spread of HIV. Among the Swazi and neighboring Nguni speakers, for example, pus discharge from the penis is widely believed to result from a type of sorcery known as *likhubalo*, perpetrated by husbands who are trying to ensure their wives' sexual fidelity when the husbands are absent. When the discharge symptoms appear, traditional rather than modern-biomedical therapies are usually sought because the cause of the affliction is thought to lie outside the domain of Western medicine (cf. Green and Makhubu 1984: 1073).

AIDS is also transmitted through means other than sexual intercourse, which may help account for the fact that overall prevalence rates in Africa may be as high for women and children as they are for men. In addition to the problem of infected blood supplies due to inadequate screening (a problem already well recognized and not really a *behavioral* problem) as well as the problem of re-use of needles and lack of adequate aseptic techniques on the part of *trained* health personnel (a financial, educational, and logistical problem for the formal health care system), behavior that places the general population of Africans at risk for AIDS includes various uses of skin-piercing implements by various people for a variety of reasons. Specifically, traditional healers and other non-biomedically trained specialists or lay-persons may be spreading AIDS through use of hypodermic needles, razor blades used for traditional vaccinations, and needles and other implements used for scarification and perhaps tatooing. There is preliminary evidence for this:

> The potential for HIV transmission by unsterilized needles...should not be underestimated, the further studies should be undertaken to assess risk associated with these factors and to develop effective means of prevention. [In a study of AIDS patients in Zaire]...twenty-nine percent of patients utilized traditional medical practitioners, and eighty percent reported receiving medical injections...The use of

unsterilized needles or other skin-piercing instruments for medical or ritual purposes (for example, scarification, tattooing, ear piercing, male or female circumcisions, blood-brotherhood ceremonies) has potential for HIV transmission.

[In a study of seropositive children in a Kinshasa hospital]...a history of scarification in the previous year was significantly more common among 40 seropositive children of 2 to 14 years old (25%) compared with 92 seronegative children of the same age and sex (25 versus 6.6%). These data suggest that injections and scarifications are associated with HIV infection, but it is difficult to distinguish whether the association is truly causal, that is, provides a means of exposure to HIV, or secondary due to treatment for early symptoms of HIV infection or other illnesses, such as sexually transmitted diseases. [Brackets (but not paren.) mine]. (Quinn *et al.*1986: 959. cf. also Liskin and Blackburn 1986: 204-4; Mann 1987: 7-8).

There are suggestions that traditional inoculation in Africa may have been responsible for the appearance of AIDS in humans (Kashamura, quoted in *The Economist* (1987:76). Whatever the possible role of unsterilized needles and other implements in HIV transmission--and the jury is still out, so to speak--the World Health Organization is implementing a strategy to "collaborate with members states to ensure the use of sterile needles, syringes and other skin-piercing implements" and it calls for surveys of "skin-piercing practices in medical and other settings" (WHO 1987: II-3-4), with "other settings" broadly referring to ethnomedical and other traditional settings.

Information concerning what is scientifically known about AIDS, including the various means of AIDS prevention, is beginning to spread in Africa. In some countries with high AIDS prevalence, information and awareness campaigns have already begun. Even in the absence of these, information of some sort is circulating about AIDS, "slim disease," or whatever the disease is locally called. In addition to sexual behavior and skin-piercing practices, there is a need for anthropologists to establish what is locally known or believed about AIDS itself, including inter-group and socioeconomic variations in such knowledge and beliefs, in order to plan and implement appropriate, culturally-tailored education and other intervention strategies. Large national surveys are not called for at the present stage; not enough is known about AIDS-related knowledge, belief, and behavior patterns to attempt to measure these patterns. Instead, qualitative data should be gathered through key-informant and indepth interviews, focus group discussions, direct observation, and other techniques anthropologists typically rely on. As with surveys--but to an even greater extent--behavioral scientists will be needed to interpret qualitative research findings and to ensure their utilization.

The Cultural Context Of AIDS-Related Behavior

Sexual behavior and indigenous health practices exist in a cultural context which--along with the behavior itself--must be adequately understood before attempting to direct behavior change. For example, in patriarchal societies where men control economic and other resources, those who control more resources are able to maintain sexual relations with a greater number of women. This includes more permanent relations with wives and mistresses, as well as less permanent ones with prostitutes, bar-girls, and casual girlfriends. In any case, men achieve status in part by the number of women with whom they maintain sexual relations. Women may be rewarded in cash or gifts for sexual favors, which does not necessarily make them prostitutes. A good deal of female sexual behavior in Africa can be viewed as economic survival and adaptation to patterns of male dominance.

Patterns of male dominance also make it possible for men to coerce women, including teen-age girls, into sexual intercourse--without much fear of having to account for their behavior so long as the woman is currently unmarried. Unmarried and younger women have little power to resist sexual advances from older men in particular, and they may have little recourse even in cases of outright rape. Most often cases of rape are settled traditionally rather than in civil courts by requiring the offending man to pay a fine to the woman's family. While some may regard this as "paying for services," the victim is certainly not a prostitute. In any case, sexual practices must be understood in their cultural context in order to understand the transmission of AIDS, the necessary intervention points to interrupt transmission, and realistic strategies for intervention.

Understanding cultural context can also help to explain recent epidemiological findings in Africa. For example, when a sample of HIV infected individuals in Zaire (Ryder *et al.*1987) was divided into groups based on sex and age, a striking difference in the female/ male ratio for carriers emerged:

Age Category	Female:male Ratio
0-15 years	1:1
15-30 years	6:1
more than 30	0.64:1

Ryder *et al* conclude, "The overall female:male infection ratio in our study (1.1:1) is similar to the figure widely used in describing the epidemiology of HIV infection in Africa. However, we found that cases of infection clustered in two risk groups, young women (ages 13-25) and middle to older aged men." In light of the earlier discussion of how younger, unmarried women are forced or coerced into sexual relations with older men, it is possible to offer some explanation for the age-specific prevalence differences found between men and women. Still, a fuller explanation should be explored through behavioral research in Africa.

The sociocultural context relating to the possible spread of HIV by contaminated needles and other skin-piercing implements must also be better understood. In the United States, outside of the high-risk group of intravenous drug-users, relatively few individuals become infected with HIV by this means. In Africa, however, people receive numerous injections for both the prevention and treatment of illness. In Zaire for example, over 80 percent of healthy children and adults have received one or more injections in a 3-year period. This frequency, combined with poor practices of sterilizing needles, may have contributed to HIV infection. As Quinn *et al.* (1986:959) note:

> The potential importance of HIV transmission by needles reflects several cultural factors in Africa that merit emphasis. Patients often express strong preference for parenteral rather than oral therapy. For example, in survey of 50 mothers in Kinshasa, 84% expressed the belief that parenteral medication is more effective than oral medication.

This preference for parenteral--or skin piercing--therapy finds expression in a variety of needle, razor blade and other therapies offered by traditional healers and other indigenous health practitioners. Details of such practices as well as their cultural context and underlying belief systems need to be understood before effective behavior change strategies can be designed. Such practices must be documented by consolidation of existing research and by a substantial amount of empirical anthropological research. Some of the questions that need to be researched are: Who gives injections and traditional vaccinations; for what reasons and how frequently are they given; how are they administered; and is anything done to sterilize needles? To what extent are needles shared and re-used? What about non-healing practices involving skin-piercing, such as scarification and tattooing?

If traditional health practitioners prove to be part of the problem of AIDS transmission, it must be recognized that they are also in a good position to become part of the solution.[1]

Identifying Necessary Behavior Change, Intervention Points And Strategies

Once the social and cultural dimensions of AIDS are better understood, it will be possible to clearly define the behavior which must be changed by a significant segment of the population, if the spread of AIDS is going to be controlled in Africa. Regarding necessary changes in behavior:

1) Both unmarried and married men will have to become monogamous or severely restrict their number of sexual partners. Women will have to be empowered to refuse sexual intercourse to a far greater extent than they are at present;

2) Practices of prostitution--different in Africa than in Western, industrial countries--will have to be radically changed;

3) Men and women with STDs--especially diseases that result in open genital lesions--will have to seek appropriate treatment, and either avoid sexual intercourse until the condition is removed or else use condoms;

4) Correct condom usage will have to be adopted on a massive scale by at least young adults and by men until late middle age;

5)   Practices relating to use of hypodermic needles, razor blades used for traditional vaccination, and traditional scarification devices--all of which may be used by traditional healers and others untrained in modern medicine--may have to be severely altered or restricted.

The consolidation of the knowledge base suggested here should provide a basis upon which to select intervention points, as well as strategies for interventions. For example, in order to change practices related to traditional vaccination and other healing practices, it will probably be necessary to collaborate directly with traditional healers. As Rogers (1983, quoted in NAS 1986: 233) correctly observes, "...research on the diffusion of innovation finds that acceptance of new ideas depends on the role of personal networks and opinion leaders who are trusted, especially when innovation requires changes in social and cultural norms."

Precedents for collaboration with traditional healers in AIDS interventions such as condom distribution can be found. In Lagos state, Nigeria, herbalists have been trained in community-based distribution of condoms in a pilot project implemented though the Lagos Board of Traditional Medicine (Green 1986). In Zimbabwe, the National Family Planning Council (ZNFPC), the Zimbabwe National Traditional Healers Association (ZINATHA), and the AID-funded Social Marketing for Change project are already planning to collaborate in condom distribution (Green 1987).

Traditional healers, including traditional birth attendants, are accessible to all Africans--wherever they live or whatever their circumstances--and are culturally appropriate and affordable. They have credibility as well as respect and prestige in local African communities; otherwise clients would not seek their advice and pay for their services. Traditional healers are in a unique position to:

-Persuade their clients or patients to adopt preventive measures such as reducing the number of sexual partners, and using condoms;
-Serve as male motivators (traditional healers, as distinct from traditional birth attendants, tend to be predominantly male);
-Provide education and condoms in areas unserved or underserved by biomedically-trained health personnel;
-Quickly learn and then communicate the facts of the AIDS disease. As established health practitioners, traditional healers

may already be advising their clients about sexually-transmitted diseases, and they already have established patient caseloads.

--Successfully carry out the entrepreneurial aspects of community-based distribution of condoms (eg., selling contraceptives at a mark-up, reinvesting part of the profits into a revolving fund, etc.), since traditional healers are already entrepreneurs by profession--and often successful ones. Because healers are already financially self- supporting, they are not forced to subsist on the meager profits from condoms sales alone;

--Motivate clients and deliver services in ways that are culturally appropriate and persuasive;

--Refer AIDS patients to modern health facilities, once healers themselves learn to identify AIDS symptoms.

Still, changes in sexual practices will be very difficult to effect. The problem should be approached from several different directions at once. Both women and men must be educated--through different channels and using different approaches and mechanisms--about sexual means of transmission, risks involved, and methods of protection. Accepted community leaders, both political and religious, ought to be educated so that they can use their positions to influence behavior. In some countries, radio programs have been successful in promoting basic awareness of AIDS. By 1986, 70 percent of the population of Rwanda was aware of the dangers of AIDS, due largely to radio education.

One intervention will certainly be testing individuals at high risk, and then counselling those who test seropositive for HIV exposure. It must be emphasized that testing alone is insufficient. Studies conducted in the United States have shown that individuals who know they are HIV-infected do not necessarily change their behavior. In a recent *Washington Post* interview, Dr. Larry Gostin of Harvard's School of Public Health noted, "There is preliminary evidence that testing can change people's behavior in a reckless way, particularly if unaccompanied by education and counselling." The perceived risk of infection has motivated behavior change among significant numbers within certain groups in the U.S., notably male homosexuals, but such motivational and decision factors are not well understood. Motivational factors relating to sexual behavior change are even less well understood for groups in Africa.

Focus group discussions and other qualitative research recommended here can shed light on these motivational and decision factors in specific social groups, providing a basis for the design of culturally meaningful counselling for those who test positive for exposure to AIDS. For example, in societies where a man may have more social and financial responsibilities for his illegitimate child than for the child's mother, awareness that the mother can infect the unborn child may be more instrumental in changing male behavior than knowing that the mother can become infected. If this were established by qualitative research--and corroborated by existing ethnographic research--effective motivational messages and strategies could be developed and used.

The Social, Economic And Institutional Impact Of AIDS

There is no question that AIDS will change the social and institutional landscape of Africa, beginning with the regions of current high prevalence in Eastern and Central Africa. AIDS is most prevalent among young adults, the most economically productive members of society and those responsible for childbearing and child rearing (Holk 1987: 7). HIV carriers also appear to predominate among the urban-based, higher socioeconomic groups. As Jonathan Mann, head of the WHO AIDS Program, observed in a recent *Newsweek* interview, "AIDS is a threat to the social shape of Africa in a way starvation and malaria aren't. It has the potential to wipe out the urban elite." He went on to call for a broad, general assessment of the sociocultural dimensions of the AIDS problem in Africa.

No sector of the economy will escape the impact of AIDS. When the virus spreads to the rural areas--beginning with areas of highest population concentration and agricultural productivity, as can already be seen in Rwanda or in the Northwest Tanzania highlands--agriculture and animal husbandry will decline markedly. With high morbidity and mortality of women and men in their most productive years, the dependent old people and children will be left to fend for themselves (Sabatier 1987; Scriabine 1987). In a continent where food production is already perilously low, the decline which will begin in the most productive areas will greatly worsen the situation, increasing rates of malnutrition, poor health and child mortality. The need for greater imports of food from abroad will strain the already low supplies of foreign exchange.

AIDS could also have devastating consequences in the industrial and commercial sectors. As a measure of probable impact, a July 1986 survey of HIV sero-prevalence rates among workers in the Zambi, a copper belt, found that 68% of HIV-infected men were skilled professionals in the copper industry (Scriabine 1987: 4). Apart from the effects of loss of manpower on output and productivity, the health benefits and other support payments paid to employees and their families will increase as more people require care. Companies may try to pay these costs with scarce funds intended for operations, research, development, etc., at least initially. Before long, however, companies will realize that AIDS-related costs will quickly lead to bankruptcy and so well-established programs of employee health benefits will likely be severely curtailed or abandoned, leaving sick and dying employees to fend for themselves.

AIDS is already sweeping through the limited pool of professional and technical elite located in urban areas. Governments are sure to lose administrators and managers, resulting in a breakdown in service delivery. The military and police forces will suffer severe attrition from sickness and death, placing national security at risk. Trained personnel in all areas of government will be lost and, with them, the time, effort and money which has been invested in their education and training--a significant amount of which has been underwritten by the U.S. government. Several African governments have expressed fear that the United States and other donor countries will discontinue their financial support for education and training if they believe their investments will be lost (Scriabine 1987).

An AIDS-Related Social And Institutional Profile (SIP) For South-Central Africa

Behavioral scientists can do more than conduct research in the battle against the spread of AIDS. For many years, but especially since the mid-1970's, anthropologists and related specialists have served as "social analysts" and social forecasters for AIDS and the World Bank, examining sociocultural consequences of planned change (Cernea 1986; Robbins 1986; Hoben 1984, Ingersoll *et al.* 1981). In these capacities they have analyzed such things as benefit incidence, impact assessment, spread effects, obstacles to change, sociocultural feasibility, changes in power and extent of local participation, as well as the diffusion, sustainability, and replicability of project benefits. A good deal of this analysis is future-oriented, requiring projection, prediction and social forecasting (van Willigen 1986: 167-70.)

In an effort to institutionalize the use of social analytic skills at an earlier stage of project development, social and institutional profiles (SIPs) began to be developed in 1980 by AID for use in project design and related planning and analytic activities (Reyna 1987; Greeley 1987; Hoben *et al.* 1983). SIPs are similar to the social soundness analyses that AID began to require of its projects in 1975 except that SIPs are more comprehensive in scope and analysis, and they contain more institutional focus.

To better understand the changes that will occur and how to cope with these changes, as well as how best to mobilize groups to respond to the challenges of preventing the spread of AIDS, an AIDS-related Social and Institutional Profile for Africa is needed. The SIP should be developed by applying the analytic and social forecasting skills of social analysts--usually anthropologists or sociologists--who have done social soundness analyses as part of the design of AID projects, in order to focus on:

(a)   *the social and institutional consequences of mass morbidity and mortality resulting from AIDS.* What will be the impact of loss of trained, productive manpower on governments (at different levels, including the military and police) and on key economic sectors such as agriculture, mining, and manufacturing? What are the implications for national security and for internal maintenance of law and order? What sort of legislative responses might result from the pandemic and what will be the response from groups--perhaps including whole ethnic groups--who feel their rights are abridged by AIDS-related laws and regulations? Might there be local or regional outbreaks of mass hysteria leading to scapegoating behavior, inter-group hostility flare-ups, witchcraft accusation and summary executions, and the like? What will be the impact on the organized, commercial sector and can business and industry play a vital role in the AIDS campaign, beginning with educating and providing condoms to their own employees?

(b)   *strategies for mobilizing groups, organizations, and institutions--including those outside the formal or modern sector--in order to break the cycle of AIDS transmission.*   Organizations might include national and local women's organizations, professional associations of traditional healers and birth attendants, churches and church-related PVO's, councils of chiefs, and any other groups (besides the obvious health personnel) who are or could be powerful opinion leaders and/or service deliverers in a campaign against AIDS.

Given the economic and other resources available in Africa, it makes sense to work with existing organizations and institutions, both modern and traditional, in a mobilization effort against AIDS. The SIP should not only identify these groups, but should also recommend specific strategies for mobilizing them against AIDS. Some examples follow.

Business And Industry

Within the modern sector, business and industry can easily be persuaded that AIDS prevention is far preferable to treatment efforts. Companies could be motivated to provide their employees with preventive education, testing, condoms, and follow-up counselling. The expense to employers of both lost productivity and health benefits related to AIDS is already becoming understood.   As early as 1983 in Zaire, a group of companies related the threat of AIDS to their very existence and took the unprecedented step of donating $100,000 to an international AIDS research program sponsored by the Zairean ministry of health (Deering, pers. com., 1987).

U.S. health firms are already collaborating with companies in Zaire and Zimbabwe in programs to distribute contraceptives and family planning information in the workplace (TIPPS 1987).   An industry-based AIDS education and prevention project could be developed and implemented without a great deal of difficulty, and the potential impact on AIDS morbidity and mortality could be enormous. The funding for industry-based AIDS education and condom distribution could be part of the employee health benefit packages provided by companies (cf. Deering 1986). In fact, unless something along these lines is developed, it is very unclear who will pay for AIDS-related services in Africa. Governments certainly cannot afford the costs that will be required for AIDS prevention, treatment and management.

Family Planning Associations

Since AIDS is sexually transmitted, family planning associations (FPAs) are obvious candidates for disseminating information and providing education, counselling, and condom distribution services in efforts to contain the spread of AIDS. A short questionnaire was recently developed by the International Planned Parenthood Federation and mailed to its affiliates around the world. Within a short time, responses were returned from FPAs in more than 70 countries, with a majority--particularly those from developing countries--expressing interest in undertaking AIDS information campaigns (Newman 1987.9). While FPAs ought to be spearheading the drive to distribute and promote condoms as one of the few effective AIDS interventions, there seems to be ambivalence in this regard at the present time on the part of FPAs. This is because such organizations have invested heavily in promoting the idea that condoms should be regarded as respectable family planning adjuncts rather as prophylactics used to prevent sexually transmitted diseases. It remains to be seen what role FPAs will play in condom promotion for AIDS prevention; in the meantime, government-sponsored AIDS programs have already begun to draw upon the experience of FPAs in targeting specific groups with educational messages relating to sexual behavior.

Church Groups

The church is another important institution through which to work. Its role in providing health services and spiritual guidance, in influencing attitudes and beliefs, and in addressing ethical issues will be central in Africa's response to the AIDS crisis. Churches have well-developed mechanisms for communication and they are linked with other institutions well-suited to providing information. In addition, churches and church-related private voluntary organizations (PVOs) are involved in relief work and in providing health care to a large proportion of Africa's population.

In February, 1987, the World Council of Churches issued a statement on AIDS, calling on churches to "...respond appropriately to the need for pastoral care, education for prevention and social ministry." By working through churches, a potential barrier to providing educational and distributing condoms can be removed. There is a need to examine more carefully the actual and potential role of Africa's churches in AIDS activities, in order to propose concrete strategies for effective mobilization of churches and church-related PVO's.

Women's Groups

Women's organizations can also be mobilized against AIDS. Formal and informal women's groups and networks exist throughout Africa, and they are typically coordinated at the national level by a national women's association. These networks can be employed and associations can be exploited in outreach efforts to educate and to motivate behavior change among women. They can also be useful in condom distribution and in legal initiatives and other efforts that would enhance women's ability to avoid unwanted sexual contacts.

Traditional Healer Associations

Effective organizations and institutions can also be found in what might be called the traditional sector. Collaboration with traditional healers, by working through professional associations of healers, is proposed as an effective intervention strategy, not only in changing healing practices that may contribute to the spread of AIDS, but also in directly educating and otherwise influencing the public, and even in condom distribution.

According to a recent WHO report, there are organized associations of traditional healers operating under official auspices in at least 24 African countries (WHO 1985). National associations of healers are usually made up of many thousands of healers, sometimes with "modern sector" advisors such as physicians, university professors or civil servants (Last and Chavunduka 1986). With such infrastructure and established channels of communication, it should be possible to "train trainers" among the leadership of these associations, who can then educate other association members (herbalists, diviner-mediums, traditional birth attendants, etc.) about recognizing and referring certain STD cases, about the dangers of using unsterilized needles, and indeed about how to recognize the symptoms of AIDS and AIDS-related complex.

The potential strengths and benefits of such a strategy can only be realized if governments are willing to officially recognize traditional healers and collaborate with them in the pursuit of public health goals.

After developing a SIP for Sub-Saharan Africa as a whole, with generalized social forecasting of the sort outlined here and attempted in the previous section but based on far more information and analysis, it would be useful to develop SIPs for culturally-meaningful subregions such as the Bantu-speaking East African highlands or Bantu-speaking Congo Basin. This would better enable public health officials and donor organizations to tailor education and other interventions to specific groups.

Conclusion

It has been suggested that behavioral scientists experienced in research, social analysis, and social forecasting in Africa could play a vitally important role in developing programs to contain the spread of AIDS. Skills and experience in primary health care, family planning, and health communications would also seem to be relevant to such an endeavor. First there is a need to establish an information base pertaining to the belief about and behavioral aspects of AIDS transmission in Africa comparable to what has been learned about child diarrhea or human reproduction. But the contribution of behavioral scientists should not end with research; they should also interpret research findings, advocate the policy and programmatic implications of such findings, and become involved in the design and implementation of intervention strategies to break the cycle of AIDS transmission. Furthermore, social and behavioral scientists are needed to provide valuable social analysis and forecasting to prepare African governments and donor organizations for the consequences of, and responses to, high morbidity and mortality from AIDS among the most economically and demographically productive groups in Africa.

Acknowledgements

The author would like to acknowledge the assistance of Barbara Wyckoff-Baird who assisted in researching some of the material for this chapter, as well as Ned Greeley and Jack Thomas who inspired some of the ideas presented here. Responsibility for any errors of fact or thought lies solely with the author.

ENDNOTE

[1]Good (in this volume) deals with this issue. The present author has recently discussed the possible role of traditional healers in transmitting HIV, and of their potential role in combating AIDS, with the chairmen of national associations of traditional healers in both Zimbabwe and Swaziland. Both chairmen expressed enthusiasm for mobilizing their organizations to cooperate with public health officials in combating the spread of AIDS.

BIBLIOGRAPHY

Cernea, Michael, M., *Putting People First*: *Sociological Variables in Rural Development*, New York: Oxford University Press, 1985.

Deering, Joseph, Personal communication, 7/15/87.

Deering, Joseph, "AIDS Concept Paper," Columbia, Md.: John Short & Associates, Dec. 1986.

Good, Charles, M., "Traditional Healers and AIDS Management in Africa." Paper presenter at African Studies Association, November 19-22, 1987, Denver.

Gostin, Larry, quoted in *The Washington Post*, 6/11/87, p. A15.

Greeley, Edward H., "Project Development in Kenya," in E.C. Green (ed), *Practicing Development Anthropology*, Boulder: Westview Press, 1986, pp. 235-46.

Green, Edward C., and L. Makhubu, "Traditional Healers in Swaziland: Toward Improved Cooperation Between the Traditional and Modern Health Sectors," *Soc. Sci. Med.*, Vol. 18, No. 12, pp. 1071-1079, 1984.

Green, Edward C., "Collaborative Programs for Traditional Healers in Primary Health Care and Family Planning in Africa." In Fyfe, C. and U. Maclean (eds) *African Medicine in the Modern World*, Edinburgh (U.K.): University of Edinburgh, Center of African Studies, 1986, pp. 115-44.

Hoben, Allan, "The Role of Anthropologists in Development Work: An Overview," in W. Partridge, ed., *Training Manual in Development Anthropology*, Washington, D.C.: American Anthropological Association, 1984, pp. 9-17.

Hoben, Allan, *Somalia: A Social and Institutional Profile*, Boston: Boston University, The African Studies Center, March, 1983.

Ingersoll, Jasper, M. Sulllivan and Barbara Lenkerd, *Social Analysis of AID Projects: A Review of the Experience*, Washington, D.C.: USAID, June 1981.

Last, M. and G.L. Chavunduka (eds), *The Professionalization of African Medicine*, Manchester (UK): Manchester University Press, 1986, pp. 1-19.

Liskin, Laurie, and R. Blackburn, "AIDS--A Public Health Crisis, *Population Reports*, Vol. XIV, No. 3, Series L, No. 6, July-August 1986.

Mann, Jonathan, "The Global AIDS Situation," *World Health*, June 1987, pp. 6-8.

National Academy of Sciences, *Confronting AIDS--Directions for Public Health, Health Care, and Research*. Washington, D.C., Institute of Medicine, National Academy of Sciences, National Academy Press, 1986.

Newman, Karen, "FPAs Take on New Responsibility," *People* (IPPF Journal), Vol. 14, No. 4 1987, pp. 9-10.

Newsweek, Nov. 24, 1986.

Nunn, Paul, "AIDS in Africa," *IPPF Medical Bulletin*, Vol. 21, No. 1, February, 1987, pp. 4-6.

Potts, Malcolm, "Preparing for the Battle," *People* (IPPF journal), Vol. 14, No. 4, 1987, pp. 3-6.

Quinn, Thomas C., J. Mann, J. Curran, and P. Piot, "AIDS in Africa: An Epidemiologic Paradigm," *Science*, Vol. 234, November 1986, pp. 955-64.

Reyna, S.P., An Evaluation of the Social and Institutional Profile Program of the Bureau for Program Review and Policy Coordination of the USAID, Washington, D.C., USAID, December 1987.

Robins, Edward, "The Strategy of Development and the Role of the Anthropologist," in E.C. Green, ed., *Practicing Development Anthropology*, Boulder: Westview Press, 1986, pp. 10-21.

Rogers, Everett, *Diffusion of Innovations*, New York: Free Press, 1983.

Ryder, Robert *et al*, "Community Surveillance for HIV Infection in Zaire," Paper presented to the Third International Conference on AIDS, Washington, D.C., June 1-5, 1987.

Sabatier, Renee, *AIDS and the Third World* (revised), PANOS Institute, published in association with the Norweigian Red Cross, March 1987.

Scriabine, Raiso, "Incurable Disease Poses Global Threat," *Frontlines*, March 1987, p. 4.

TIPPS (Technical Information on Population for the Private Sector), *Semi-Annual Report #4*, Columbia, MD.: JSA, inc., Sept. 1987.

van Willigen, John, *Applied Anthropology*, South Hadley, MA.: Bergin & Garvey Publishers, 1986.

WHO, Special Programme on AIDS. Strategies and Structure, Projected Needs. Geneva, March 1987.

WHO, "Report of the Consultation on Approaches for Policy Development for Traditional Health Practitioners, Including Traditional Birth Attendants." Geneva, 1985.

EVALUATING SOCIAL SCIENCE DATA RELATING TO AIDS IN AFRICA

Francis Paine Conant*

SUMMARY: Social science data on African peoples can help inform strategy to control transmission of the human immunodeficiency virus (HIV) as well as suggest ways to care for those already ill with the acquired immunodeficiency syndrome (AIDS). Ethnographies are rich in detail on the rules and institutions governing marital (and often extramarital) relationships, and since HIV is spreading primarily through heterosexual intercourse in Africa, these sources can help identify intermarrying groups and population sectors at risk to the further spread of the virus. For ethnographic data to be useful, however, they must be evaluated for their reliability. This can be done by estimating scale factors, elapsed time, and major events for a given region or rural area.

Introduction

The social sciences are perceived [12,18] as having an important potential in understanding the present threats posed by AIDS (acquired immune deficiency syndrome) as well as the further spread of HIV (the human immunodeficiency virus). This paper is on the need for evaluating the existing social science literature on topics relevant to the study of HIV transmission and the expression of AIDS in Africa. The emphasis here is on the ethnographic and anthropological literature as found in books, monographs, journal articles, and the archives of government and voluntary agencies. The topics these sources contain relate to the sexually transmitted nature of AIDS, but by no means should be thought of as relating only to the details of sexual behavior. Sexology, in fact, may have less to contribute to controlling the HIV epidemic than sociology or anthropology.

*Francis Paine Conant, Ph.D., directs the Human Ecology and Remote Sensing Laboratory, Department of Anthropology, Hunter College, City University of New York (CUNY). He has worked in both West and East Africa, from 1957 to the present with research support from the Ford Foundation and the National Science Foundation, and currently the Wenner-Gren Foundation for Anthropological Research and PSC-CUNY Research Awards program.

This is so because sexual relations everywhere, and no less so in Africa, are constrained by culturally based expectations on the part of the actors as well as by the rules and institutions governing the relationships between groups. Thus the topics relevant to AIDS begin but by no means end with normative patterns of gender acquisition and sexual maturation, and reproductive and non-reproductive sexual behavior. If HIV is mainly or even only sexually transmitted then a number of additional topics are involved: kinship restrictions on sexual behavior, rules of exogamy and endogamy regulating marriage, belief systems, perceptions of health and disease, and support systems for the care of the desperately sick and dying. There are whole sets of behaviors that initially perhaps appear only remotely connected to sexual behavior but are nonetheless there as constraints on, or as inducements to, particular patterns of sexuality, gender behavior and gender relations. In dealing with AIDS we are not just dealing with sex; we are dealing with lifeways and complex culture patterns.

The procedures suggested here are designed to assist in surveying, gathering, and evaluating social science data on African peoples and populations so that these data become more readily accessible to those concerned with (a) identifying population sectors at risk to the further spread of HIV, (b) the maintenance and support systems available to those already suffering from AIDS, and (c) designing education programs which are culturally sensitive and locally informed. As Africanists we have important information relating to HIV transmission which is only recently coming to the attention of epidemiologists, health professionals, and those agencies helping to set strategy and fund the struggle against AIDS. However, while there is recognition that efforts to contain HIV via education programs must take cultural differences into account [3,32] much greater use could be made of what is already known of African peoples and cultures. We must make it very clear to epidemiologists that even though the words "sex" or "sexuality" do not often appear in our titles of abstracts we have much to offer in regard to research on the sexual transmission of HIV. Sexual behavior is governed by rules, and quite a lot is known about these rules.

Initially perhaps there was a tendency to dismiss most social science sources and data, especially in ethnographies, as "non-quantitative," "impressionistic" and therefore "unverifiable" and unusable. More recently, however, there seems to be some reconsideration of this attitude and statisticians, epidemiologists and others associated with the health sciences may now be seeing the merit of working with data which can be cast in the form of norms of behavior and the extremes of divergence from these norms. However, even though the ethnographic data are generally of high quality, they are not uniformly so, and, furthermore, the data can be too generously interpreted and too widely applied without adequate attention to their reliability in terms of contemporary African conditions. This is particularly true in rural areas which are emerging as a focus in the control of HIV and the care of those with AIDS in Africa.

Rural Areas And Rural-Urban Links

Rural areas are important because studies of the HIV epidemic and the expression of AIDS in Africa thus far have focused almost exclusively on *urban* populations [3,23,28]. Given the intensity of relations between urban and rural populations [4,34,35], however, it is becoming imperative to carry sociological, serological and epidemiological studies into the countryside. Rural populations, however, can be as varied as those in urban areas, and perhaps more so. There are large differences in rural demographic variables such as population density, reproduction rates and population growth. There are considerable cultural differences as well, some of which are of great historical time depth, and others of only recent origin.

In addition, peoples in rural areas are likely to contrast with each other according to (a) *environmental* factors such as seasonal food deprivation, malaria, and schistosomiasis, for example [16,24], which may well effect the way in which AIDS develops and is expressed clinically; (b) *technology* relating to sexual matters (abortifacients, hygiene) and personal and/or ritual body modifications (via circumcision, clitoridectomy, scarification [28]), which may affect HIV transmission via contact with contaminated blood; (c) *social practices* as in exogamous/endogamous relations, preferential marriage patterns, incidence of polygyny and other types of unions [24] which place a group or a population at greater or lesser risk to the spread of HIV; and (d) *ideology* or *belief systems* such as perceptions of health and disease causality which may affect the maintenance and care of the ailing and terminally ill [1].

Given all the above considerations, especially as found among rural peoples, an approach which draws upon as many *evaluated* data sources as possible seems essential in the study of AIDS in the African countryside. Surveying and evaluating the existing literature within broadly defined geographic regions brings with it several benefits. For each region it will help guide decisions not only as to *where* further fieldwork is needed but also as to which *topics* potentially relevant to the spread of HIV in the region are *well* understood, and which are *least* understood. Thus with a regional literature survey and an evaluation of each source in hand, additional fieldwork, if necessary, can be undertaken more efficiently, at less cost, and in less time.

Adopting a regional or spatial orientation at the outset allows quick identification of areas where information on one or more topics is "thick" and where it is "thin". Analysis of the spatial distribution of culture traits and patterns has an honorable tradition in anthropology [2,11,20,21,38]. A further advantage in a regional or spatially oriented approach is that ethnic groups can be referenced by geographic rather than cultural or political markets. AIDS research has been marred everywhere, not just in Africa, by the effects of inappropriate ethnic labeling [13,17]. Some of these labeling errors also result from the misapplication of the ethnographic data and from inadequate attention to evaluating the reliability of the data sources.

Rating Sources For Their Reliability

Evaluating the quality of social science sources has received considerable attention in anthropology and related fields [6, 10, 20, 27]. The question of quality, however, is somewhat different from the matter of applicability or *reliability*. Reliability is crucial in the context of the HIV epidemic because lives are at stake. This means we are less interested in estimating the elegance, in social science terms, of a particular source than we are in establishing for it a *reliability rating* (RR), a score which represents, in effect, the confidence we can place in a given source and its relevance to contemporary peoples and conditions. The RR is estimated first in a general way for a given source, and then for the particular topics of interest found within that source. The procedure outlines here can no doubt be improved upon, and if changes are to be made it is urged they are made in the direction of further simplification. The proposed system derives from a long-term interest and involvement with developing a regionally or spatially oriented "cultural data management system" [6-10]. The present objective is to suggest several clearly stated rules so that health officials, planners, and personnel in government and non-governmental agencies, as well as social scientists, will be able to arrive at RRs for a particular source or a number of sources and the topics they cover. In short, the rating system should be such that, armed with paper and pencil, and whether a social scientist or not, a teacher, planner, a health official, should be able to arrive at a fair estimate of the reliability of the social science information on topics in the literature bearing on HIV transmission and AIDS expression in African populations, especially in rural areas.

The most important factors affecting an RR include considerations of scale, field methods and the nature of the data, the amount of time which has elapsed since the fieldwork was undertaken, and the kinds of events taking place in the area subsequent to fieldwork and publication or archiving of the data. In what follows, a procedure is suggested for rating or scoring the effect each of these factors may have on the reliability of the data. In real time it takes about three hours to rate the reliability of a single source and an additional hour per topic within that source. With practice and with growing familiarity of the literature available for a region, the time needed for estimating reliability of the sources may be reduced.

The scoring system is based on points deducted rather than points awarded; the maximum number of disallowed points is 20. The cut off point at which a given source or a topic covered within a source is considered unreliable should be set only after the limits of the epidemic research area have been set and the extent of ethnographic or other social science sources has been estimated. Obviously, if a suspected epidemic area has been only lightly studied and only a few sources of information exist then a very low cut- off point may be desirable at least until further data become available. If an epidemic research area is rich in published or achieved materials then higher cut-off points can be set. Scoring proceeds as follows:

Scale

a. In the original source, what area is covered by the author's fieldwork? If a figure is not given, can an estimate be given [7,8]?

b. To what extent does an author extrapolate from the area of original or primary area of observation to a larger area of interpretation or generalization?

c. In using this source for HIV/AIDS research within a given area or region, how large is the epidemic research area and what is the ratio of it to the source's original fieldwork area or larger area of interpretation and generalization?

Scoring: If no geographic or cultural delimiters are given in the original source and none can be estimated, deduct 4 points, and proceed to subsequent sections of rating and scoring. Deduct 1 point if the ratio of the area of original investigation to the area of generalization or interpretation is greater than 1:5; deduct two points if the ratio of the epidemic research area is equal to two to three times the area of ethnographic generalization; deduct four points if the epidemic area is five times (or more) the area of ethnographic interpretation.

Fieldwork and Field Data

a. Was the field work a solo or team effort?

b. Was research carried out in the local language or lingua franca?

c. Were the investigators competent in this language?

d. If translators were used, is it stated what checks were made on the accuracy of the translations?

e. Is there likely to have been a "gender effect" leading to a bias in one or more of the topics being investigated?

f.   For a given topic, are the data quantified?

g.   If not, can "normative" and "exceptional" or "variant" patterns of behavior be identified and ranked in terms of frequency?

Scoring: Deduct one point if the fieldwork was a solo effort; deduct another point if research was NOT carried out in a local language or lingua franca, and additional points (one each) if no statement is made on the linguistic competence of the investigator, if no controls existed for verifying translations, if there is a mismatch of genders between the investigator or translators and informants giving information on sexual behavior, reproductive histories and other topics likely to be affected by gender mismatching. Deduct one point if the data on a given topic are non-quantified and two points if they cannot be restated in normative or variant terms.

Time and Events

a.   In what year was the fieldwork carried out?

b.   In what year published?

c.   Was there ever a restudy? If so when, and what changes were noted?

d.   Do these changes concern topics relating to HIV transmission or the expression of AIDS?

e.   In the ethnographic or the epidemic areas, has there been serious famine, flood, drought?

f.   Raiding, war?

g.   Extensive development of new services (health, educational)?

h.   Major development projects (i.e., roads, dams or irrigation, resettlement schemes)?

i.   If any of the foregoing, at what intervals between events?

j.   Which topics would this chronology of events seem to most likely affect?

Scoring: Deduct 1 point if the time between fieldwork and publishing is greater than 10 years; deduct 1 point if there was no restudy and the time since the original fieldwork is greater than 20 years; if changes are known to have taken place in topics relevant to HIV transmission or AIDS expression, deduct 1 point for each topic so affected by any of the events cited in (e) through (h); if the interval between any of these events is less than 10 years, deduct an additional point per topic.

Summary And Discussion

There is a real need for a regionally oriented approach for evaluating cultural practices thought to be involved in the efficient transmission of HIV in rural Africa. In the system proposed here, a score is assigned each topic and an overall reliability rating assigned each information source. Thus the epidemiologist, health officer, or research agency can be assisted in most efficiently allocating scarce resources for further studies in the field *as needed* and as indicated by making maximum use of the existing information sources on African rural populations at risk to the further spread of HIV. Further, in applying information obtained from ethnographic sources, the user is made fully aware of the relative reliability of the source itself as well as the topics it contains.

Abbreviations

A	*Africa*
AA	*American Anthropologist*
AAAS	American Association for the Advancement of Science
ARA	*Annual Reviews in Anthropology*
ASA	African Studies Association
AT	*Anthropology Today*
CA	*Current Anthropology*
CDC/A	Centers for Disease Control/Atlanta
CUP	Columbia University Press
FAO/UN	Food and Agriculture Organization/ United Nations
HO	*Human Organization*
HRAF	Human Relations Area Files
IAI	International African Institute
JAMA	*Journal of the American Medical Association*
L	*Lancet*
MMWTR	*Morbidity and Mortality Weekly Report.* CDC/A
N	*Nature*
NAS	National Academy Science
OUP	Oxford University Press
PERS	*Photogrammetric Engineering and Remote Sensing*
ROAPE	*Review of African Political Economy*
S	*Science*
SSM	*Social Science and Medicine*
SSRC	Social Science Research Council
UCP	University of California Press
WER	*Weekly Epidemiological Record.* WHO/UN
WHO/UN	World Health Organization/United Nations

ENDNOTES

1. Ademuwagun, Z . A. J. Ayoade, I. Harrison, D. Warren, eds.,
   "1979 African Therapeutic Systems." Waltham, ASA, Crossroads Press.

2. Baumann, H.
   "1928 The Division of Work According to Sex in African Hoe Culture." A, 1:289-319.

3. Biggar, Robert J.
   "The AIDS Problem in Africa." L, 11 January 1986, pp. 79-83.

4. Caldwell, John C.
   1969 African Rural-Urban Migration. NY. Columbia University Press.

5. Chrisman, Nicholas R.
   "1987 Design of Geographic Information Systems Based on Social and Cultural Goals." PERS 53.10:1367-70.

6. Conant, Francis Paine
   "1984 Remote Sensing Discovery and Generalizations in Human Ecology." In E. Moran, ed., *The Ecosystem Concept in Anthropology*. Westview Press.

7. "1984a Cultural values, Landuse and Environmental Perceptions." PSC-CUNY Research Grant 664302.

8. "1982 Strength, Reproductive Capacity and the Division of Labor in East Africa." In Edgerton & Kennedy, eds., *Cultural Ecology: eclectic perspectives*. AA Special Publication 15, pp. 26-55.

9. "1981 Five cultural contexts for a Geographic Information System." *Proceedings*, NASA Conference on Remote Sensing of the Environment. Purdue.

10.   Conant, Francis Paine, Peter Rogers, Marion Baum-
      Gardner, Cyrus McKell, Raymond Dassmann, Priscilla
      Reining, eds.,
              "1983 Resource Inventory and Baseline Study
              Methods for Developing Countries." Washington
              D.C., AAAS.

11.   Driver, Harold
              1966 "Geographical-historical vs. psycho-
              functional explanations of kin avoidances."
              CA 7:131-48.

12.   Ergas, Yasmine
              1987 "The Social Consequences of the AIDS
              Epidemic." *Items*, 41,3/4: 33-39.

13.   Feldman, Douglas A.
              1985 "AIDS and Social Change." HO 44,4: 343-
              8.

14.   Glass, Roger I.
              1986 "New Prospects for Epidemiological In-
              vestigations." S, 234: 951-4. 21 November.

15.   Glick, Barry
              1979 "The Spatial Autocorrelation of Cancer
              Mortality." SSM 13d: 123-30.

16.   Hartwig, G. & K. D. Patterson, eds.
              1978 *Disease in African History*. Durham.
              Durham University Press.

17.   Herdt, Gilbert
              1987 "AIDS and Anthropology." AT, 3,2: 1-4.

18.   Institute of Medicine
              1986 "Confronting Aids." NAS, Washington, DC.

19.   International Business Machines
              1985 *The Guide to Software for Developing
              Countries*. IBM South, Neuilly sur Seine.

20.   Jorgensen, J. G.
              1979 "Cross-cultural Comparisons." ARA 8:
              309-31.

21.   Kroeber, Alfred
              1939 *Cultural and Natural Areas of North
              America*. Berkeley, UCP.

22.   Latham, M. C.
        1975 *Human Nutrition in Tropical Africa*.
        Rome, FAO/UN.

23.   Mann, Jonathan M., H. Francis, T. Quinn, *et al*.
        1986 "Surveillance for AIDS in a Central
        African City." JAMA 255,23: 3255-9.

24.   May, Jacques
        1958 *The Ecology of Human Disease*. New York.
        MD Publications.

25.   May, Robert M. and Roy M. Anderson
        1987 "Transmission Dynamics of HIV Infection."
        N 326: 137-142. 12 March.

26.   Murdock, G.P.
        1959 *Africa*. NY, McGraw-Hill.

27.   Naroll, Raoul
        1973 "Data Quality Control" In Naroll & Cohen,
        eds., *A Handbook of Method in Cultural Anth-
        ropology*. NY, Columbia University Press.

28.   Quinn, Thomas C., J. Mann, J. Curran, P. Piot
        1986 "AIDS in Africa: an Epidemiological
        Paradigm." S, 234: 955-63. 21 November.

29.   Robinson, Vincent B. and Andrew U. Frank
        1987 "Expert systems for Geographic Infor-
        mation Systems." PERS 53,10: 1435-41.

30.   Robinson, V. B. and J. C. Coiner
        1986 "Characteristics and Diffusion of a
        Microcomputer Geoprocessing System: the
        Urban Data Management System." *Proceedings*,
        Urban and Regional Information Systems Assoc-
        iation, pp. 214-226.

31.   Robinson, V. B. and A. H. Strahler
        1984 "Issues in Designing Geographic Infor-
        mation Systems under Conditions of Inexact-
        ness." *Proceedings*, 10th International
        Symposium on Machine Processing of Remotely
        Sensed Data. Purdue.

32.   Schoepf, Brooke Grundfest
        "Women and AIDS in Africa: An Action Research
        Perspective." Forthcoming in H. Tierney, ed.,
        The Study of Women: Views from the Sciences.
        Greenwood Press.

33.   1986 "Primary Health Care" in Zaire. ROAPE 36.

34.   Simms, Ruth P.
              1965 *Urbanization in West Africa*. Evanston,
              Northwestern University Press.

35.   Smith, M. G.
              1960 *Government in Zazzau*. London, OUP for
              IAI.

36.   Tegnaes, Harry
              1952 *Blood Brotherhood*. NY. Philosophical
              Library.

37.   Thomas, David Hurst
              1986 *Refiguring Anthropology*. Prospect
              Heights, Waveland Press.

38.   White, Douglas R., M. L. Burton and M. Dow
              1981 "Sexual Division of Labor in African
              Agriculture: a Network Autocorrelation
              Analysis." AA 83: 824-849.

AIDS AND SOCIETY IN CENTRAL AFRICA: A VIEW FROM ZAIRE

Brooke Grundfest Schoepf
Rukarangira wa Nkera
Claude Schoepf
Walu Engundu
Payanzo Ntsomo*

Introduction

This article presents an anthropological perspective on the epidemiology of AIDS in Central Africa.[1] It draws upon enthnographic research conducted by members of the CONNAISSIDA Project since February 1985 in Zaire.[2] The project aims to develop a broad understanding of the spread of infection and the ways that AIDS is perceived and reacted to by the population, as well as to suggest culturally appropriate means of limiting the epidemic.

AIDS, a new lethal communicable disease syndrome, has rapidly developed into a pandemic affecting more than 125 countries. The human immunodeficiency virus (HIV) which causes AIDS is transmitted from infected persons by sexual contact, inoculations of contaminated blood and transplacentally from mother to foetus.[3] Insects and close household contact do not transmit the virus.[4] In Central Africa, infection occurs primarily as a result of heterosexual intercourse with an infected partner. Cities contain the highest concentration of diagnosed AIDS patients and of seropositive people, that is, those whose blood contains antibodies to the HIV virus.

Research conducted in Zaire since late 1983 indicates that the major focus of infection is in Kinshasa, a city of more than three million people.

*Brooke Grundfest Schoepf, Ph.D., and Rukarangira wa Nkera, D.V.M. are Co-Directors of the CONNAISSIDA Project. Payanzo Ntsomo, Ph.D., is Graduate Professor of Sociology at the University of Kinshasa. Claude Schoepf lives in Woods Hole, Massachusetts, U.S.A., Walu Engundu is a Research Associate at the Centre de Recherche en Sciences Humaines (CRSH), in Kinshasa. Lachung Amen, Eke Tukumbe and Pika Nianga, Research Assistants at the CRSH, contributed to the field research which includes more than 600 individual and group interviews conducted between February 1985 and November 1987. The project acronym combines the French word *connaitre* (to know), with the acronym SIDA (AIDS).

About 5% of the general population and 8 to 10% of sexually active adults in the capital probably were infected in 1987. Low levels of HIV infection have been identified in Kinshasa and some rural areas from the mid-1970s (Biggar *et al.* 1985b; Forthal *et al.* 1986; De Cock 1986; De Cock *et al.* 1987; Desmyter *et al.* 1986).[5] Infection rates appear to be rising rapidly in market towns situated on major trade and labor migration routes (Aktar *et al.* 1987; De Lalla *et al.* 1987; Surmont and Desmyter 1987).

Sexual transmission of HIV has been found to occur both from males to females and from females to males (Cameron *et al.* 1987; Clumeck *et al.* 1983; Melbye *et al.* 1986; Peterman *et al.* 1988; Piot *et al.* 1984; Van de Perre *et al.* 1984). Male to female transmission may be more efficient, as in the case of gonorrhea (Friedland and Klein 1987). However, the efficiency of transmission is markedly less than in the case of other sexually transmitted diseases (hereafter STDs). Nevertheless, while some regular partners of infected persons remain disease-free after years of sexual relations, others become infected after a single episode (Peterman *et al.* 1988). Transmission appears most likely to occur immediately following seroconversion and again when HIV infection reaches high levels in the blood during clinical disease. STDs, especially genital ulcers, significantly increase the risk of HIV infection (Greenblatt *et al.* 1987; Quinn *et al.* 1986).

In the assessment that follows, we first review epidemiological studies carried out in Zaire by members of an international biomedical research team, Project SIDA. Thereafter we summarize our data on social conditions, sexual behavior and reactions to AIDS in Kinshasa. Finally, we explore issues of AIDS prevention and technology transfer and sociocultural change.

Risk Among Women And Children

Laymen tend to perceive AIDS as a threat mainly to elite or wealthy men, and many emphasize the role of women as transmitters of disease.[6] This perspective is similar to the lay view of other STDs. In fact, women tend to predominate both among the ill and among infected persons. Thus women and children together comprise the majority of persons affected by AIDS in Zaire.

213

Among the first 500 AIDS cases diagnosed in Kinshasa from August
to December 1985, 55% were female (Quinn *et al*. 1986:958 fig.2). Women
aged 20 to 29 constituted 24.1% of patients, while men of that age were only
7.4%. The age group most represented, 30 to 39 year olds, was nearly evenly
divided between men and women and made up 38.8% of patients. While
women with AIDS were more likely than men to report that they were
unmarried (61%:36%), this figure is close to that reported for a survey of
hospital workers in which 67% of women said they were unmarried.[7]

Serological studies of healthy persons also indicate a preponderance
of women among those infected. Among 2,384 hospital workers tested in
October 1984, 8.1% of women and 5.2% of men were infected. Younger
women aged 20 to 29 years had a rate of 13.9% (Mann *et al*. 1986). In 1986,
8.4% of those individuals still working at the hospital were reported
seropositive (N'galy *et al*. 1987).

Tests of 5,099 healthy Kinshasa residents conducted in 1985 found the
highest percentage of positives (10.3%) among women aged 20 to 29 years,
while 9.8% of women aged 15 to 19 were positive (Quinn *et al*. 1986). Men
in the corresponding age groups had rates of 4.4 and 3.7%, respectively.
Among 30 to 39 years old the sexes had nearly equal rates of infection, just as
among the patient population described above; 6.8% of men and 6.1% of
women were infected. Among 40 to 49 year olds, women showed somewhat
higher rates than men (6.3%:5.0%), while at 50 years and older, infected men
maintained the 5% rate and significantly outnumbered women, among whom
only 1.6% were seropositive. This is the only age group in which men's
seroprevalence exceeded that of women. Sampling characteristics and
technical difficulties of the early serotesting may eventually cause figures on
general levels of infection to be revised downward (*Lancet* 1986; Biggar
1987). Nevertheless, women in the childbearing years are at increasing risk.
This is demonstrated by studies of pregnant and parturient women and their
infants in three Kinshasa hospitals. Blood samples of pregnant women
stored from 1970 and 1980 show levels of .25 and 3% respectively (Desmyter
et al. 1986). These are used by Biggar (1987) to estimate a doubling time for
HIV infection of 4.7 years.

In 1986 the seroprevalence among 6,000 women delivering at Mama Yemo Hospital (MYH), the government hospital serving the poor and working classes of Kinshasa, is reported at 5.7% (Nsa *et al.* 1987). Nearly half (45.7%) of the 349 seropositive mothers who delivered at MYH had ARC symptoms, and 12% were sick with AIDS. Over 70% of the infants of seropositive mothers delivered at this hospital were infected, and 30% died by the age of one year (Ryder 1988).

At the private Ngaliema Hospital, serving mainly the upper middle class, 6.7% of 2,574 prenatal patients were seropositive (Bayende *et al.* 1987; Nzila *et al.* 1987). The percentage age of seropositive mothers was higher at Ngaliema Hospital, but the women tended to be in less advanced stages of disease. Thirty percent of the 54 mothers had ARC symptoms and 1.5% full-blown AIDS; their babies were more likely to live into the second year. In other words both mothers and babies were sicker at MYH. Some of the differences may be attributable to the small sample; however, the possibility of different rates of exposure to co-factors concomitant with economic differences should be investigated. Infected women were more likely to have had previous obstetrical incidents, including spontaneous abortions and neonatal deaths. Moreover, pregnancy may increase the speed at which seropositive women progress to clinical disease (Tshibangu, Kayembe *et al.* 1986).

New studies confirm that AIDS is becoming a significant public health and development problem. In January 1986, 33% of 174 in-patients on the medical wards of MYH were seropositive (Colebunders *et al.* 1987). Moreover, the sex ratio may be even further skewed in the direction of women. The average ages of 89 female and 85 male patients were not significantly different (x=36 and 39 years, respectively). However, 42% of the women were seropositive compared with 25% of the men. For both sexes seroprevalence was highest among patients 30 to 39 years. By the end of 1986, at least 25% of adult deaths at this 2000 bed hospital, were seropositive (Quinn *et al.* 1986).

Although infection is not confined to any special population group, women with multiple sexual partners are most at risk of becoming infected. Twenty-seven percent of a sample of women soliciting in Matonge bars were found to be seropositive in 1985 (Mann *et al.* 1986b). This level is lower than infection rates among poor prostitutes in Nairobi--61% in 1985 and 88% in 1986 (Kreiss *et al.* 1986; Plummer *et al.* 1987). Nevertheless, it is cause for grave concern. Low income prostitutes who report the highest frequency of encounters are most at risk.[8] This is also the cohort most likely to have a history of recurrent STD episodes, particularly genital herpes and chalmydia which cause open sores (D'Costa *et al.* 1985).

Economic And Social Issues In The Aids Crisis

AIDS has emerged and spread in Central Africa as a result of a set of historically specific economic and social relations. Many areas of sub-Saharan Africa have experienced severe economic crisis, including declining per capita food production and widening income disparities over the past decade. The crisis includes the decline of family farming, exodus to cities already crowded with unemployment, soaring food prices and increasing hunger in both urban and rural areas. About 40% of Zaire's more than 33 million population is urban and sex ratios are nearly equal, with 51% males and 49% females in most large cities (GOZ 1984). The feminization of poverty, observed throughout the developed West and the Third World, is not well documented for Zaire. Nevertheless we expect the crisis to be experienced most severely by poor women and their children, who are most at risk for malnutrition and related diseases. The impact of the crisis upon women helps to explain the rapid spread of AIDS.

As figures presented above indicate, young women constitute the major risk group for AIDS in Central Africa. Professional prostitutes who make their livelihood mainly from the sale of sexual services to multiple partners are not the only women at risk.[9] Many other types of multiple partner relationships, with varying degrees of social recognition and legitimacy exist among people of all social classes and ethnic origins. Some types are new versions of old forms of structured interaction; others, like prostitution, have emerged with the incorporation of African societies in the modern world system of capitalist markets and industrial production (Dirasse 1978). While there are people who avoid pre-marital and extra-marital sex on moral and religious grounds, there are also those for whom multiple partners are a form of recreation, a source of prestige and/or a source of income. Polygyny continues widespread in all social classes, and neglected wives may seek compensation elsewhere.[10] Even polygynous husbands do not always restrict their activities to socially recognized partners. Moreover, recognized relationships may be of relatively short duration. As in the West, young people and those who are divorced or separated may experiment with a series of casual partners before settling down.

It is useful to draw attention to the role of urban labor migration in destabilizing family relationships throughout Africa (Quinn *et al.* 1986). However, it is unwise to assume that people living in rural areas are free from the danger of infection. Although the precolonial societies of Central Africa often made rules about sex, they seldom prescribed lifetime exclusivity for either men or women. Some cultures included a variety of acceptable partners for married or unmarried people, and "rules-for-breaking-rules" abounded. Moreover, warfare, armed occupation, trade and labor migration have all transformed social relationships in many rural areas to the extent that traditional normative sanctions no longer serve as deterrents. For some people, Christian precepts have reinforced or replaced indigenous African proscriptions. The percentages of couples practicing monogamously exclusive relationships and of celibate unmarried people are not known.

Although no statistics exist, observers generally agree that multiple partner relationships appear to be increasing as a result of the economic crisis which affects many women somewhat differently than men. Gender role ideology inherited from the colonial period emphasizes female dependency and male responsibility. It masks the extent to which urban women have been major providers of their own support and that of family members (Bernard 1972; Comhaire-Sylvain 1968; Schoepf 1978; Schwartz 1972; Walu 1987; Wilson 1982). Although sex discrimination is illegal, the mass of women without school diplomas is virtually excluded from formal sector employment. The expectation of frequent child bearing constitutes an additional disincentive for employers in a stagnant economy. This situation is common throughout Central and East Africa (Bujra 1986; Mbilinyi 1984; Obbo 1981; White 1980; government of Zimbabwe 1982). As a result, women engage in a variety of self-employed income-generating occupations. These include gender-typed activities such as food processing, petty trade, sewing, hair dressing, and market gardening. While some--generally those with family capital and connections--succeed (MacGaffey 1986a,b), most remain impoverished (Schoepf 1978; Walu 1987).

Deepening crisis, propelled by the debt service burden, continuing inflation and rural exodus, has rendered the already crowded formal economic sector increasingly less profitable. Poor women traders report sharply declining incomes over the past three years, and failures are common. Moreover, those who in the past could rely on contributions to household expenses from a steady male partner now report that the men are providing less and less. Men acknowledge that they are cutting back on the amount of support they extend to plural households.

Extended families are reported unable to provide as much financial assistance as formerly. Women say that consequently now more than ever they need to find "spare tires" (*pneus de rechange*), that is, men to whom they offer sexual services when they need ready cash to obtain health care for a sick child or to meet social obligations.[11] The actual monetary value of any single sexual liaison may be very low, [12] yet poor female- headed households cannot survive without them. Now more than ever traders and women with clerical and professional jobs need the protection, networks and gifts that high status men can provide (Schoepf 1978; Schuster 1979).

The health consequences of multiple partner strategies, risky in the past, have become much more so over the past decade. It is the fact of multiple partners, rather than the type of relationship, however socially categorized and labelled, which puts people at risk. AIDS now has transformed what appeared to be a survival strategy into a death strategy.

In addition to the tragic consequences for individuals, AIDS presents enormous challenges for the survival of social systems. Other authors deal with demographic and development implications. An additional consideration is not to be neglected. In the past, disease pandemics and economic crises have given rise to scapegoating and witch-hunting in Africa as in the West. In the US, the stigma of AIDS has compounded existing prejudices against minorities. In a number of other African countries, urban women, including prostitutes, traders and others who escape male control, have been deported to rural areas. Where AIDS is blamed on women, the conjunction of economic crisis and a lethal sexually transmitted disease may give rise to untoward consequences.

Technology Transfer And AIDS Control

Apart from action by health care providers to screen blood supplies and sterilize equipment, the only immediate hope of limiting HIV transmission is to devise intervention strategies that effectively induce substantial numbers of people to change their behavior. Celibacy and a single lifetime partner are not realistic options for many people. Reduction in the number of partners will require institutional as well as behavioral change. Risk-reducing technology may be more readily accepted.

Although condoms are by no means a panacea, correctly used they have been found to lower the risk of sexual transmission (Kreiss *et al*. 1986; Mann *et al*. 1987; Ngugi *et al*. 1987). Latex condoms not only block the passage of HIV in intercourse; they help to check sexually transmitted diseases which appear to act as co-factors. They also prevent repeated infection by different strains of the rapidly mutating virus. In addition they eliminate the deposition of semen which, even when not infected, may lower resistance to infection and facilitate the replication of HIV in infected persons (Turner *et al*. 1987).[13] People with multiple partners or whose partners have multiple partners may reduce their risk of infection by using or convincing all partners to use condoms during every sexual encounter. Prevention of pediatric AIDS also requires primary prevention of HIV infection among women and girls.

Much more than a simple transfer of material culture is involved in the process of condom adoption, for there are powerful sociocultural and psychological constraints to overcome. To many people condoms are an unnatural, uncongenial foreign import. A survey conducted in the port of Matadi, downriver from Kinshasa, found that among couples already practicing some form of birth spacing, condoms were the least acceptable technology (Bertrand and Niandu, 1985).[14] We found most adolescents and many adults unfamiliar with condoms.

Ideological issues also need to be addressed. In Zaire nationalist sentiment currently links contraception and condom use to western population control strategies, which are viewed as a form of imperialism. Some husbands also view contraception as an encouragement for wives' extra-marital sexual relations. Elsewhere in Central Africa, as well, politicization of contraception has made it difficult to gain acceptance for birth spacing (Schoepf 1983b). These considerations suggest that it may be preferable to separate AIDS prevention from birth control efforts, rather than to place responsibility for AIDS interventions within family planning programs.[15]

Condoms are somewhat socially acceptable to men who purchase the services of prostitutes. However, social acceptability is not the same as psychological acceptability. Even more problems surround condom use with regular partners, including spouses. Depth interviews revealed other factors in the resistance to condoms. These include beliefs about the contribution of semen to women's health and reproduction; fear that condoms may injure women, and even cause sterility; suspicion and hostility believed likely to result from proposing condom usage to a regular, or even a casual, partner; difficulties with in-laws over condom use with a spouse, and other fairly-level conflicts. In addition to cognitive and sociocultural constraints, both men and women cited psychological obstacles.

Men who have tried condoms object to the loss of sensation that results from wearing a sheath. Others say that they would miss the gratification obtained from knowing that they are depositing semen inside a woman. A few say that they fear that semen remaining in a condom might be used for sorcery. Some men in our study report that even after repeated trials, they are unable to ejaculate.

Complex non-verbal communication follows coitus among people whose emotions are engaged in a sexual relationship. Women say they feel rejection, resentment and sadness if a partner withdraws immediately following ejaculation. A woman whose partner has left her unsatisfied may use the ability to control her vaginal muscles to expel a flaccid penis in an expression of displeasure and contempt. Condom protection, which requires the women to remain passive and the man to withdraw before losing his erection, interferes with post-coital expressivity.[16] Male informants reported that women refuse condom protection; numerous women who are aware of the risk say that they would like their partners to use them and explain why they feel unable to introduce the subject.

Women who openly acknowledge their main source of livelihood comes from sex with multiple partners have been among the first to change their behavior in favor of condom use. Mann and co-workers reported that only 8 of 85 women used condoms with more than half of their clients in 1985 (Mann *et al.* 1987). Most prostitutes whom we interviewed in mid-1986 similarly scoffed at condoms, and many were unfamiliar with them. Sixteen months later, knowledge had increased and attitudes and practices had changed significantly, particularly among the women with wealthy clients. By mid-1987 a few reported that they required clients to use condoms, carried their own and would send away any man who refused because "we don't want to die." Some, to whom AIDS was equally real, said that they proposed condoms but could not reject clients who refused because they needed the money. Most merely reported that they would accept a condom if the client supplied it. By the end of 1987, some of the poorest, illiterate women who originally had repulsed a CONNAISSIDA interviewer asked the project to provide information and condoms. They reported the clients increasingly initiated condom use.[17] In addition, since neighbors began to accuse them of spreading AIDS, the women inquired whether serotesting could be used to prove them disease-free. Although these women have a special stake, they are not the only ones who have begun to make changes. What has triggered the beginnings of wider change?

Seeking Solutions:
Changing Behavior And The CONNAISSIDA Project

In the interim the level of AIDS awareness in Kinshasa grew. Many people who previously had dismissed AIDS as an imaginary syndrome invented by Europeans to discourage African lovers[18] became convinced of its reality of AIDS. The dense rumor network of the "sidewalk radio" (*radio trottoir*) spread news of deaths of prominent people from AIDS. Some people watched relatives and acquaintances waste away. Health officials, including the Minister and biomedical researchers, confirmed the danger and advised the public on prevention (see Tshiani *et al.* 1986; Tshimanga 1984). Radio and television programs and print media publicized the information (see Loseke and Amulo 1986).

By early 1987, school children were heard taunting one another with carrying the stigmatized "dirty disease." In May the National Committee to Fight AIDS (established by the government in 1985) issued a leaflet in French and Lingala.[19]   At the same time the popular singer Luambo Makiadi (Franco), released a cassette of detailed information and advice set to music. Broadcast on the national radio and played in bars, taxis and shops, the news was difficult to avoid. The Government, which heretofore had concentrated its efforts in Kinshasa, launched a national information campaign in June 1987. In September the popular television group, *Théâtre de Chez Nous*, broadcast a comic sketch about AIDS and multiple partners. Church groups and other non-governmental organizations took up the challenge, printing leaflets and holding meetings for their members. In November the Catholic Archdiocese of Kinshasa devoted the four weekly meetings of its 1,000 community groups to discussions of AIDS. The pamphlet distributed to group leaders, prepared by CONNAISSIDA's Rukarangira wa Nkera, includes advice about condoms.

As a result of the multi-media information campaign people interviewed in Kinshasa in June 1987 knew that AIDS is fatal and transmitted by sex and blood. Although some said that they did not know much about it they appear to have been expressing feelings of powerlessness and/or seeking to avoid reality. Interview texts show that many informants followed their profession of ignorance by asking the researcher when a cure or vaccine would be found.

While some people in Kinshasa continue to deny the danger, denial has become more difficult. Increasing AIDS awareness led some people to change; most did not. However, it produced a readiness which allowed CONNAISSIDA to field test its community based training design. Based on group dynamics principles and using structured exercises, experiential training allows participants to reflect together in depth and engage in problem-solving on matters of common concern. Active teaching methods demonstrate to participants their capacity to take control of their situation. Work began with a group of prostitutes. They had come to realize that they must find ways to convince clients to use condoms. The training designed by CONNAISSIDA includes practice in helping recalcitrant men to change. Informed that untreated STDs increase their risk of infection, the women exchanged experiences about the health care available in their community. They identified a need for accessible and affordable services where qualified health workers would treat them courteously rather than stigmatizing or abusing them.

Married women increasingly perceive themselves to be at risk because they know, assume or suspect that their husbands have multiple partners. Some informants said that they wished their husbands would use condoms but were reluctant to introduce the subject because they believed that their husbands would not listen to them and that conflict would result. When news of CONNAISSIDA's group sessions with the prostitutes spread, a neighborhood churchwomen's club requested training as well. Eighty women attended training sessions at the church. Acting in their capacity as primary health care providers to their households, they also sought information for their husbands, siblings and adolescent children. As with most informants interviewed in earlier waves, the possibility of maternal-fetal transmission was virtually unknown to the women in these groups.

Predictably, that information strengthened the participants' resolve to convince partners and children of the danger. The women also requested training sessions for husbands and older children in order to reinforce their own efforts. different sex and age groups are particularly indicated for such sessions in light of the constraints in many cultures on explicit discourse about sex across gender and/or generation lines within the immediate family. The women suggested that discussing other modes of transmission could attenuate the climate of guilt and suspicion aroused among spouses by discussions of sexual transmission. One participant related her experience in observing health care workers and making polite inquiries about sterilization of syringes and cutting instruments. Although most of the women do not own watches, they do have an idea of the time it takes to boil rice; twenty minutes of boiling will also sterilize health care equipment.

Noting that several members were former prostitutes who feared that deepening poverty would force them back to the profession, the group's president pointed to the need for income-generating activities to enable women to reduce their number of partners. The group asked CONNAISSIDA to help them discover informal sector opportunities that might offer dependable sources of income. The group meetings show how people place AIDS in a wider context in which poverty, getting enough to eat and malaria are their biggest problems. They also indicate that local community groups and social networks are concerned about AIDS and can be mobilized to support behavioral change. Group dynamics methods can be taught to members of community groups for use on AIDS and other primary health care problems that require community mobilization.

Conclusion

In Africa, as well as in the developed countries, the AIDS epidemic "quickens social apprehensions." Governments are concerned both to change behavior and to avoid public panic. There is a pressing need to reach the general population of Central African cities with intervention strategies that can effectively support sexual risk reduction behavior. Zaire and other countries have many formal mass media channels and informal ones as well. Mass media education campaigns and leaflets are raising levels of AIDS awareness. These types of interventions have seldom proved effective by themselves (Rogers 1976). Particularly in the case of sexual behavior, more than increased knowledge is required to produce widespread, rapid change. CONNAISSIDA seeks to develop community-based interpersonal communication strategies with methods and materials that can be used not only by workers in community health facilities but by local level organizations and social networks as well. These strategies would not replace mass media campaigns but would be used in conjunction with them to provide continuing the encouragement, support and reinforcement that most people will need to sustain change.

The two community groups with which we worked--the first an informal network, the second a local voluntary organization--have been invaluable in helping us to understand the social context and changing reactions to AIDS. With them we were able to try out an experiential training design intended to engage people directly in solving the problem of AIDS prevention in their own lives. The training sessions provide creative ways to approach AIDS education and to obtain further information on the cultural construction of AIDS. The action-research also has other benefits. The rapport generated in these sessions makes it possible to conduct depth interviews with individuals and small groups on sensitive subjects such as sexuality. This method appears likely to yield more reliable information than that obtained from questionnaire surveys without requiring the extensive preparations involved in ethnographic community studies.

Like so many other diseases produced by rapid urban growth and by socioeconomic and political conditions, AIDS is a disease of "development" (Hughes and Hunter 1970), a biological event magnified by the current world economic crisis. Our data suggest that behavior change will be best achieved by integrating preventive efforts into primary health care instead of creating costly new vertical programs. This view is shared by Dr. G. Monekqasso, WHO Regional Director for Africa (cited in Kingman 1987) and by Piot and co-workers (1987). However, since community participation in health promotion is the weakest aspect of many PHC programs, these cannot be relied upon at present to meet the immediate challenge posed by the AIDS pandemic. For this reason, a combination of vertical and horizontal programs is needed to generate widespread immediate action. If AIDS control strategies can be reoriented toward genuine community health action, they might play a transformative role of the type envisioned by WHO leaders and member states, which in 1978, established the utopian development goal of "health for all by the year 2000." Without rapid community mobilization, the future of Central Africa may be grim indeed.

The initial impression that heterosexual transmission of AIDS in Central Africa "represents a new epidemiological setting" (Piot *et al.* 1994:64) remains correct. However, the prevalence of multiple sex partners and untreated STDs among adolescents and young adults in western societies leaves no room for complacency or invidious comparison. Africa may simply be twenty years ahead of the US with respect to heterosexual transmission (Dr. Scott Halstead, personal communication, December 1986). Unless behavior changes before HIV infection becomes widely established in heterosexual populations in other countries, Central Africa's health and development of the 1980s may turn to be a harbinger, a grim model of the West at the dawn of the twenty-first century.

[1]This article is based on a colloquium presented by B.G. Schoepf and Payanzo at the CRSH, November 13, 1987.

[2]Projet CONNAISSIDA, located at the CRSH received funding in 1987 from the Conseil Executif (Government) of Zaire, the Rockefeller Foundation and OXFAM(UK). The authors wish to express their gratitude to the above institutions for their support, which does not constitute endorsement of the findings. Responsibility for interpretation and conclusions rests solely with the authors.

[3]Although infection may occur perinatally (during birth) and through breast milk, the situation is unclear, as yet few cases have been documented in which these constitute the sole risk factor. Parenteral transmission (by injections or cuts made with contaminated instruments) appears to depend upon the amount of inoculate (infected material) that is transferred.

[4]Neither casual contacts nor insects are implicated in HIV transmission, nor is malaria a co-factor predisposing to HIV infection (Nguyen-Dinh et al. 1987). However, unless malaria can be prevented, or treated in early stages, until blood supplies can be screened, the treatment of severe malaria-related anemia will continue to be an important factor in transmitting HIV infection to children. Greenberg and co-workers (1987) reviewed the records of 1,000 pediatric patients. Transfusions were ordered for 480 children. Of these, 69.2 percent suffered from malaria-related anemia. Nearly all the 392 malaria patients who were transfused (97.3 percent) had hematocrits of 25 percent or less, and immediate transfusions were judged necessary to save their lives.

[5]Urban rates in neighboring countries probably are considerably higher (Dr. Scott Halstead pers. comm. December 30, 1987), and rural infection is reported high around the Great Lakes (Serwadda et al. 1985). The earliest identification of an HIV has been made on a blood sample drawn in Zaire in 1959 (Nahmias et al. 1986).

[6]Some biomedical researchers and program officers in several funding agencies shared this view in 1986 and early 1987. Requests for support were rebuffed on the grounds that the organizations focus primarily on maternal-child health programs.

[7]What percentage were cohabitating with stable partners in "free unions" is not specified. Some of those in the "unmarried" category were in this situation (Mann et al. 1986a); others may have been in plural marriages without legal sanction but nevertheless, formally recognized by their families and sanctioned by bridewealth.

[8]A group of poor women reported 2 to 7 encounters daily (interviews November 1987).

[9]Prostitutes include the *londoniennes*, peripatetic hookers who regularly stand along thoroughfares in the city center or solicit in gambling casinos, high-priced night clubs and hotels. There are also those who sit outside their rooms in the popular quarters or who make nightly rounds of the inexpensive beer parlors. Interviews in several networks indicate that

members serve an overlapping pool of clients. Many women who go to dancing clubs to seek partners on weekends are not professional prostitutes. Rather, they are more like western habitues of middle class singles' bars, except that, given the low-wage economy, they depend upon gifts of cash for clothes and other expenses. Women in these roles generally do not provide domestic services other than sex. However, they may also have a regular partner to whom they supply domestic services.

[10]The notion that African women do not or should not expect sexual satisfaction from marriage (Caldwell and Caldwell 1981) does not apply to most cultures in this area, and some traditions include special ways to help women realize their potential for enjoyment.

[11]Funeral contributions are most often cited in the latter context.

[12]A rapid encounter in a poor Kinshasa neighborhood cost 50 to 60 zaires in July 1987. This was equivalent to US$.50 and would purchase a large bowl of cassava meal, a beer, an onion or three eggs.

[13]Researchers have suggested that the time of conversion from HIV infection to clinical disease in male homosexuals is shortened by receiving repeated doses of semen, whether infected or not (Turner *et al*. 1987). They report that human seminal plasma contains immunosuppressive agents that inhibit normal immune response against viral infection. In addition semen contains the prostaglandin E_2, which *in vitro*, facilitates the replication of HIV. Their suggestions should be equally relevant to women partners of heterosexual males. If their hypothesis is confirmed, then repeated deposition of seminal fluid within the body would constitute a risk factor for both women and homosexual men. This would mean that an infected woman herself is in need of protection, not only from possible reinfection with new HIV strains but from uninfected semen.

[14]The study reported that family planning met a cool reception, even when health workers accompanied house-to-house contraceptive distribution with community education meetings.

[15]Informants report that the Tahiti condoms currently distributed by USAID are too small and inelastic. Condoms which hurt their wearer or break during normal use may limit the effectiveness of AIDS prevention efforts.

[16]Discussion with Citoyenne Bisumbukuboko helped to focus on these questions.

[17]Similar findings are reported by Ngugi and colleagues (1987) working with a cohort of prostitutes in Nairobi. They compared the effects of two types of health education. Among those who attended mass meetings 85 percent report using condoms. Individual counseling increased the rate to 90 percent. 65 percent of controls who received no education but shared in the free condoms supplied to all women in the experiment also reported using condoms. The abstract does not specify what level of use is involved, that is, what proportion of encounters among the condom users are covered by condoms. Nor does it indicate whether the cohorts were spacially and socially isolated from one another. Prostitutes in Kinshasa and Lubumbashi tend to participate in far-flung social networks; such segmentation as exists is ethnic rather than spacial.

[18]The acronym SIDA (AIDS in French) is popularly known as *Syndrome Imaginaire pour Décourager les Amoureux.*

[19]This leaflet, printed with funds from OXFAM/UK, is the first official public information document to be widely distributed.

BIBLIOGRAPHY

Aktar, L. *et al.* 1987. "Distribution of Antibodies to HIV-I in an Urban Community (Aru, Zaire)." II International Symposium on AIDS and Associated Cancers in Africa. Naples, October 7-9. Abstract TH 34.

Bayende, E. *et al.* 1987. "Congenital Transmission in an Upper Middle Class Hospital in Kinshasa." II International Symposium on AIDS and Associated Cancers in Africa. Naples, October 7-9.

Bernard, Guy. 1972. "Conjugalité et Role de la Femme à Kinshasa," *Canadian Journal of African Studies* 6, 2:261-74.

Bertrand, Jane T. and Nlandu Mangani. 1985. "Family Planning Operations Research: The PRODEF/Tulane Project in Base-Zaire." Final Report (February).

Biggar, Robert J. 1986a. "The AIDS Problem in Africa." *The Lancet* I:79-82.

Biggar, Robert J. 1986b. "The Clinical Features of HIV Infection in Africa." *British Medical Journal* 293,6560:1453-54.

Biggar, Robert J. 1987. "AIDS and HIV Infection: Estimates of the Magnitude of the Problem Worldwide (1985-1986)." *Clinical Immunology and Immunopathology* 45:297-309.

Biggar, Robert J. *et al.* 1985b. "HTLV Retrovirus Antibody Reactivity Associated with Malaria and Immune Complexes in Healthy Africans." *The Lancet* 2,8454 (Sept. 7):520-23.

Booth, W. 1987. "Another Muzzle for AIDS Education?" *Science* 248, 4830:1036.

Briggs, Asa. 1961. "Cholera and Society in the Nineteenth Century." *Past and Present* 19 (April):76-96.

Bujra, Janet M. 1975. "Women Entrepreneurs of Early Nairobi." *Canadian Journal of African Studies* 9, 2:213-34.

Caldwell, P. and J.C. Caldwell. 1981. "The Function of Child-Spacing in Traditional Societies and the Direction of Change." In *Child-Spacing in Tropical Africa*, ed. Hilary J. Page and Ron Lesthaeghe. Academic Press.

Cameron, D.W. *et al.* 1987. "Female to Male Transmission of HIV Infection in Nairobi." Poster MP 91. III International Conference on AIDS, Washington, DC.

Colebunders, Robert, Henry Francis *et al.* 1987. "Evaluation of a Clinical Case-Definition of Acquired Immunodeficiency Syndrome in Africa." *The Lancet* I, (February 28):492-94.

Colebunders, R., H. Francis, J.M. Mann, K.M. Bila, L. Izaley, L. Kimputu *et al*. 1987. "Persistant Diarrhea, Strongly Associated with HIV Infection in Kinshasa, Zaire." *American Journal of Gastroenterology* 82, 9:859-64.

Clumeck, N. *et al*. 1983. "Acquired Immune Deficiency Syndrome in Black Africans" (letter). The *Lancet* 8235-642.

Comhaire-Sylvain, Suzanne. 1968. *Femmes de Kinshasa Hier et Aujord'hui*. Paris: Mouton.

D'Costa, L.J., F.A. Plummer, I. Bowmer, L. Fransen, P. Piot, A.R. Ronald, Nsanze. 1985. "Prostitutes are a Major Reservoir of Sexual Transmitted Diseases in Nairobi, Kenya." *Sexually Transmitted Diseases* 12:64-67.

De Cock, Kevin M. 1986. "Infection par le Virus de l'Immunodeficience Humaine dans la Région de l'Equateur." Unpublished manuscript.

De Cock, Kevin M., N. Nzilambi, D. Forthal *et al*. 1987. "Stability of HIV Infection Prevalence over 10 years in a Rural Population of Zaire." Poster WP.43, III International conference on AIDS, Washington, DC.

De Lalla, F. *et al*. 1987. "Rapid Spread of HIV Infection in a rural District in North Uganda." Abstract 84:177, III International AIDS Conference. Washington, DC. June.

Desmyter, J., P. Gouban, S. Chamaret, L. Montagnier. 1986. "Anti-LAV/HTLV-III in Kinshasa Mothers in 1970 and 1980." (Abstract-Communication 110:S17g). II International Conference on AIDS. Paris 1986:106.

Dirasse, Laketch. 1978. "The Socioeconomic Position of Women in Addis Ababa: The Case of Prostitution." Ph.D. Dissertation, Department of Anthropology, Boston University. Ann Arbor, MI: University Microfilms.

Dunne, Richard. 1987. "AIDS in New York City: Policy and Planning." Bulletin NY Academy of Medicine 63, 7:673-78.

Fisher, E.J. 1987. AIDS Update (review). *Henry Ford Hospital Medical Journal* 35, 1:5-16.

Forthal, Donald M. *et al*. 1986. "Antibody to HTLV-III/LAV in Sera collected in 1976, Equateur Region, Zaire." Abstract of paper presented at International AIDS Conference, Paris, June 23-25.

Friedland, G.H. and R.S. Klein. 1987. "Transmission of the Human Immunodeficiency Virus." *New England Journal of Medicine* 317 (Oct. 29):1125-35.

Government of Zaire. 1984. *Recensement Scientifique de la Population*. Kinshasa: Départment du Plan.

Government of Zimbabwe. 1982. *Report on the Situation of Women in Zimbabwe*. Harare: Ministry of Community Development and Women's Affairs.

Greenberg, Alan E. *et al*. 1987. "The Association Between HIV Seropositivity, Blood Transfusion and Malaria in a Pediatric Population in Kinshasa, Zaire." III International Conference on AIDS, Washington, DC. June. Abstract M. 8.5.

Greenblatt, R.M. *et al*. 1987. "Genital Ulceration as a Risk for Human Immunodeficiency Virus Infection in Kenya." Poster 68. III International Conference on AIDS, Washington, DC.

Hughes, Charles C. and John M. Hunter. 1970. "Disease and 'Development' in Tropical Africa." *Social Science and Medicine* 3:443-93.

Kingman, Sharon. 1987. "AIDS Monitor: Africa Blames the Urban Lifestyle." *New Scientist* (15 October):26.

Kreiss, J.K., D. Koech, F.A. Plummer *et al*. 1986. "AIDS Virus Infection in Nairobi Prostitutes: Spread of the Epidemic in East Africa." *New England Journal of Medicine* 314:414-18.

Laga, M. and P. Piot. 1987. "The Struggle Against AIDS in Africa: A Public Priority" (La Lutte contre le SIDA en Afrique: Une Priorité de Santé Publique). *Annales Société Belge de Médecine Tropicale* 67:1-6.

Lancet, 1986. Editorial: An Unexpected New Human Virus. *The Lancet* II, 8521-22:1430-31.

Lancet. 1987. Editorial: AIDS in Africa. *The Lancet* II, 8552:192-94.

MacGaffey, Janet. 1986a. "Fending for Yourself: The Organization of the Second Economy in Zaire." In the *Crisis in Zaire: Myths and Realities* (141-56) ed. Nzongola-Ntalaja. Trenton, NJ: Africa World Press, Inc.

MacGaffey, Janet, 1986b. "Women and Class Formation in a Dependent Economy: Kisangani Entrepreneurs." In *Women and Class in Africa* (161-77) ed. Claire Robertson and Iris Berger. New York: Africana Publishing Company.

Mann, Jonathan M. *et al*. 1986a. "Surveillance for AIDS in a Central African City: Kinshasa, Zaire." *Journal of the American Medical Association* (JAMA) 255,23:3255-59.

Mann, Jonathan M. *et al*. 1986b. "Sexual Practices Associated with LAV/HTLV-III Seropositivity Among Female Prostitutes in Kinshasa, Zaire." Presented at the II International Conference on AIDS, Paris (June 23-25).

Mann, Jonathan *et al*. 1986c. "Association Between HTLV-III/2AV Infection and Tuberculosis in Zaire (letter)." *Journal of American Medical Association* 256-346.

Mann, Jonathan M. *et al*. 1986d. "Prevalence of HTLV-III/LAV in Household Contacts of Patients With Confirmed AIDS and Controls in Kinshasa, Zaire." *JAMA* 256,6:721-24.

Mann, Jonathan M. *et al*. 1986e. "Risk Factors for Human Immunodeficiency virus Seropositivity Among Children 1-24 Months Old in Kinshasa, Zaire." *The Lancet* (Sept. 20):654-56.

Mann, Jonathan M. *et al.* 1986f. "Natural History of Human Immunodeficiency Virus Infection in Zaire." *The Lancet* (Sept. 27):707-9.

Mann, Jonathan M. *et al.* 1986g. "Human Immunodeficiency Virus Seroprevalence in *Pediatric* 2 to 14 Years of Age at Mama Yemo Hospital, Kinshasa, Zaire." Pediatrics 78, 4:673-77.

Mann, Jonathan M. *et al.* 1986h. "HIV Seroprevalence Among Hospital Workers in Kinshasa, Zaire: Lack of Association With Occupational Exposure." *JAMA* 256,22:3099-3102.

Mann, Jonathan M. *et al.* 1987. "Condom Use and HIV Infection Among Prostitutes in Zaire (letter)." *New England Journal of Medicine* 316,6:345.

Mbilinyi, Majorie. 1984. "Women in Development Ideology: The Promotion of Competition and Exploitation." *The African Review* 2, 1:14-33.

Mudimbe, V.Y. 1981. "Signes Thérapeutiques et Prose de la Vie en Afrique Noire." *Social Science and Medicine* 15B:195-211.

Nahmias, A.J., J. Weiss, X. Yao, F. Lee, R. Kodsi *et al.* 1986. "Evidence for Human Infection with an HTLV-III/LAV like Virus in Central Africa (letter). *Lancet* 1:1279-80.

Nelkin, Dorothy. 1987. "AIDS and the Social Sciences: Review of Useful Knowledge and Research Needs." *Reviews of Infectious Diseases* 9, 5 (Sept.-Oct.):980-86.

N'galy, B., R.W. Ryder, B. Kapita, H. Francis, T. Quinn, J. Mann. 1987. "Continuing Studies on the Natural History of Human Immunodeficiency (HIV) Infection in Zaire." (Abstract) *American Journal of Epidemiology* 126, 4 (Oct.):757.

Ngugi, E.N. *et al.* 1987. "Effects of an AIDS Education Program on Increasing Condom Use in a Cohort of Nairobi Prostitutes." III International Conference on AIDS, Washington, DC. June. 5:157.

Nguyen-Dinh, Phuc *et al.* 1987. "Absence of Association Between HIV Seropositivity and *Plasmodium falciparum* Malaria in Kinshasa, Zaire." III International Conference on AIDS, Washington, DC. MP.73 (p. 22).

Nsa, W., R. Ryder, H. Francis and D. Utshudi. 1987. "Congenital Transmission in a Large Urban Hospital in Kinshasa." II International Symposium on AIDS and Associated Cancers in Africa. Naples, October 7-9. Abstract F1.

Nzila, N., R.W. Ryder, F. Behets, H. Francis *et al.* 1987. "Perinatal Human Immunodeficiency Virus (HIV) Transmission in Two African Hospitals." (Abstract) *American Journal of Epidemiology* 126, 4 (October):757.

Obbo, Christine. 1981. *African Women, Their Struggle for Economic Independence.* London: Zed Press.

234

Payanzo, Ntsomo. 1987. "Structure, Organisation et communication dans la Ville de Kinshasa." Two lectures, CONNAISSIDA Action-Research Training Program. Kinshasa: Centre de Recherche en Sciences Humanines, July.

Piot, P. *et al.* 1984. "Acquired Immunodeficiency Syndrome in a Heterosexual Population in Zaire." *The Lancet* II, 8394:65-69.

Piot, P., R. Colebunders, M. Laga *et al.* 1987. "AIDS in Africa: A Public Health Priority." *Journal of Virol. Meth.* 17, 1-2 (August):1-10.

Quinn, Thomas C., Jonathan M. Mann, James W. Curran, Peter Piot. 1986. "AIDS in Africa: An Epidemiologic Paradigm." *Science* 234, (Nov. 21):955-63.

Rogers, Everett M. (ed.). 1976. *Communication and Development: Critical Perspectives.* Beverly Hills: Sage.

Rukarangira wa Nkera. 1987. "Evolution de l'Economie Informelle dans le Sud-Est du Shaba." Research report, World Bank, Kinshasa, May. Forthcoming in *The Second Economy of Zaire*, ed. J. MacGaffey.

Schoepf, Brooke G. 1978. "Les Femmes dans l'Economie Informelle à Lubumbashi." Paper presented at the IV International Congress of African Studies, Kinshasa, December.

Schoepf, Brooke G. 1982. "Technology Transfer, Values and social Relations in Health." In *Proceedings of the Tuskegee Institute Inaugural Symposium*, ed. Paul Wall. Tuskegee Institute: Carver Research Foundation.

Schoepf, Brooke G. 1983. "Health for Rural Women." *Community Action* (Zimbabwe) I:26-27.

Schoepf, Brooke G. 1985. "The 'Wild,' the 'Lazy' and the 'Matriarchal': Nutrition and Cultural Survival in the Zairian Copperbelt," Michigan State University, Women in International Development, working Papers No. 96 (September) 22pp.

Schoepf, Brooke G. 1986. "Primary Health Care in Zaire." *Review of African Political Economy* 35 (September):54-58.

Schoepf, Brooke G. in press. "Women, AIDS and Economic Crisis in Central Africa." *Canadian Journal of African Studies.*

Schuster, Ilsa. 1979. *The New Women of Lusaka.* Palo Alto, CA: Mayfield.

Schwartz, Alf. 1972. "Illusion d'une Emancipation et Aleénation Réelle de l'Ouvriére Zaïroise." *Canadian Journal of African Studies* 6, 2:183-212.

Surmont, I. and J. Desmyter. 1987. "Urban to Rural Spread of HIV infection in Dungu, Zaire." II International Symposium on AIDS and Associated Cancers in Africa, Naples, Oct. 7-9, Abstract TH 3.

Tshibangu, Kataka K. Kayembe *et al.* 1986. "Feto-Maternal Risk During Acquired Immunodeficiency Syndrome." Poster 87, II International Conference on AIDS. Paris, June 23-25.

Turner, M.J., J.O. White and W.P. Soutter, 1987. "AIDS Incubation Period in Male Haemophiliacs." (Letter) *Nature* 330 (24/31 December):702.

Van de Perre, P. *et al.* 1984. "Acquired Immunodeficiency Syndrome in Rwanda." *The Lancet* II, 8394:62-65.

Van de Perre, P., N. Clumeck, M. Caraél *et al.* 1985. "Female Prostitutes: A Risk Group for Infection with Human T-cell Lymphotropic Virus Type III." *The Lancet* 1985, ii:524-26.

Vincke, Edouard. 1980. "Problémes Transculturels dans l'Enseignement de la Biologie et des Disciplines connexes." In *La Dépendance de l'Afrique et les Moyens d'y Remédier* (316-23), ed. V.Y. Mudime, Paris: Berger-Levraut.

Walu Engundu. 1987. "Les Femmes dans l'Economie Informelle de Kinshasa." Report on women's household budgets prepared for the World Bank, Kinshasa (May).

White, Luise. 1980. "Women's Domestic Labor in Colonial Kenya: Prostitution in Nairobi, 1909-1950." Boston: Boston University African Studies Center, Working Paper No. 30.

Wilson, Francille. 1982. "Reinventing the Past and Circumscribing the Future: *Authenticité* and the Negative Image of Women's Work in Zaire." In *Women and Work in Africa* (153-70), ed. Edna G. Bay. Boulder, CO: Westview Press.

PART V

**Resource Material
for the Study of AIDS in Africa**

RESOURCES ON THE SOCIAL IMPACT OF AIDS IN AFRICA

Nancy J. Schmidt*

The resources discussed and listed in the following pages provide background information on the social impact of AIDS in Africa. It is a working bibliography because there has not been time to conduct exhaustive bibliographic research. The bibliography is divided into two sections: one focuses on social science publications and the other on African press reports. There has been relatively little social science research on AIDS. However, African newspapers and news magazines regularly report on both the social and medical aspects of AIDS.

There are two other bodies of literature about the social impact of AIDS in Africa which are not represented in the following bibliography. Literature on the medical aspects of AIDS is covered by published indexes and bibliographies, as well as the Medlars and Public Health and Tropical Medicine online databases. Social science literature on Africa about marriage, migration, rituals and a host of other social factors that provide the context in which AIDS exists is not easily accessible, although several scholars are currently compiling bibliographies on this literature.

Social Science Publications

Since there has been little social science research on AIDS in Africa, there is relatively little published material on the social impact of AIDS. The literature consists of short articles and letters to editors, primarily on four topics: the public awareness of AIDS in Africa, the political aspects of AIDS in Africa, the epidemiology of AIDS in Africa and pleas for the involvement of social scientists in research on AIDS, including suggestions for the kinds of research needed.

---

*Nancy J. Schmidt , Ph.D., an anthropologist, is African Studies Area Specialist, Indiana University Library, Bloomington, Indiana.

Some of the articles are based on observations by social scientists resident in Africa (e.g. Feldman, 1987 and Klovdahl, 1985). However, most articles are based on secondary published data, primarily that of the World Health Organization. Only the article by Fortin (1987) gives serious consideration to African print media as a source of information.

Articles that plead for the involvement of social scientists in AIDS research, such as that by Herdt (1987) directed to anthropologists, are followed by replies, such as Payne (1987), indicating that research is in process and suggesting the need for coordination of research and the development of networks of researchers engaged in AIDS research. American anthropologists have responded to the need for networking through establishing an AIDS interest group within the American Anthropological Association at its 1987 annual meeting and through a USAID contract project at the Institute for Development Anthropology at SUNY-Binghamton.

Media Reports

African newspapers and news magazines are one source for obtaining information about the social impact of AIDS in Africa from African perspectives. Therefore, a survey was made of the coverage of the social impact of AIDS in Africa in 37 African newspapers and news magazines published in Africa or published in Europe based on first hand reports from Africa. The news sources surveyed are listed at the end of the bibliography. They were selected for their accessibility for regular examination. While they do not represent a systematic survey of Sub-Saharan perspectives, they do reflect African perspectives that should be given attention in social science research in Africa. Although the generalizations that follow are expressed in continental terms, they should be understood to apply only to the countries in which print media were surveyed.

African newspapers initially denied the existence of AIDS in specific countries (e.g., the country in which the newspaper was published). At the same time the newspapers included short articles about AIDS elsewhere in the world, including other countries in Africa. Once deaths from AIDS were recorded in a country, newspapers regularly carried articles about AIDS in the country of publication as well as elsewhere in the world.

African newspapers and news magazines regularly carry articles on health issues and problems including malaria, cholera and infant diarrhea among others. AIDS has been added to the health issues that are regularly discussed, but it has not eclipsed them. Newspapers and news magazines emphasize that far more people die daily from other diseases than AIDS and editorialize that their countries cannot give all their attention to AIDS when there are other diseases that must be dealt with.

African newspapers and news magazines print informative articles aimed at educating the literate public about AIDS. A few newspapers and news magazines have regular columns that provide information about AIDS such as "AIDS Aid" in the *New African*. Most of the articles have straightforward descriptive titles, although a few have such eye-catching titles as "Your Next Sexual Partner Could Be That Very Special Person" (*Voice of SADCC/PTA*) and "AIDS: Express Train to Death" (*New Nigerian*). The articles are all factual in content, often quoting local medical personnel and providing information about the disease and how to avoid contracting it. Photographs of persons with AIDS often accompany magazine articles adding powerful illustrations of the personal impact of AIDS.

A few newspapers have been used as part of the national AIDS information campaign (e.g., Anti-AIDS Campaign, *Herald*). Newspapers and news magazines report on national AIDS campaigns conducted on radio and television, in rural and urban areas and in the national and vernacular languages. Most information campaigns have been directed at adults, but one in Zimbabwe was for secondary school students (e.g., Pupils in Danger of AIDS, *Herald*). The enlistment of Christian and Muslim clergy in AIDS campaigns also is reported, as is the failure of AIDS campaigns. For example, in Nigeria and Zimbabwe the failure of AIDS campaigns was attributed primarily to the difficulty of quickly changing people's attitudes and behavior, and suggestions were made for different approaches needed in AIDS campaigns.

A part of the regular coverage of AIDS is reporting on progress in medical research on AIDS. Research conducted by African doctors is emphasized in this context, and in a few cases differences in perspectives between African and Western scientists have been noted. The extent of testing for AIDS carriers within individual countries also is regularly reported.

Reports in African newspapers and news magazines make it clear that AIDS is a political issue of major importance in three general areas:

First, racism in the attribution of the origin of AIDS to Africa, when AIDS is found throughout the world and is more prevalent in many other parts of the world. Outrage has been expressed at some European press reports about the origin of AIDS, especially the one in France that attributed the origin of AIDS to a man in Zaire sodomizing a green monkey.

Second, racism is found in the expulsion of Africans who test positive for AIDS or the forced testing for the AIDS virus in countries in Europe, Asia and Egypt. In Kenya there was the additional incident of British sailors not being permitted to go ashore. The Kenyan legislature has been especially active in discussing this kind of racism and in lodging protests with the appropriate political authorities.

Third, controlling AIDS within specific African countries is an issue. There are numerous issues involved including what to do about prostitutes, how to allocate AIDS testing equipment within the country, whom to test, how much of the national budget to spend on AIDS relative to other priorities, and whether to enlist external aid and from whom. The World Health Organization is a relatively uncontroversial source of assistance, and articles report on WHO seminars held in various countries. The major political issue over external aid is that African countries want to maintain control over AIDS prevention and treatment and not be dictated to or taken over by foreign groups with their own agendas.

In addition to these political issues news reports indicate other social issues that need further research and solutions. For example, women in Zaire are said to be developing a psychosis related to the fear of sex as a result of the prevalence of AIDS. Villages in some regions of Uganda are being depopulated. In some countries AIDS is affecting young and middle-aged professionals more than other segments of the population, and there has been an increase in the number of orphans because of the death of their parents from AIDS.

Letters to the editors, opinion articles and some news reports indicate confusion and misunderstanding about AIDS. Articles try to sort out facts and fiction about AIDS and alert readers to "scare tactics" regarding AIDS. Some examples of misunderstanding about AIDS include the report in the *Cameroon Outlook* that AIDS is not related to sexual intercourse, the refusal of a few Nigerian athletes to attend the All Africa Games because of the prevalence of AIDS in Nairobi, the belief that having sex with fat women is all right since they cannot have the "slim disease" (the local name for AIDS in parts of Uganda), the belief that AIDS can be contracted from toothbrushes and any blood shedding. The latter belief led to some barbers in Zimbabwe refusing to give shaves. In Nigeria the sales of condoms increased as a result of the AIDS information campaign, but in some areas they were not used because of the belief that anyone using a condom must be an AIDS carrier.

As this summary shows, African newspapers and news magazines provide information about the social impact of AIDS which can be investigated by social science research. However, since the majority of the population of Sub-Saharan Africa is not literate, radio, television and other oral means of communication in vernacular as well as national languages also must be monitored by social scientists as background for their research.

SOCIAL IMPACT OF AIDS IN AFRICA

A Working Bibliography

Introduction

This bibliography covers social science and media reports on the social impact of AIDS in Africa, and a limited number of medical citations, primarily on epidemiology, that refer to the social implications of AIDS. The media sources listed at the end of the bibliography were systematically examined only for articles about AIDS in Africa or for educating Africans about AIDS. Articles about AIDS in other parts of the world that appeared in African newspapers and news magazines have not been included in the bibliography. Because complete runs of African newspapers are not available for examination, the citations from the sources listed at the end of the bibliography cannot be considered exhaustive.

Social Science Publications

Achkar, J. AIDS: Origin in Africa? *The Medic* (Accra) June (1986) 2. (Editorial).

Achkar, J. and J. Appia-Kusi. HLTV III and AIDS. *The Medic* (Accra) June (1986) 20-21.

Acquired immune deficiency syndrome (AIDS). Legislation. Zimbabwe. *Weekly Epidemiological Record* Jan. 17 (1986) 18.

Acquired immunodeficiency syndrome (AIDS). Plan of action for control in the African region. *Weekly Epidemiological Record* Mar. 28 (1986) 93-94.

Acquired immunodeficiency syndrome (AIDS) Global Data. *Weekly Epidemiological Record* (Statistical reports at least monthly from Nov. 1986 include African data.)

Acquired immunodeficiency syndrome. Contraceptive methods and human immunodeficiency virus (HIV). *Weekly Epidemiological Record*. Aug. 14 (1987) 244.

Acquired immunodeficiency syndrome. Meeting of the WHO collaborating centres on AIDS. *Weekly Epidemiological Record* July 24 (1987) 221-23.

Africa: fighting AIDS without resources. *Third World* 9 (1987) 7.

AIDS and the Third World. London Panos Institute, 1987, Chp. 5. Africa: AIDS and the shrinking development dollar.

AIDS update. *Zimbabwe Science News* 21, 9/10 (1987) 129-130.

Barker, Carol and Meredeth Turshen. AIDS in Africa. *Review of African Political Economy* 36 (1986) 51-54.

Biggar, Robert J. The AIDS problem in Africa. *The Lancet* Jan. 11 (1986) 79-82.

Burton, Mike. AIDS and female circumcision. *Science* Mar. 14 (1986) 1236. (Letter).

Butorin, Pavel. AIDS spreads in Africa: an overview. *Development Forum* 14,9 (1986) 4-5.

Chouinard, Amy. AIDS in Africa: a deadly shadow. *IDRC Reports* Jan. (1987) 16-17.

Coker, W.Z. AIDS virus and mosquitoes, in *Medical entomologist's contribution towards health for all by the year 2000*. An inaugural lecture delivered at the University of Ghana, Legon on 17th April, 1986. Accra: Ghana Universities Press 1986. pp. 42-43.

Dickson, David. Africa begins to face up to AIDS. *Science* Oct. 30 (1987) 605-7.

Epstein, P. and R. Packard. Ecology and immunology: the social context of AIDS in Africa. *Science for the People* 19, 1 (1987) 10-19.

Feldman, Douglas. Anthropology AIDS and Africa. *Medical Anthropology Quarterly* 17, 2 (1986) 38-40.

Feldman, Douglas *et al*. Public awareness of AIDS in Rwanda. *Social Science and Medicine* 24,2 (1987) 97-100.

Fortin, Alfred J. The politics of AIDS in Kenya. *Third World Quarterly* 9,3 (1987) 906-19. (Includes citations to medical articles and articles from the media).

Georges, Alain. AIDS in Africa. *World Health Forum* 6,4 (1985) 334.

Gras, Claude, Jean-Claude Cuisinier-Raynal and Pierre Aubry. Le SIDA en Afrique. *Afrique contemporaine* 143 (1987) 21-34.

Herdt, Gilbert. AIDS and anthropology. *Anthropology Today* 3,2 (1987) 1-3.

Hooper, Ed. AIDS hits villages. *Development Forum* 14,9 (1986) 1,4. (Uganda).

Hrdy, Daniel B. Cultural practices contributing to the transmission of human immunodeficiency virus in Africa. *Reviews of Infectious Diseases* 9, 6 (1987) 1109 -19.

Imperato, Pascal J. The epidemiology of the acquired immunodeficiency syndrome in Africa. *New York State Journal of Medicine* Mar. (1986) 118-21.

In the heart of the plague. *Economist* Mar. 21 (1987) 45. (Uganda).

International Symposium on African AIDS, Brussels 22 & 23 November 1985, Programme and Abstracts. Brussels: SDR Associated, 1985. (Esp. relevant: Overview of the AIDS epidemic and its African connection 02/1; Socio-Cultural factors in relation to HTLV-111/LAV transmission in urban areas in Central Africa 05.1; Epidemiological studies of HTLV-111/LAV infections in Southern Africa P05; AIDS virus infection in Nairobi prostitutes: spread of the epidemic to East Africa P4; The spectrum of HTLV-111/LAV infection in gay men in Johannesburg P5).

Isaacs, G. and D. Miller. AIDS: its implications for South African homosexuals and the mediating role of the medical practitioner. *South African Medical Journal* 68, 5 (1985) 327-30.

Kapita, B.M. AIDS in Africa. Paper presented at the Second International Conference on AIDS. Paris, June 23-25, 1986.

Kibedi, Wanume. AIDS: an African viewpoint. *Development Forum* 15,2 (1987) 1,6.

Kingman, Sharon, ed. AIDS monitor: Uganda acts to stem epidemic. *New Scientist* Mar. 19 (1987) 21, (Uganda).

Kitchen, Lynn W. AIDS in Africa: knowns and unknowns. *CSIS African Notes* 74 (July 17, 1987) 1-4.

Klovdahl, A.S. Social networks and the spread of infectious disease: The AIDS example. *Social Science and Medicine* 21, 11 (1985) 1203-16.

Konotey-Ahulu, F.I.D. AIDS in Africa: misinformation and disinformation. *Lancet* 2, 8552 (1987) 206-7.

248

Kreiss, Joan K., *et al.* AIDS virus infection in Nairobi prostitutes. *The New England Journal of Medicine* Feb. 13 (1986) 414-18.

Leishman, K. AIDS and insects. *The Atlantic Monthly* Sept. (1987) 56-72.

Mann, Jonathan M. AIDS in Africa. *New Scientist* Mar. 26 (1987) 40-43.

Mann, Jonathan M. The global AIDS situation. *World Health Statistics Quarterly* 40, 2 (1987) 185-92.

Mann, Jonathan M. Surveillance for AIDS in a central African city. Kinshasa, Zaire. *Journal of the American Medical Association* June 20, (1986) 3255-59.

Neequaye, A.R. *AIDS - fact and fiction.* Accra: Ghana Universities Press, 1986.

Newmark, Peter. AIDS in an African context. *Nature* Dec. 18-25 (1986) 611.

Norman, Colin. Politics and science clash on African AIDS. *Science* Dec. 6 (1985) 1140, 1142.

Padian, Nancy S. Heterosexual transmission of acquired immunodeficiency virus: international perspectives and national projections. *Reviews of Infectious Diseases* 9,5 (1987) 947-60.

Padian, Nancy S. and John Pickering. Female to male transmission of AIDS: a reexamination of the African sex ratio of cases. *Journal of the American Medical Association* Aug. 1 (1986) 590. (Letter).

Payne, Kenneth and Stephen O. Murray. AIDS. *Anthropology Today* 3,2, (1987) 19-20. (Letter responding to Herdt article).

Quinn, Thomas C. *et al.* AIDS in Africa: an epidemiological paradigm. *Science* Nov. 21 (1986) 955-63.

SIDA. L'OMS fait le point. *Famille et développement* 45 (1987) 15-20.

Sida et tiers mode. *Environment africain* 118-19 (1987).

Tinker, John and Renée Sabatier. AIDS the hidden enemy. *Development International* 1, 1 (1987) 22-27.

Uganda acts to stem epidemic. *New Scientist* Mar. 19 (1987) 21.

Warren, D.M. *et al.* Ghanaian national policy toward traditional healers: the case of the Primary Health Training for Indigenous Healers (PRHETIH) program. *Social Science and Medicine* 18 (1984) 374-85.

Media Reports

Abu, Sully. AIDS: Nigerian break-through? *African Guardian* June 18 (1987) 30.

Action at last. *Weekly Review* Jan. 23 (1987) 15.

Adekambi, Jerone. Le SIDA en question. Se serrer les coudes face la maladie. *Fraternité Matin* Apr. 4-5 (1987) 10.

Adesida, E.O. Cure for AIDS. *New Nigerian* Mar. 9 (1987) 4.

Adinoyi-Ojo, Shaibu. AIDS scare saga on as 'victim' heads for Benin. *Guardian* Nov. 20 (1986) 1-2. (Nigeria).

Adinoyi-Ojo, Shaibu. Four-day AIDS scare is a hoax says victim. *Guardian* Nov. 21 (1986) 1-2. (Nigeria).

AFP. Burundi. Le SIDA inquiète: 54 cas déjà! *L'Union* June 10 (1986) 9.

AFP. Neuf états pour une stratégie de lutte contre le syndrome. *L'Union* Oct. 26-27 (1985) 15. (Symposium in Bangui).

AFP. New AIDS plan for Africa announced. *Daily Nation* Mar. 19 (1987) 2.

AFP. Propagation préoccupanté du virus en Afrique centrale? *L'Union* Nov. 22 (1985) 8.

AFP. SIDA on en parle en Afrique. *L'Union* Apr. 28 (1986) 10. (East African countries).

AFP/NAN. AIDS not from Africa. *New Nigerian* Aug. 9 (1987) 6.

Afrani, Mike. AIDS claims 107 victims. *African Concord* 133 (1987) 20. (Ghana).

Africa and the AIDS stigma. *Guardian* Mar. 11 (1987) 8. (Editorial).

African experts asked to find cure for AIDS. *Daily Times* Oct. 15 (1987) 2. (Nigeria).

Africans for AIDS test in Belgium. *Daily Times* Apr. 2 (1987) 3.

Agbabiaka, Tunde. The AIDS pestilence in Africa. *African Concord* 123 (1987) 21-26.

Agbabiaka, Tunde. 'Racist bigotry on AIDS.' *African Concord* 143 (1987) 25. (Uganda).

Ahonto, Lucien. SIDA, un million ou soixante-quinze millions? *Afrique-Asie* 401 (1987) 44.

Ahua, Bernard. Le Ministre Djédjé Mady: le SIDA ne doit pas nous affoler. *Fraternité Matin* Feb. 12 (1987) 2-3. (Côte d'Ivoire).

Ahua, Bernard. SIDA la peur de l'inconnu. *Fraternité Matin* Mar. 18 (1987) 4-5. (Côte d' Ivoire).

Ahua, Bernard. SIDA les enquêtes sérieuses restent à faire. *Fraternité Matin* Apr. 9 (1987) 29.

Ahua, Bernard. SIDA pas de panique, mais... *Fraternité Matin* Apr. 15 (1987) 2-3.

AIDS: Are you at risk? *Moto* 38 (1985) 3.

AIDS: Babangida absolves Africans. *New Nigerian* Sept. 8 (1987) 16.

AIDS: Fear is the cure. *New Nigerian* Sept. 2 (1987) 5.

AIDS: India's policy amounts to racism. *Daily Nation* Mar. 16 (1987) 6. (Editorial).

AIDS: no-one wants to talk. *African Concord* 141 (1987) 20. (Nigeria).

AIDS: 3 students deported. *Daily Nation* Mar. 30 (1987) 2.

AIDS aid. *New African* 236 (May 1987) 24-25. (Zambia protects its babies; Kenya spreads facts, not fear; India's medical apartheid; Rural areas safer than Kampala; Tests for Africa; AIDS reported cases.)

AIDS aid. *New African* 237 (June 1987) 25. (Uganda's death village; New virus discovered; Kaunda knows the danger; Chinese introduce AIDS test).

AIDS aid. *New African* 238 (July 1987) 38. (Nigeria faces up to reality; Uganda prepares to fight AIDS; New campaign financed by UK).

AIDS aid. *New African* 239 (Aug. 1987) 18. (Nigeria investigates harmless variant; Cameroon's one man war; Weeding out Zambian AIDS patients; Kenyan screening machines in place).

AIDS aid. *New African* 240 (Sept. 1987) 32. (Zimbabwe tackles AIDS; Criticism of Nigerian AIDS education; Zambian ban on information for foreign press).

AIDS aid. *New African* 241 (Oct. 1987) 46. (AIDS revelations taken lightly in Tanzania; Zambian dentists make policy; Resistance to Nigerian medics).

AIDS and condoms. *Weekly Review* June 12 (1987) 2-3. (Three letters about AIDS article in May 29th issue).

AIDS carriers live close to our borders. *New Nigerian* May 16 (1987) 13.

AIDS claims 3 more lives. *Daily Times* Aug. 4 (1987) 16. (Nigeria).

AIDS may kill 1m Africans in 10 years. *Herald* Nov. 26 (1986) 1,7.

AIDS not spread by sexual intercourse. *Cameroon Outlook* 17,4 (Dec. 4-11, 1986) 1,4.

AIDS panel members on study tour of East Africa. *Guardian* May 23 (1987) 13.

AIDS panel to organise seminar for journalists. *Daily Times* Oct. 5 (1987) 11. (Nigeria).

AIDS phobia. *African Guardian* May 14 (1987) 25.

AIDS prejudice claim. *Weekly Review* (Nairobi) Apr. 3 (1987) 9-10. (In India).

AIDS questions and answers. *Moto* 53 (1987) 25.

AIDS report. *Africa Research Bulletin, Political Series* 24,4 (1987) 8487-89.

AIDS reported in Kenya. *Guardian* Jan. 21 (1985) 5.

AIDS scare. *Herald* June 7 (1987) 8. (Editorial).

AIDS screening tool functions soon. *Daily Times* Sept. 4 (1987) 10. (Nigeria).

AIDS screening tools soon for all states. *Daily Times* Oct. 14 (1987) 17. (Nigeria).

AIDS spreads in Africa - report. *Daily Nation* May 23 (1987) 2.

AIDS tests rile African students. *Daily Nation* Dec. 15 (1987) 24. (Finland).

AIDS update. *Weekly Review* Mar. 20 (1987) 13-14.

AIDS worldwide, not African problem. *Guardian* Nov. 24 (1986) 5.

Ajayi, Dupe. Egypt seeks AIDS free papers from Nigerians. *Guardian* Mar. 4 (1987) 1-2.

Ajayi, Femi. AIDS: big scare, big politics. *Daily Times* May 6 (1987) 5.

Ajayi, Femi. The problematic war against AIDS. *Daily Times* Apr. 29 (1987) 5.

Ajayi, Iolu. The truth about AIDS. *Daily Times* May 27 (1987) 9.

Akinbami, Gbolahan. Politics of AIDS. *Daily Times* May 28 (1987) 9. (Nigeria).

Akinwande, Olufemi. Kaduna and the AIDS syndrome. *Guardian* Apr. 17 (1986) 11. (Nigeria).

Akinyebo, Toyin. Antidote to spread of AIDS, by Okogie. *Guardian* Mar. 30 (1987) 1-2. (Nigeria).

Allen, Caroline. Killer AIDS sweeps Africa. *Prize Africa* Oct. (1986) 12-13.

Altman, Lawrence K. Is AIDS really an African disease? *Guardian* Nov. 15 (1985) 7. (Culled from International Herald Tribune).

Amurun, Omafume. 2 committees to assess extent of drug abuse. AIDS infection. *New Nigerian* July 4 (1987) 16. (Nigeria).

Andriamirado, Sennen. SIDA avant de mourrir, un congolais a décrit sa longue agonie. *Jeune Afrique Magazine* 41 (Oct. 1987) 82-83.

Anti-AIDS Campaign: Avoiding AIDS. *Herald* July 21 (1987) 5.

Anti-AIDS Campaign: HIV infection in children. *Herald* July 16 (1987) 5.

Anti-AIDS Campaign: Only treatment is prevention. *Herald* July 18 (1987) 5.

Anti-AIDS Campaign: Prevention is main priority. *Herald* July 23 (1987) 11.

Anti-AIDS Campaign: Transmission of HIV virus. *Herald* July 17 (1987) 11.

Anti-AIDS programme: EEC-APC cooperation. *Telex Africa* 297 (Feb. 17, 1987) 17-18.

Anuforo, Emeka. AIDS: the Nigerian connection. *New Nigerian* May 25 (1987) 5.

AP. 14 cases of AIDS reported in SA. *Daily Nation* Dec. 3 (1986) 2.

APS. L'hépatite "B" tue plus que le SIDA. *Le Soleil* Apr. 27 (1987) 8.

Aregbesola, Ayodeji. Living at the mercy of AIDS. *Daily Times* May 28 (1987) 9.

Assi, Amedie. Des recherches sur le SIDA enterprises dans notre pays. *Fraternité Matin* Jan. 19 (1987) 10.

Atenega, Henry. No AIDS in Nigeria? *Daily Times* June 29 (1987) 15.

Attai, Victor. Adverse publicity on AIDS can ruin any country - Dr. Okupe. *New Nigerian* July 28 (1987) 10.

Avance notable dans la découverture d'un medicament contre le SIDA. *Bingo* 413 (1987) 13.

Awotusin, Tayo and Toyin Akinyebo. Ministry to conduct studies on AIDS disease. *Guardian* Oct. 31 (1985) 3. (Nigeria).

Ayo-Thompson, Ajayi. American embassy won't demand AIDS proof from Nigerians. *Guardian* May 8 (1986) 10.

L'AZT combat le SIDA. *Bingo* 406 (1986) 29. (AZT = azidothymidine.)

B.A. SIDA. L'Offensive de l'OMS commence. *Fraternité Matin* Apr. 9 (1987) 28.

Baba, A.M. AIDS: Kenyan fury at press campaign. *African Concord* Feb. 19 (1987) 50.

Baiye, Edwin and Mike Adonu. Stop AIDS with God's word. *Guardian* May 2 (1987) 7. (Nigeria, Uganda).

A baleful shadow, Kenyan Catholic bishops condemn condom use. *Weekly Review* May 29 (1987) 37.

Battling the spread of a deadly virus. *Weekly Review* Jan. 16 (1987) 8-15.

Bazie, Jacques Propper. SIDA entre nous. *Sidwaya* Feb. 13 (1987) 4.

Bey, Faycal. SIDA afin que nul ne meure. *Jeune Afrique* 1381 (1987) 44.

Bey, Faycal. Vaccin anti-SIDA: l'espoir vient du Zaire. *Jeune Afrique* Mar. 25 (1987) 17-18.

Blampain, Rogers. Une attention particulière accordée à l'évolution du SIDA. *L'Union* Nov. 30 - Dec. 1 (1985) 15. (Meeting of OCEAC - Organisation de coordination pour la lutte contre les endémies en Afrique centrale).

Boekkooi, Jaap. Major row between AIDS experts on prevalence of viruses in SA. *Star International Airmail Weekly* Sept. 23 (1987) 8.

Bond, Catherine and Riba Linden. AIDS: race against mounting odds. *South* Apr. (1987) 109-12.

Boscaini, Elio. L'AIDS de Enzo Biage. *Nigrizia* 105,4 (1987) 84.

Carim, Enver and Graham Hancock. AIDS and the nations of the South. *New Internationalist* 169 (1987) 8-9.

Catley-Carlson, Margaret. AIDS: Global action, not global panic. *Afrika* 7-8 (1987) 8.

Chako, Arun. AIDS: Expulsion causes furor. *Daily Nation* Jan. 10 (1987) 24. (India).

Chako, Arun. Kenyan held over AIDS protest march. *Daily Nation* Feb. 28 (1987) 24.

Chimbano, Chola. Zambia panics as AIDS cases run at twenty a week. *Prize Africa* Oct. (1986) 12-13.

Chine, Alain. Quelle relation entre le timbre-poste et le SIDA Fraternité Hebdo May 7 (1987) 38. (Letter).

Chirimuuta, Richard, Rosalind Harrison and Davis Gazi. AIDS, The spread of racism. *West Africa* Feb. 9 (1987) 261-263.

Comité de Redressement de l'Information. A propos du SIDA. *Ehuzu* Mar. 9 (1987) 1. (Benin).

Comparou SIDA à lepra. *Domingo Actualidade* May 10 (1987) 1.

Une conférence à Dakar sur le SIDA. *Bingo* 411 (Apr. 1987) 24-27.

D.W. Genital ulcers, oral contraceptives may increase risk of AIDS; scientists question new anti-viral drug due for clinical trials. *Chronicle of Higher Education* June 10 (1987) 8-9.

Dagunduro, Sehinde. FG sets aside N1.5m to combat AIDS. *New Nigerian* June 23 (1987) 1, 13.

Daily Times Opinion. Public campaign against AIDS. *Daily Times* May 14 (1987) 8.

Dangana, Suleiman. WHO, nurses associations plan comprehensive course on AIDS for nurses. *New Nigerian* May 17 (1987) 4.

Dankoko, Boubacar Samba. SIDA Reponse à Sabou Traore et Mamadou Amath. *Le Soleil* May 7 (1987) 6. (Response to T.V. debate by intern in Urology Clinic).

Denton, Anthony. AIDS: Troop ban remains. *Daily Nation* Jan. 15 (1987) 24.

Denton, Anthony. UK ministries in row over AIDS ban. *Daily Nation* Jan. 14 (1987) 1,28.

Di ro de Lisboa, O cancro é contagioso. *Domingo* June 28 (1987) 11.

Diaw, Far. Le SIDA a nos portes affirment des specialists. *Le Soleil* Apr. 9 (1987) 2. (Senegal).

Diaw, Far. Le SIDA n'est pas une preoccupation majeure en Afrique de l'Ouest. *Le Soleil* Dec. 11 (1986) 3. (Interview with Souleymane Mboup, Director, Laboratoire de Virologie et de Bacteriologie).

Diaw, Far. SIDA on fait le point à Dakar. *Le Soleil* Dec. 5 (1986) 4.

Dickson, Daivd. AIDS: Racist myths, hard facts. *AfricAsia* 41 (1987) 50-53.

Diop, Jean. SIDA ruée vers un vaccin. *Afrique Nouvelle* Mar. 4 (1987) 12-13.

Don gives recipe on AIDS. *Daily Times* July 25 (1987) 2. (Nigeria).

Doudou, Venance. Les ivoiriens face au SIDA entre la capote et la fidélité. *I.D.* 840 (Mar. 15, 1987) 8-9.

Eboh, Camillus. Now that AIDS is here. *New Nigerian* Apr. 16 (1987) 12.

Ellis, Susan. 'Senegal virus' may check AIDS. *New Nigerian* Mar. 8 (1987) 9.

Emenari, Ransom. Govt. plans surveillance group on AIDS. *Guardian* Dec. 5 (1986) 3. (Nigeria).

Emeruwa, John O. AIDS and prostitution in Nigeria. *Daily Times* Apr. 16 (1987) 8.

Enagnon. Qui a peur du SIDA? *Ehuzu* Mar. 2 (1987) 1,8.

Enouan Ezando, Stanislas. SIDA: que d'exagération? *Fraternité Matin* Mar. 14-15 (1987) 21.

Escoffier-Lambiotte. Africa confrontada como SIDA. *Domingo* Mar. 9 (1986) 5.

Everett, Richard. Suspected AIDS carriers avoid police in Senegal. *Herald* May 14 (1987) 4.

Ezeigbo, Edmund. AIDS: fancies and the facts. *Daily Times* May 20 (1987) 9.

Le fils du président Kenneth Kaunda mort du SIDA. *Ehuzu* Oct. 7 (1987) 3. (Zambia).

First AIDS death. *West Africa* May 4 (1987) 885-86. (Nigeria).

4 African nations to get N 50 m for anti-AIDS programmes. *New Nigerian* Aug. 8 (1987) 8. (Ethiopia, Kenya, Uganda, Tanzania)

France ignores AIDS report. *Daily Nation* Feb. 10 (1987) 28. (Kenya).

Gambanga, John. AIDS publicity campaign has long way to go. *Herald* May 22 (1987) 10. (Zimbabwe).

Le gouvernment décide la création d'un laboratoire de depistage du SIDA. *Fraternité Matin* Apr. 9 (1987) 32. (Côte d'Ivoire).

Government to conduct national AIDS survey. *Herald* July 2 (1987) 1. (Zimbabwe).

Griot, Marc. Trafic du sang: le SIDA en prime. *Croissance des jeunes nations* 297 (Sept. 1987) 16-18.

Guetney, Jean-Paul and Faycal Bey. SIDA le maître mot la prevention. *Jeune Afrique* Mar. 18 (1987) 10-16.

Guimaraes, Rui. SIDA em Africa um virus different. *Africa Hoje* 22 (1987) 65,71.

Harden, Blaine. AIDS may replace famine as the continent's worse blight. *Washington Post National Weekly* June 15 (1987) 16-17.

Harden, Blaine. Countries in Africa resent the reports that it all started there. *Washington Post National Weekly* Mar. 30 (1987) 10-11.

Health Minister's meeting (Cairo). *Africa Research Bulletin Political Series* 24, 5 (June 1987) 8520-21.

Herald Correspondant. "All doctors can now test for AIDS" *Herald* July 20 (1987) 5. (Zimbabwe).

Herald Reporter. AIDS campaign taking stock. *Herald* Apr. 22 (1987) 3.

Herald Reporter. AIDS on rise in Africa. *Herald* June 2 (1987) 1.

Herald Reporter - Ziana. New AIDS data show rise of killer disease. *Herald* June 3 (1987) 1. (Zimbabwe).

Hey, Robert P. Conferees hear of spread, but note corrective steps. *Christian Science Monitor* June 3 (1987) 3. (Kenya, Uganda).

Hooper, Ed. AIDS ravaging Africa. *Africa Now* 66 (1986) 34-36.

Hooper, Ed. Le SIDA au village. *Africa International* 190 (1987) 63-64. (Uganda).

IPS. No funds for information. Medical congress in Zimbabwe discusses precautions against AIDS. *Afrika* 7-8 (1987) 9.

IPS. Zambia: church weddings only after AIDS test. *Afrika* 7-8 (1987) 9.

Ibrahim, Abdullahi. How to best cure AIDS. *New Nigerian* Sept. 9 (1987) 4. (Letter).

Igbinoba, Ikpo. AIDS scare threatens games. *Daily Times* May 3 (1987) 20. (All Africa games in Kenya).

Ikhurionam, Ebhohon. WHO chief calls for task force on AIDS. *Guardian* Apr. 10 (1986) 9. (Nigeria).

I'm ignorant says AIDS researcher. *Daily Times* June 4 (1987) 1,12.

Impressed. Article on AIDS commendable. *Sunday News* Mar. 29 (1987) 4. (Comment on letter by Faustin Muntu).

Les insectes africains et le SIDA. *Bingo* 405 (1986) 14-15. (Le SIDA frappe a l'est; Le SIDA et la tuberculose; Un medicament contre le SIDA; 664 morts en Tanzanie).

Interromperam gravides por causa do SIDA. *Domingo* Feb. 16 (1986) 4.

Irabor, Nduka. AIDS: before a cure comes. *Guardian* Mar. 22 (1987) 4.

Jackson, Helen. AIDS victims need acceptance not blame, rejection. *Herald* July 19 (1987) 10-11.

Kaigarula, Wilson. AIDS: mere tip of iceberg. *Sunday News* Oct. 4 (1987) 8.

Kambou, Sansan. SIDA: plus de panique que de mal au Burkina. *Carrefour africain* 980 (1987) 13-14. (Interview with Azara Bamba, Minister of Health).

Kapalala, Novatus. Nani ana AIDS nani hana? *Radi* 1 (Nov. 1985) 29-31.

Karoro, Godfrey. Crise económica dificulta luta contra SIDA. *Africa Hoje* 25 (1987) 43.

Karoro, Godfrey. Religion beats AIDS. *African Concord* 145 (1987) 33. (Somalia).

Kaunda's son died of AIDS. *Daily Times* Oct. 6 (1987) 23. (Zambia).

Kerdellant, Christine. SIDA préservons-nous du mal. *Jeune Afrique* 1373 (Apr. 29, 1987) 50.

Kibedi, Wanume. AIDS: an African Viewpoint. *New Nigerian* Aug. 16 (1987) 12.

KNA. Shun propaganda on AIDS, says Moi. *Daily Nation* Feb. 7 (1987) 1,24.

Kone, Samba. SIDA et tuberculose à Abidjan. *Fraternité Matin* Apr. 9 (1987) 32. (Côte d'Ivoire).

Kpatindé, Francis. SIDA: les enfants aussi. *Jeune Afrique* 1399 (1987) 58-60.

Kuti's Cure. *New Nigerian* Mar. 25 (1987) 5. (Nigeria).

Lead anti-AIDS fight, MPs urged. *Herald* Aug. 21 (1987) 13. (Zimbabwe).

Leo, D.K. AIDS: who are the victims? *Concord Weekly* 29 (Feb. 25, 1985) 40-41.

Let's have the real facts on the AIDS scare. *Daily Nation* Jan. 14 (1987) 6. (Editorial).

Lima-Ayite, Brigid de. AIDS scare: doctors disagree. *Guardian* Nov. 3 (1985) 12. (Nigeria).

Linden, Reba. Medical safari in Kenya. *New Internationalist* 169 (1987) 9-11.

Lingane, Duma. SIDA em Africa. Mais uma preocupacao a somar às existentes. *Domingo* June 14 (1987) 12.

M.S.T. 2000 - SIDA psychose ou réalité. *Bingo* 415 (1987) 15.

Malheiros, José Victor. SIDA Africano: o virus esquecido. *Domingo Actualidade* May 10 (1987) 5.

Martin, Daniel. AIDS hits Africa's professional élites. *Washington Times* Aug. 10 (1987) D3.

Massai, N.A. Media show the way in AIDS campaign. *Daily Nation* Mar. 24 (1987) 14.

Matsiendi, Paul Mbadinga, Claude Massavou and Ngoyo Moussavou Bikoko. SIDA: la psychose. Restons calmes. Menace, mais pas danger. Ignorance et exagération. *L'Union* Nov. 9-10 (1985) 16-17.

Mehta, J.M. No racism in India's AIDS policy. *Daily Nation* Mar. 19 (1987) 7. (Letter).

La meilleure lutte contre le SIDA demeure la prévention. *Ehuzu* July 24 (1987) 4.

Minister advocates research for AIDS diagnosis. *Guardian* Apr. 11 (1986) 7. (Nigeria).

Minister seeks priests' support to battle AIDS. *Guardian* Mar. 27 (1987) 16.

Misser, Francois. Africa not interested in EEC help on AIDS. *New African* 235 (Apr. 1987) 16. (On WHO programs, problem of spread with vaccinations).

Misser, Francois. L'AIDS sono gli altre. *Nigrizia* 105,4 (1987) 22-24. (Review of Panos Dossier).

Misser, Francois. La connection Africana. *Nigrizia* 104,4 (1986) 6-8.

Monkey-eaters 'risk catching AIDS.' *Daily Nation* Feb. 18 (1987) 2.

Morinet, Frédéric. L'Afrique noire et le SIDA. *Aujourd'hui l'Afrique* 33 (1986) 22-23.

Moussavou, Claude and Olivier Mouchetou. SIDA: la psychose. Ignorance et exagération. Terreur et panique. *L'Union* Nov. 16-17 (1985) 19.

Moyo, Dave. Fighting AIDS in Africa. *AfricAsia* 41 (1987) 54-55. (Zambia).

Mpassi-Muba, Auguste. SIDA, l'Afrique bouc emissaire. *Sidwaya* Feb. 4 (1987) 9.

Mshindi, Tom. AIDS: Envoy explains troops ban. *Daily Nation* Jan. 13 (1987) 24.

Mulaki, Gideon. AIDS scare hits tour industry. *Daily Nation* Jan. 12 (1987) 24. (Kenya).

Muntu, Faustin. The costly prolonged agony of AIDS. *Sunday News* Feb. 22 (1987) 4. (Letter).

Munyakho, Dorothy Keveyu. AIDS spread facts, not fear. *African Concord* 134 (1987) 34-35.

Musandu, Obilo, Sakala Ambetsa and Motanya Moture. AIDS tests on Africans unfair. *Daily Nation* Apr. 15 (1987) 7. (India).

NAN. Ministry to verify claim on AIDS cure. *New Nigerian* Aug. 10 (1987) 17.

Ndamba, Jean Louis. SIDA: demain l'apocalypse? *Africa International* 190 (1987) 62-64.

Ndlovu, Saul. AIDS. *Prize Africa* Feb. (1986) 8-9.

Nduati, Samuel and Gideon Mulaki. AIDS: Mabiba hits at Europe's attitude. *Daily Nation* Jan. 16 (1987) 32.

Ngoya Moussavou Bikoko. SIDA: quel danger pour le Gabon? *L'Union* Nov. 5 (1985) 6.

Nguesso flays West for tracing AIDS origin to Africa. *Guardian* May 21 (1987) 5.

Njoku, Amby. AIDS soon in yam and banana. *Daily Times* July 19 (1987) 7.

No AIDS fear at Kenya '87. *Daily Times* May 10 (1987) 19.

Nwosu, Salome Chiduzie. AIDS: self-discipline is the only known prevention as of now. *Daily Times* June 21 (1987) 13.

Nyamora, Pius. From aid to AIDS: MPs tackle itchy problems. *Daily Nation* Dec. 6 (1986) 6.

Ochillo, Sams. Spare the poor carriers of AIDS. *Daily Nation* Feb. 18 (1987) 7.

Odemwingie, Tommy. Kenya: AIDS aside. *Guardian* Mar. 28 (1987) 7.

Odunjo, Lekan. 10,000 persons tested for AIDS. *New Nigerian* Oct. 7 (1987) 9. (Nigeria).

Ogunsade, D. and F. Opadina. Closer look at Gallo's outburst on AIDS. *Daily Times* June 13 (1987) 7. (Response to June 4 article).

Ogunseitan, Seun. AIDS: a cure? *African Guardian* May 21 (1987) 32.

Ogunseitan, Seun. AIDS: Different experts, different views. *Guardian* Dec. 22 (1985) 8.

Ogunseitan, Seun. AIDS cited as cause of 6 deaths at UCH. *Guardian* Dec. 15 (1985) 1,12. (Nigeria).

Ogunseitan, Seun. AIDS viruses found in 86 people by 1984, says report. *Guardian* Apr. 24 (1987) 1-2,17. (Nigeria).

Ogunseitan, Seun. Harmless AIDS virus found in West Africa. *Guardian* Apr. 11 (1987) 1-2.

Ogunseitan, Seun. Malaria and AIDS: an incomparable pair. *Guardian* May 12 (1987) 13.

Ogunseitan, Seun. Nigerian AIDS researcher identifies likely carriers. *Guardian* Jan. 25 (1987) 10.

Ogunseitan, Seun. Two AIDS victims treated at LUTH. *Guardian* Apr. 26 (1987) 1-2. (Nigeria).

Ogunseitan, Seun. Variant of AIDS virus: experts to find out cause of immunity. *Guardian* Mar. 22 (1987) 1,10. (Nigeria).

Okafor, Basil. AIDS: the horrifying fact. *Daily Times* July 19 (1987) 14-15.

Okpara, Dr. Robert A. and Dr. Eka A. Williams. AIDS: African link not proven. *Guardian* Dec. 12 (1985) 9.

Okuleye, Yewande. AIDS: the wages of sin. *Daily Times* Dec. 12 (1987) 9.

Oladepo, Wale and Sam Loco Smith. Nigerians dare AIDS. *Quality* (Ikeja) Sept. (1987) 8-9.

Omoro, Ben. AIDS spread affecting social life. *Daily Nation* Dec. 3 (1986) 15.

Onim, Radiala. AIDS furor. *New African* 234 (Mar. 1987) 25-26.

Ononuju, Ernest U.K. AIDS: Express train to death. *New Nigerian* Mar. 25 (1987) 12 and Apr. 2 (1987) 12.

Onyando, Joseph. The folly of those wild AIDS claims. *Daily Nation* Feb. 6 (1987) 7.

Opebiyi, Aishatu. AIDS: Should I tell? *Guardian* Apr. 21 (1987) 9.

Opebiyi, Aishatu. How to avoid AIDS. *Guardian* Mar. 25. (1987) 9; Mar. 26 (1987) 11.

Orere, Onajomo. AIDS: Panel boss says none in Nigeria. *Guardian* Feb. 18 (1987) 16.

Orere, Onajomo. AIDS, the deadly plague, is not here. *Guardian* Aug. 22 (1986) 1-2. (Nigeria).

Orere, Onajomo. 8 centres to test Nigerians for AIDS. *Guardian* Mar. 26 (1987) 1-2.

Orere, Onajomo. More AIDS testing kits in Lagos soon. *Guardian* Apr. 30 (1987) 24. (Nigeria).

Orere, Onajomo. Panel monitoring spread of AIDS inaugurated. *Guardian* June 25 (1986) 1-2. (Nigeria).

Orere, Onajomo. Panel spells out do's and don'ts on AIDS. *Guardian* Apr. 25 (1987) 1-2.

Orere, Onajomo. 2 women become 'first' AIDS victims. *Guardian* Mar. 18 (1987) 1-2,11. (Nigeria).

Osuntokun, B.O. The occurrence of AIDS. *Guardian* Dec. 28 (1985) 13. (Nigeria).

Ottih, Stella. Solutions to AIDS. *New Nigerian* Aug. 21 (1987) 4.

Oubdd, Dieudonné. Connaître le SIDA pour mieux l'éviter. *Carrefour africain* 1004 (1987) 20-21.

Our Reporter. WHO test for AIDS cure "feat." *Daily Times* Aug. 10 (1987) 28. (Nigeria).

Owuor, Otula. 'Avoid pious attitude towards AIDS.' *African Concord* 139 (May 7, 1987) 31-33. (Kenya).

Owuor, Otula. Don't allow foreign AIDS tests in Kenya. *Daily Nation* Feb. 12 (1987) 15.

Ozoagu, Anene. Foundation proposed for victims of cancer, AIDS. *New Nigerian* Mar. 31 (1987) 11. (Obazee Research Institute, Lagos)

Palaver. *New African* 233 (Feb. 1987) 30. (Includes two short articles: Man claims prayer healed AIDS; Libreville's apostle of AIDS).

PANA/NAN. AIDS: Nguesso disagrees with western nations. *New Nigerian* May 21 (1987) 8.

Pekkanen, John. SIDA a Africa ameacada. *Africa Hoje* 24 (1987) 50-55.

Plan d'urgence francais pour la lutte contre le SIDA en Afrique. *Ehuzu* Mar. 19 (1987) 8.

The Politics of AIDS in Kenya. *Weekly Review* Sept. 4 (1987) 11-13.

Pouyfaucon, Héléne. L'Afrique Centrale livrée au SIDA? *Croissance des jeunes nations* 293 (Apr. 1987) 8-9.

Le Professeur Monékosso favorable à une action concretée contre le SIDA. *Ehuzu* Oct. 2 (1987) 4.

Programme spécial de l'OMS sur le SIDA. *Ehuzu* Oct. 16 (1987) 4. (Benin).

Pupils in danger of AIDS. *Herald* Sept. 3 (1987) 4. (Zimbabwe).

P.W. La lutte contre le SIDA. *Bingo* 410 (1987) 31-33.

Ransome Kuti: 'AIDS is not here.' *Guardian* Dec. 5 (1985) 7. (Nigeria).

RIK. Musicians now sound the AIDS alert. *Daily Nation* Feb. 14 (1987) 15. (Peter Mwambi, Kyanganga Boys and Ngoleni Brothers "Muthelo AIDS, the warning" in Kenya; Hilarion Ngnema in Zaire; The syndrome invented to discourage lovers).

263

Row over anti-AIDS campaiagn. *New Nigerian* June 10 (1987) 8. (Zambia).

Rule, Sheila. Frank talk on AIDS brings praise for Uganda. *New York Times* Nov. 1 (1987) 8.

Runyowa, Dr. P.K. AIDS and Zimbabwe. *Herald* Apr. 23 (1987) 12.

Rustic Realist. Simplify anti-AIDS campaign. *Herald* Aug. 25 (1987) 4. (Zimbabwe).

Ryan, Miriam. AIDS. Branding suspect genes. *South* 83 (1987) 103.

Ryan, Miriam. AIDS virus spreads its tentacles. *South* Feb. (1986) 61-62.

Sarr, S. A propos du SIDA. *Le Soleil* Mar. 7 (1985) 6.

Saxon, Andrew. AIDS jitters for barbers? *Herald* Sept. 27 (1987) 11. (Zimbabwe).

Sense and nonsense on AIDS (Editorial) *West Africa* Feb. 9 (1987) 247.

70 African students held in AIDS protest. *Herald* July 14 (1987) 2.

Sharp increase in AIDS numbers. *Weekly Review* Aug. 7 (1987) 7. (Kenya).

Shilts, Randy. Fear of epidemic in the mud huts. *San Francisco Chronicle* Oct. 5 (1987) A5-A6. (Uganda, Rwanda, Zaire, Tanzania, Zambia).

Shilts, Randy. Uganda in desperate pursuit of runaway AIDS. *San Francisco Chronicle* Oct. 6 (1987) A8-A9.

SIDA: ce que vous ne pouvez plus ignorer. *Jeune Afrique Magazine* (1987) 14-19. (Detailed review of book *Le SIDA en questions* by Francoise-Barré-Sinoussi, J.C. Chermann and Willy Rozenbaum with comments on prevention).

SIDA: epidemie au Zaire. *Bingo* 403 (1986) 7.

SIDA: propagation vertigineuse en Afrique. *Bingo* 418 (Nov. 1987) 17.

"SIDA," a doenca que gerou pânico. *Domingo* Feb. 5 (1984) 10.

SIDA comenca a preocupar Zambia. *Domingo* Jan. 19 (1986) 11.

SIDA comment il tue. *Jeune Afrique Magazine* 41 (Oct. 1987) 78-81.

SIDA disposta a apoiar Mocambique revela o seu director-geral adjunto. *Domingo* Nov. 4 (1984) 2.

SIDA e a medicina. *Domingo* Nov. 25 (1984) 11.

SIDA esta a gerar pânico desenfreado. *Domingo* Apr. 27 (1986) 5.

Le SIDA se propage à grande vitesse en Afrique. *Bingo* 415 (1987) 11. (Uganda)

SIDARAMA. *Le Soleil* Apr. 19-20 (1987) 23. (Senegal, Cameroun, Gabon).

SIDARAMA. Plus de 1000 nouveaux cas. *Le Soleil* May 28-31 (1987) 28. (Les directives de l'OMVS; La Chine barricade; Solidarité Nord-Sud).

Sidley, Pat. Our cure for migrants' AIDS: Kindly go home. *Weekly Mail* Sept. 4-10 (1987) 2. (South Africa).

Sogolo, Godwin. Getting aid from AIDS. *Guardian* May 4 (1987) 11. (Nigeria).

Special health checks on some Africans for AIDS likely in UK. *Guardian* Sept. 22 (1986) 1-2.

Special report on AIDS. *African Concord* Jan. 15 (1987) 21-26.

Special SIDA. *Jeune Afrique Magazine* 34 (Feb. 1987) 82-93.

S.T. Un contraceptif anti SIDA. *Sidwaya* Feb. 11 (1987) 10.

Student deported following false AIDS accusation. *Daily Times* Sept. 9 (1987) 5. (Congo student from China).

Sunday Mail Reporter. Survey reveals poor response to AIDS awareness campaign. *Sunday Mail* Aug. 23 (1987) 1,4. (Zimbabwe).

Taketa, Mari. AIDS scare spurs new laws, fear of foreigners in Asia. *Daily Nation* Apr. 10 (1987) 9.

3 African students in Bulgaria deported over AIDS. *New Nigerian* Mar. 31 (1987) 8.

3 Nigerians die of AIDS. *Daily Nation* Apr. 25 (1987) 2.

Tiendrebeogo, Dr. Hilaire. Le SIDA en question. Gardons la tête froide. *Carrefour africain* 1003 (Sept. 11, 1987) 17-18.

Traore, Bougary M. Origin of AIDS. *West Africa* July 13 (1987) 1350-52.

Ubwani, Zephania. News blackout on AIDS. *African Concord* 138 (1987) 25. (Tanzania, 1st reports 1983).

Uganda: Minister refuses to "shy away" from AIDS. *Africa Now* July (1987) 14.

Ugoh, Vitalis. AIDS: Religious leaders urged to educate followers. *New Nigerian* Mar. 27 (1987) 1, 13.

Ugoh, Vitalis. Suspected AIDS victims healthy. *New Nigerian* Mar. 18 (1987) 3.

Umaru, Richard. AIDS: Scientists in dilemma. *African Guardian* Mar. 12 (1987) 18.

Videhouenou, S. Remise d'un lot de materiel de depistage du SIDA. *Ehuzu* Oct. 19 (1987) 1, 8. (Benin).

WHO gives AIDS top priority. *Daily Times* May 4 (1987) 2.

WHO to help in AIDS, cancer screening. *Daily Times*_Sept. 8 (1987) 13. (Nigeria).

WHO to spend N136m on AIDS. *New Nigerian* May 14 (1987) 1.

WHO's equipment on AIDS arrives. *Daily Times* June 10 (1987) 12. (Nigeria, diagnostic equipment).

Who's afraid of AIDS? *Moto* 43 (1986) 16.

Y. N. Etudiants d'aujourd'hui: la peur du chômage et du SIDA. *Fraternité Matin* Apr. 2 (1987) 2-3. (Côte d'Ivoire).

You could be carrying AIDS. *Moto* 53 (1987) 4.

Your next sexual partner could be that very special person. The Voice of SADCC/PTA 1, 4/5 (1987) 4.

Zambia criticises alien press over AIDS. *Daily Nation* Mar. 21 (1987) 2.

Zambian leader says his son died from AIDS. *Chicago Tribune* Oct. 5 (1987) 12.

Ziana. AIDS outbreak in prisons. *Herald* Aug. 28 (1987) 1. (Zimbabwe).

Ziana. Use religion in combating AIDS. *Herald* Aug. 20 (1987) 7. (Zimbabwe).

Ziana. IPS. Churches in row over AIDS. *Herald* June 10 (1987) 2. (Zambia).

Ziana-AP-Nan-Bopa-Pana. AIDS deaths reported in U.S., Botswana, U.K. *Herald* May 9 (1987) 2.

African Newspapers and News Magazines Consulted

Africa Hoje (Lisbon)

Africa International (Dakar)

Africa Now (London)

African Concord (London)

African Guardian (Lodon)

AfricAsia (Paris)

Afrique-Asie (Paris)

Afrique Nouvelle (Dakar)

Bingo (Dakar)

Cameroon Outlook (Limbe)

Carrefour Africain (Ouagadougou)

Daily Nation (Nairobi)

Daily Times (Lagos)

Domingo (Maputo)

Ehuzu (Cotonou)

Fraternité Hebdo (Abidjan)

Fraternité Matin (Abidjan)

Guardian (Lagos)

Herald (Harare)

I.D. (Abidjan)

Jeune Afrique (Paris)

Jeune Afrique Magazine (Paris)

Moto (Harare)

New African (London)

New Internationalist (London)

New Nigerian (Kaduna)

Nigrizia (Verona)

Prize Africa (Harare)

Sidwaya (Ouagadougou)

Soleil (Dakar)

South (London)

Star International Weekly (Johannesburg)

Sunday News (Dar es Salaam)

Union (Libreville)

Weekly Mail (Johannesburg)

Weekly Review (Nairobi)

West Africa (London)

SEXUALLY-RELATED ILLNESS IN EASTERN AND CENTRAL AFRICA: A SELECTED BIBLIOGRAPHY

Tom Barton, M.D.[*]

SUMMARY: As AIDS is a sexually transmitted disease, it would be expected that many of the people at risk for AIDS will also be those who have been most susceptible to other STD's. The objective of this bibliography is to provide an understanding of sexuality and sexually transmitted diseases in Central East Africa within which information about AIDS can be contextualized. The source articles come from a variety of disciplines and have been thoroughly annotated to facilitate their use as an independent resource where library facilities are limited. This material is excerpted from a book-length bibliography in progress.

Introduction

Other chapters in this book attest to the high levels of public and scientific attention being focused on the biologic origins of AIDS, its current status and potential future course. Information and resources in this chapter are included with the objective of increasing understanding about the context of sexuality and sexually-related illness in Central East Africa where AIDS is most prevalent. This material is part of a larger work in progress, a book-length annotated bibliography of some 2000 references on sexuality and health in sub-Saharan Africa.

There has been little concerted effort to study the full range of sexuality and health in sub-Saharan Africa generally, or Central East Africa specifically. Information about sexual beliefs, behaviors, and related illness conditions is widely scattered. Some material is found in ethnographies of initiation rites and marriage forms and some is to be found in sociologic studies of labor migration, urbanization, and prostitution. Religious and political histories have also occasionally provided some useful information about missionary and colonial influences.

---

[*] Tom Barton, M.D., is currently completing a Ph.D. program in medical anthropology at the University of California (Berkeley and San Francisco). His earlier work included primary health care delivery and primary health care teaching in Botswana and the USA.

The medical literature of sexually transmitted diseases, infertility, and family planning in Africa yields much useful information, within certain limitations. For example, most of the literature is found in poorly distributed regional journals - a situation which compounds the difficulties of serious comparative study in the developing world (Adwok, 1986). Another limitation is the dearth of social information in much of the medical literature. Only a few studies such as those by Dodge, *et al.* (1963), and Bennett (1962) extensively describe the ethnic groups involved in populations with sexually-related illnesses. While such a practice may be defended as culturally sensitive and not stigmatizing particular groups, it limits the usefulness of the data for health educators, policy makers, and other researchers. It becomes difficult to integrate useful information from other bodies of literature, such as anthropology, which can contribute to understanding beliefs and behaviors that affect prevention and treatment.

A further caution concerns the content of the articles as several authors have commented on the frequent unreliability of African data about sexually-related conditions. Verhagen and Germert (1972) point out that official statistics include variable standards of recording, exclusion of data from private practitioners, and computation on the basis of sometimes inaccurate census data. Patient questionnaires/interviews may be skewed by inhibitions about discussing conditions which may be stigmatized or illegal such as prostitution and adultery. Lack of laboratories in rural areas and lack of staff adequately trained in sexually transmitted diseases results in a common pattern of misdiagnosis (Arya and Lawson, 1977)[1]. Too often, almost all cases of urethritis and vaginitis are attributed to gonorrhea, and all genital sores are diagnosed as syphilis. Furthermore, overcrowded clinics and lack of privacy contribute to a situation where cases are sometimes diagnosed and treated only on the basis of a brief history without a physical examination.

Several major trends are observable in this bibliography. Rural areas constitute a huge and important reservoir of sexually transmitted diseases. The average rural population is sufficiently affected by the prevalence of STD's that fertility in many parts of Central East Africa is generally lower than elsewhere in Africa. High levels of antibiotic resistant strains of gonorrhea in both urban and rural areas suggest an active exchange of disease organisms between the two areas. Self-medication is frequently reported, in part because STD's are not believed to be "serious" by many people. The minimizing of "seriousness" seems to contribute to a lack of stigma for STD's, in spite of scientific understanding about its correlation with infertility. Condom use is noted by several authors to be uncommon and considered undesirable by both men and women.

The annotations in this chapter are actually new abstracts, with an emphasis on information of relevance to current studies of AIDS and other sexually-related conditions. Pertinent results and authors' conclusions are extracted for the annotations. The intent is to provide a resource that will be usable with or without access to research libraries. Selection of references has been guided by a desire for information from a wide variety of sources that would help understand current sexual attitudes and practices in East Central Africa. Space has also been the major factor in deciding to include only journal resources and leave out books and monographs.

Bibliography

Adwok, J.A. Urethral strictures at the Kenyatta National Hospital. *East African Medical Hospital* 63, 3 (March 1986) 175-181.

A prospective study conducted with 77 male urethral stricture patients over the course of one year in Nairobi, Kenya. The etiology was post-inflammatory in 71%; which is contrasted to 50% or less in European countries. The duration of time between urethritis and structure symptoms averaged 5 years. Urethritis patients reported that they generally were untreated or did not seek treatment for a long period of time. More than 45% of the post-inflammatory stricture patients gave a history of more than one episode of urethritis. It is suggested that the majority of post-inflammatory strictures are due to gonorrhea; however, the design of this study is not able to confirm this association. Trauma accounted for 27% of this series and iatrogenesis for only 1%. The author indicates that post-prostatectomy patients were not included, contributing to significant under-representation of the iatrogenesis category.

Arya, O.P. Changing patterns in the organization of the venereal diseases
and treponematoses service in Uganda. *British Journal of Venereal
Disease* 49 (1973) 134-137.

Sexually transmitted diseases have been an issue in Uganda since the
earliest medical observations a century ago. Around the turn of the century
chiefs were very conscious of venereal diseases and lent their support to
venereal disease treatment programs. About this time a venereal disease
hospital and a series of rural clinics were constructed. These units later
evolved into the national reference hospital (Mulago Hospital in Kampala)
and the rural network of primary health clinics.

Venereal disease incidence data are reviewed for university students
in Kampala (25% of all male students per year) and VD clinics in Kampala
(2000 cases of early syphilis in 1971). The prevalence of long-term
consequences of venereal diseases are reviewed: female infertility (up to
50% of women in some areas), urethral stricture in males (389 new cases at
Mulago Hospital in 1971), and gonococcal ophthalmia neonatorum ("not
uncommon"). The author discusses the importance of the cultural milieu,
with labor migration, urbanization, and the presence of prostitution as
determining factors for the prevalence of venereal diseases. He also
mentions self-medication with capsules purchased in the marketplace as an
issue.

Arya, O.P. and Bennett, F.J. Venereal disease in an elite group (university
students) in East Africa. *British Journal of Venereal Disease* 43 (1967)
275-279.

A quarter (28%) of all male visits to the student health service during
the previous year at Makerere University in Kampala, Uganda, were for
sexually related conditions. Out of a total student population, 340 students
accounted for 476 attacks of venereal disease. Gonorrhea was the most
common disorder (47% of total VD episodes), followed by non-gonococcal
urethritis (40%). Syphilis and chancroid were seen much less often (6.1%
and 2.3% respectively). The authors note that VD ranks with upper

respiratory conditions and psychoneurosis as the main causes of morbidity in this population.

Incidence data are classified in terms of ethnic origin, age, year in school, marital status, and course of study. There were some gradients in all of these dimensions, but the most significant was year in school. The most affected group was freshmen students, 23% of whom got venereal disease in their first semester at school. This pattern is explained in terms of few female students on campus, the students having to rely on prostitutes and good-time girls from the surrounding town for companionship. Another factor appears to be a combination of immaturity, distance from family and its social rules, and loneliness. Ethnic groups that were less likely to get gonorrhea had more permanent friendships and stronger prohibitions about visiting prostitutes.

Arya, O.P. and Bennett, F.J. VD control: a case study of university students in Uganda. *International Journal of Health Education* 27, 1 (1974) 53-65.

This paper describes a sexual health education program for students at Makerere University, Kampala, Uganda. The basic method of the program included prepared talks, discussion groups, and a pamphlet to be read before the presentations. The behavioral objectives promoted: a) premarital abstinence; b) if sexually active, then limited contacts; c) use of condoms; d) examination for symptoms; e) follow prescribed treatment if disease occurs; f) cooperate to get all relevant partners treated; g) refrain from excessive alcohol in sexually permissive situations; h) avoid self-medication; and i) obtain further information from reliable sources if uncertain about any aspects of sex or VD.

A survey of the program was done soon after the talks, and again with students presenting in the clinic with VD. The survey yielded information about the sexual beliefs and practices of the students. Many students were using self-medication (up to 41% of the males with a history of VD). Condoms were infrequently used; student attitudes about the sheath are included in the article. A number of ineffective beliefs held by students about ways to select "safe" partners are presented, as are student rationalizations for not informing their partners after getting VD (only 10% of students with VD brought their partners in for care). Male student statements about intercourse indicate that some students associate extensive sexual experience with mental health.

A lower percentage of female than male students know that women could have symptomatic venereal disease. More women used precautions before sex than men, and 60% of women students abstain from premarital sex compared to 9% of men.

Arya, O.P.; Taber, S.R.; and Nsanze, H. Gonorrhea and female infertility in rural Uganda. *American Journal of Obstetrics and Gynecology* 138, 7 part 2 (Dec. 1, 1980) 929-932.

Large variations in levels of fertility had been previously recorded in certain districts of Uganda, e.g., Teso with low fertility (crude birth rate of 37/1000) and Ankole with a high fertility (55/1000). In Teso the authors examined 343 women (history, physical exam, and laboratory), and 250 in Ankole. Gonococcal cervicitis and clinical evidence of salpingitis occurred significantly more frequently in the women of Teso (18.3% and 19%, respectively) than in Ankole women (2.4% and 5.9). In both districts almost half the women were in polygamous marriages, less than 10% were single, and about 17% were divorced, separated, or widowed. Though current marital status was not significantly different, the amount of serial marriage was much higher in Teso than in Ankole (32.7% versus 9.6).

The authors note that the prevalence of pelvic inflammatory disease is very different between the two districts and correlates well with the levels of fertility. They also point out the gonococcal infection is common and highly correlated with both PID and infertility. Confirming data is presented on the levels of gonorrhea among the husbands of Teso district; husbands of infertile women versus fertile women showed higher prevalence rates for active gonorrhea (24.5% versus 6.7%), for past history of urethritis (75.5% vs. 57.7%), and for thickened epididymides (18.4% vs. 5.8%). Chlamydia was not studied in this project.

Bennett, F.J. The social determinants of gonorrhea in an East African town. *East African Medical Journal* 39, 6 (June 1962) 332-342.

The author studied 1406 men diagnosed with gonorrhea at the Mulago Hospital in Kampala, Uganda. Half of the men came from the surrounding rural areas as the radius of daily movement extended to nearly 30 miles. Cases are classified by urban or rural residence, tribal origin, and age. Eight cases studies are presented to illustrate common patterns.

Urban prostitution is discussed, including the note that condoms were actively rejected by women in Kampala. The author mentions that until recently the Baganda traditionally attached no stigma to acute gonorrhea. The three main categories of prostitutes in Kampala at the time of the study included Haya women from Tanzania who generally stay in their rooms and charged time-related fees. Their clients were largely single immigrant men, especially members of the Nilotic and Nilo-Hamitic ethnic groups. Next were the more numerous group of beer- and dancehall prostitutes, mainly Ganda, Toro and Ruanda, with some Luo and Teso who kept to their own ethnic groups. The third group were sophisticated Ganda and Toro women who worked the hotels and upper-class bars. Difficulties in differentiating lover relationships, free marriage, concubinage, and good-time girls from prostitutes are mentioned. A small category of homosexual young men catering to European clients was also briefly noted.

Bennett, F.J. The social, cultural, and emotional aspects of sterility in women in Buganda. *Fertility and Sterility* 16, 2 (Mar.-April 1965) 243-251.

This article is based on a series of interviews with 17 female patients who were referred to Mulago Hospital for evaluation of sterility in Kampala, Uganda. Production of a child is important for establishing a Ganda woman's right to qualify as an adult and as an asset for her husband and society. The commonest self-perception about the etiology of sterility was a traditional Ganda disease known as *Ekigalanga*. This illness is characterized by sterility, abdominal pains, weakness, poor vision, and a small, thin voice. The causative factor is thought to be a spirit; herbal medicines are the usual treatment. Other etiologies ascribed by the women were venereal disease and excessive intercourse when young.

Almost all the women had received some form of traditional treatment. All but one woman had obtained some form of Western diagnosis and treatment; many of them had received numerous courses of injections and tablets. Marital histories are presented and document a number of serial marriages, though they may not be higher than the averages for the Baganda as a whole. Two cases histories are presented, and a good table of the consequences of sterility in Buganda. This table lists reactions of patients, husbands, co-wives, and the relatives.

Bewes, P.C. Urethral stricture. *Tropical Doctor* 3 (April 1973) 77-81.

At the time of this report urology clinics were necessary three times per week at the national hospital in Kampala, Uganda, due to the numbers of patients with urethral stricture. Mulago Hospital recorded 1500 new cases of urethral stricture during 1970-1972. The majority of these cases were presumably caused by gonorrhea, some of which was attributed to inadequate dosage of penicillin at hospital clinics in the past. Attempted self-treatment and its consequences are described; some patients attempted self-boundinage with grass stems and aggravated their condition. Presenting symptoms, diagnostic and therapeutic procedures are detailed in the article.

Bhagwandeen, B.S. and Naik, K.G. Granuloma venereum (granuloma inguinale) in Zambia. *East African Medical Journal* 54, 11 (Nov. 1977) 637-642.

Forty cases of granuloma inguinale (or donovanosis) were seen over a three and a half year period in Zambia. This disease is one of low virulence but a confusing clinical picture. It is sometimes mistaken for syphilis in the early stages and malignancy in the later, more developed lesions. The confusion with malignancy is significant in Zambia where cancer of the genital tract is reported to be the commonest cancer in the country. Failure to make the correct diagnosis may result in considerable tissue destruction and mutilation. There was no evidence of geographic clustering, patients being referred from all over the country. Five were men and 35 were women, the males presenting with lesions on the prepuce and the women with a less predictable pattern. The age of only 24 of the patients was recorded, and 46% (11/24) were under the age of 20 years.

Caldwell, John C. and Caldwell, Pat. The demographic evidence for the incidence and cause of abnormally low fertility in tropical Africa. *World Health Statistical Quarterly* 36 (1983) 2-21.

This comprehensive review article provides a thorough analysis of explanatory mechanisms for female sterility (used as a marker for infertile couples) in Sub-Saharan Africa. The limitations of any study in Africa relying on personal reports about stigmatized conditions like fetal loss and sterility is discussed. The major area of high sterility (low fertility) in Africa is centered around upper Zaire. Historical evidence demonstrates the relatively recent course of this development within the last 100 years. Primary sterility is ethnic group-specific and related to different cultural attitudes about adolescent sexual activity. No correlation exists with levels of health care or other indices of mortality.

There is a connection between secondary sterility and prolonged post-partum sexual abstinence. The Central African forest ecology has a limiting effect on the protein adequacy of the mother's diet. In a low-protein situation, the health of the living child is least at risk with a long period of breast feeding. Abstinence thereby reduces the risk of an early conception and its hazards for the child, mother and fetus. Male promiscuity generally increases with prolonged spousal abstinence, with a parallel increase in the risk of bringing home a sexually transmitted disease. Changes in sexual practices with education and urbanization are noted. The authors carefully discuss the various roles of both sexes in introducing and maintaining the levels of sexually transmitted disease (especially gonorrhea) necessary to explain the observed patterns of primary and secondary sterility.

Carty, M.J.; Nzioki, J.M.; and Verhagen, A.R. The role of gonococcus in acute pelvic inflammatory disease in Nairobi. *East African Medical Journal* 49, 5 (May 1972) 376-79.

Fifty-eight consecutive patients admitted with pelvic inflammatory disease were examined and tested for gonorrhea. Half of these women had already received some form of treatment prior to the exam for this research. In spite of the prior treatment cultures were positive for gonorrhea in 43% and the smear was suspect positive in a further 10% of those with negative cultures. This study contributes to the accumulating body of information about salpingitis and gonorrhea as causative factors for infertility in Kenya, as well as suggesting the inadequacy of treatment regimens in the community at that time.

Chhabra, S.C.; Uiso, F.C.; and Mishiu, E.N. Phytochemical screening of Tanzanian medicinal plants. I. *Journal of Ethnopharmacology* 11 (1984) 157-79.

There are four main types of traditional healers in Tanzania: herbalists, herbalists-ritualists, ritualist-herbalists, and spiritualists. Among the herbalists are specialists of different kinds including obstetric and gynocological disorders and traditional birth attendants. Conditions distinguished include gonorrhea, primary and secondary syphilis, and scabies. The vernacular name, family/botanical name, part used, preparation of remedy and medicinal uses are listed for 52 plants. Of these plants, 11 are used in the treatment of gonorrhea, syphilis, genital ulcers, or scrotal swelling. Five other plants have been used as aphrodesiacs. Women's menstrual disorders (dysmenorrhea, menorrhagia, etc.) are treated with six plants, two for female infertility, and one to prevent miscarriage.

Cooper-Poole, B. Prevalence of syphilis in Mbeya, Tanzania - the validity of the VDRL as a screening test. *East African Medical Journal* 63, 10 (Oct. 1986) 646-550.

Testing was done on 6989 sera from people in four groups: antenatal patients (AC), outpatients (OPD), blood donors (BD), and newborns. Positive screening syphilis tests (VDRL) were subsequently checked with the treponemal hemagglutination test (TPHA). Specificity of 94-97.5% was found with the VDRL if retesting was done for weakly positive results. The syphilis rates were: ANC 16.4%, OPD 13.2%, donors 8.6%. The overall syphilis rate for Mbeya town is 15.1%. Rates are compared to Dar es Salaam (ANC 5.2%, OPD 3.7%) and Lusaka where the incidence of congenital syphilis is high. The newborns tested were only ones showing signs of congenital syphilis in the hospital, of which 9 out of 20 were positive.

D'Costa, L.J.; Plummer, F.A.; Bowmer, I.; Fransen, L; Piot, P.; Ronald, A.R.; and Nsanze, H.   Prostitutes are a major reservoir of sexually transmitted disease in Nairobi, Kenya. *Sexually Transmitted Disease* 12, 2 (April-June 1985) 64-67.

Prostitutes from low, middle, and upper socio-economic strata were studied for the prevalence of STDs and their rate of reinfection with gonorrhea after treatment. The mean number of sex partners per day was significantly greater for middle and lower social strata prostitutes (5.0 and 5.6) versus 0.3 for the upper strata. Many women attempted some form of prophylaxis against STDs, such as external cleansing of the genitals or taking antibiotics. Condom use is not mentioned by the authors. Self-care practices apparently did not affect the high levels of STDs; up to 70% of the prostitutes have at least one STD. Social strata was negatively correlated with the prevalence of gonorrhea, which affected 16% of the upper strata, 28% of the middle, and 46% of the lower strata. In a group of 97 lower strata prostitutes followed longitudinally, the mean time to reinfection of gonorrhea after treatment was 12 days. As the authors state, this is an "astounding rate" and highly significant for any kind of STD health care planning.

Dodge, O.G; and Linsell, C.A. Carcinoma of the penis in Uganda and Kenya Africans. *Cancer* 16, 10 (Oct. 1963) 1255-1263.

Cancer of the penis is the most common cancer in African male Ugandans and accounts for 12.2% of all cancers in male patients. Incidence data are presented by district and tribal group. At the time of writing this article, the rate in and around Kampala was 4.7 per 100,000 per year. This was ten times higher then the rate in Norway during a comparable time. The most affected group were the Ganda (52.2% of cancers, 16.5% of the population). Circumcision was not generally practiced in most of Uganda.

The apparent incidence of penile cancer was much less in Kenya where penile cancer accounted for only 1.9% of all male cancers. The majority of cases (63%) occurred in the Luo (14.5% of the population), and only one case came from the largest ethnic group, the Kikuyu. Virtually all male Kikuyu are circumcised; the trend is toward operation in the hospital at a younger age than the former tradition of surgery at late adolescence. The Luo do not practice circumcision, nor do the Turkana, the other Kenyan ethnic group with a relatively high incidence of penile cancer. Brief mention is made of a possible connection to venereal disease rates, especially considering the high prevalence in Uganda of post-infective urethral stricture.

Griffith, H.B. Gonorrhea and fertility in Uganda. *The Eugenics Review* 55, 2 (July 1963) 103-108.

This study was the first to extensively document the correlation between gonorrhea levels and fertility rates in Uganda. Fertility data were drawn from the 1959 census and disease incidence data came from the annual returns for all Government and Mission Hospitals and dispensaries for 1959-1961. In the least fertile districts half the women have become sterile by the age of 30 years. Griffith includes a good table of the results with data broken out by district and sub-district. The Teso sub-district had the lowest fertility at 115 births per 1000 women of reproductive age, and the highest incidence rate of gonorrhea at 50.1% of all men in the sexually most active years (age 15-34). Kigezi subdistrict had the highest fertility rate (431/1000 reproductive age women) and the lowest gonorrhea rate (1.0% of sexually active age men). The author notes that the Baganda do not seem to attach any stigma to venereal disease. As a historical footnote, he relates a hit of folklore about gonorrhea in Uganda. After the Baganda king, Mutesa the First, contracted gonorrhea in the 1870's, men with gonorrhea were known as "Amazira" or the "Brave Ones." Griffith wonders if some of the same attitude is still prevalent.

Hautvast, J.G.A.J. and Hautvast-Mertens, M.L.J.   Analysis of a Bantu medical system: a Nyakyusa case-study (Tanzania). *Tropical and Geographical Medicine 24* (1972) 406-414.

Among the Nyakyusa the profession of medicine is usually learned in dreams from an ancestral spirit.   Traditional healers are concerned with explaining the cause of illnesses, as well as their treatment.   Diseases are distinguished into the following categories: diseases caused by a supernatural being (disease of god), witchcraft, and sorcery.   Physical examinations are seldom performed, though female healers sometimes make a vaginal examination in cases of infertility.   Home care and family involvement in decisions about the care of the sick family member are presented.   Specific diseases recognized and treated include syphilis and infertility.   Formerly autopsies were performed on the newly dead, at which time a condition compatible with pelvic inflammatory disease was one of the lesions distinguished.   Ascites was attributed to illicit sexual intercourse; and a distended gall bladder to the patient taking too many kinds of traditional medicine that counteracted one another.

Hira, P.R.   Observations on *Trichomonas vaginalis* infections in Zambia. *Journal of Hygiene, Epidemiology, Microbiology, and Immunology* 21, 2, (1977) 215-224.

The sample population in this study was drawn from the clinics and wards of the University Teaching Hospital in Lusaka, Zambia.   Of the prenatal patients, 38.5% were positive on culture or microscopy for trichomonas, the highest percentage occurring in the youngest age group (15-19 year old, 53.6% positive).   Similar results were noted in the gynaecology clinic patients, (31.4% positive), and the highest concentration in adolescents (57.8%).   General outpatients were screened only with urine microscopy; males showed 4.8% with trichomonas, females with 8.2%.   Similar screening of inpatients showed males with 2.3% positive, and females with 7.5%.

Asymptomatic and symptomatic cases were noted in the study, dysuria and abdominal pain are the most common presenting symptoms. The primary mode of passage is sexual, but other potential mechanisms are discussed. A brief discussion of urethritis due to schistosomes also is included.

Hira, S.K.; Ratnam, A.V.; Sehgal, D.; Bhat, G.J.; Chintu, C.; and Mulenga, R.C. Congenital syphilis in Lusaka - I. Incidence in a general nursery ward. *East African Medical Journal* 59, 4 (April, 1982) 241-246.

Screening was done for syphilis on 233 consecutive infants under 3 months of age who were admitted to the University Teaching Hospital in Lusaka, Zambia. Congenital syphilis was presumed for 20 infants who had positive serologies. The clinical picture showed hepatosplenomegaly in 90%, pallor in 50%, and skin lesions in 40%. X-rays of the long bones showed periosteal changes in all 20 infants. Congenital syphilis ranked fourth in total mortality at 6 deaths (after respiratory infections 20, tetanus 18, and septicemia 8 out of 65 total deaths) and fourth in mortality rate or lethality per diagnosis at 30% (after tetanus 81.9%, meningitis 50%, and septicemia 47.1%).

The mothers of the infants with congenital syphilis are profiled: low socioeconomic status and multiparity were noted in 89% and home delivery in 56%. Inadequate prenatal care was also mentioned. The authors believe that the high incidence of congenital syphilis confirms that there is a very large reservoir of infection due to unidentified infections as well as delayed diagnoses. It is suggested that increased promiscuity among men during their wives' pregnancies may increase the maternal risk of acquired venereal infection in the prenatal period. They also point out that a high index of suspicion is needed to uncover congenital syphilis in the sick child under 6 months of age because of the high number of home deliveries, frequent lack of antenatal care, variable clinical picture, and high mortality rate.

Hopcraft, M.; Verhagen, A.R.; Ngigi, S.; and Haga, A.C.A. Genital infections in developing countries: experience in a family planning clinic. *Bulletin of the World Health Organization* 48 (1973) 581-586.

Female genital infections with candida, trichomonas, and gonorrhea were investigated at clinics in Nairobi, Kenya. The authors had observed that women or their health care providers frequently blamed contraceptives for physical symptoms without considering the possibility of venereal disease. The study population was composed of 200 urban women divided into groups of 50 according to marital status and contraceptive history. Fewer than half of the women (46%) had no infections, 40% had 1, 12% had 2, and 2% had all 3 infections. Candidiasis was found most often (27.5%), with the highest rates in women using hormonal contraceptives. Trichomonas was next (26%), and both trichomonas and candida were slightly elevated in women who had gonorrhea. Gonorrhea was found in 17.5% of all urban subjects and was more common in the unmarried.

Another 50 women presenting for the first time at a rural family planning center also were studied for comparison. In the rural group at Kiambu, gonorrhea was found in 14%. The authors felt this was important since this area of the country reports few cases of gonorrhea and the majority of these women were stable, married agricultural workers.

In follow-up interviews, most women were unable to name a specific adverse effect of venereal diseases. Only one woman mentioned condoms as a preventive for venereal disease. Treatment is rarely sought, probably because of minimal symptoms for many women. Social factors such as distance to travel for care, cost, and embarrassment about a stigmatized condition may also intervene. The author stresses that an important finding of this study is that the rate of infection between women using contraceptives and the new clinic attenders is very similar, indicating that women are not becoming more promiscuous as a result of the availability of contraceptives.

Kibukamusoke, J.W. Venereal disease in East Africa. *Transactions of the Royal Society of Tropical Medicine and Hygiene* 59, 6 (Nov. 1965) 642-648.

A thousand consecutive venereal disease patients of the urban Mulago Hospital in Kampala were studied. Acute gonorrhea accounted for 54%, urethral stricture 9%, and other late gonorrheal manifestations 3%. Ten percent of the patients had chancroid, 4% had primary syphilis, 4% had nonspecific urethritis, and another 4% had lymphogranuloma venereum. Genital neurosis was noted in 5%, especially manifesting as anxiety and impotence. The high numbers of urethral stricture patients are related to the history of gonorrhea in Uganda. Apparently the disease arrived in the Buganda region some 20 years before it reached the Eastern Region. Female sterility is also purportedly high in that area, 31% of women over the age of 45 have never had a living child.

In a section on the social background of venereal disease in Uganda, the author mentions a legend which says that gonorrhea was introduced to the country and the Ganda by Arab slave traders. The reiging king was said to have acquired the disease and, in order to remove the stigma associated with it, proclaimed that "he who was without gonorrhea was impotent." Current Ganda attitudes and behaviour in relation to sex and venereal disease, in the author's opinion, may be tied to that past.

Laurie, William. A pilot scheme of venereal disease control in East Africa. *British Journal of Venereal Disease* 34 (1958) 16-21.

The author notes that venereal diseases were second only to malaria as a cause of ill-health in East Africa during 1950. Some history of sexually transmitted diseases in East Africa is given, mostly about syphilis. The focus of this particular study are the Bahaya of Bukoba District in Tanganyika. They were studied because of fertility rates that were much lower than average for the East African region and venereal diseases that were very common in an earlier prevalence study (gonorrhea "very high" and syphilis 15%).

The research study population was non-random, representing a self-selected group of venereal disease patients who consented to the exams. Thirty percent of 1,017 males were syphilitic. Sixteen percent had both syphilis and gonorrhea, and 46% had only gonorrhea. Chancroid and urethritis composed the remainder. Nineteen percent of females had gonorrhea, 6% had syphilis and gonorrhea, and 55% had syphilis (mostly by serology). The rural/urban dimensions of the population are not discussed. Prostitution (not defined) was noted to be common, even in rural areas.

Mandara, N.A.; Takulia, S.; Kanyawana, J.; and Mhalu, F. Symptomatic gonorrhea in women attending Family Planning Clinics in Dar es Salaam, Tanzania: results of a pilot study. *Tropical and Geographical Medicine* 32 (1980) 329-332.

Family Planning Clinics evaluate and treat infertile women as well as those seeking help with family spacing. From this population, the authors obtained a random sample of 405 women (341 for family planning, 64 for infertility). A total of 7.1% were positive for gonorrhea, 7.6% of the FP women and 4.7% of the infertile patients, none of whom was symptomatic. Of the positive cases (29), twenty showed up for treatment. Only four of their male partners subsequently came in for treatment. Costs are calculated for the evaluation and laboratory per individual and for the country as a whole (no calculation for treatment cost). Also noted is a prevalence rate of 3% positive syphilis serologies in Dar es Salaam, but no information is given about the population studied.

Meheus, A.; Delgadillo, R; Widy-Wirski, R.; and Piot, P. *Chlamydial ophthalmia neonatorum* in Central Africa. *Lancet* ii (Oct. 16, 1982) 882.

All babies seen at a maternal and child health clinic in Bangui, Central African Republic, were carefully examined for conjunctivitis. Of the 27 found to have conjunctivitis (278 examined) the average age was 14 days (range 7-30). Gonorrhea was found in 26%, chlamydia in 19% and there were no combined infections. At a minimum, this suggests at least a 5% STD infection rate in the mothers, if the risk of spread by other means is considered small. Concern is expressed about the gonorrhea prevalence rates considering the frequency of penicillinase producing gonorrhea (PPNG) in Africa (up to 50% of gonorrheal strains in Nigeria are PPNG's). Prenatal screening and case-finding capabilities of developing countries like the Central African Republic are limited, but prophylaxis with silver nitrate is still considered effective and encouraged.

Mirza, N.B.; Nsanze, H; D'Costa, L.J.; and Piot, P. Microbiology of vaginal discharge in Nairobi, Kenya. *British Journal of Venereal Disease* 59 (1983) 186-188.

During a two week period in 1982, research was conducted with 122 consecutive women patients who presented at an urban STD clinic complaining of vaginal discharge. Gonorrhea was cultured in 32 (26%), most frequently in women under 20 years of age (13%). Gardnerella was present in 75%, genital mycoplasmas in 47%, trichomonas in 34%, and candida in 24%. Chlamydia was found in only 7%. A quarter of the women had two or more organisms present. The low prevalence of chlamydia is surprising to the authors considering the high rate of gonorrhea. Serologic evidence from various groups of women in Nairobi showed that 90% of these urban women had antichlamydial antibodies, indicating that these infections are actually quite common in this population.

Piot, P.; van Dyck, E.; Colarert, J; Ursi, J-P; Bosmans, E.; and Meheus, A. Antibiotic susceptibility of Neisseria gonorrhea strains for Europe and Africa. *Antimicrobial Agents and Chemotherapy* 15, 4 (Apr. 1979) 535-539.

Antibiotics were tested against 268 gonorrheal strains from Belgium, rural Rwanda, Swaziland, and urban Zaire. While 46% of 54 Swazi strains show relative resistance to penicillin, 85% of 41 Rwandan strains demonstrated a comparable level of resistance. Only five strains were tested from Zaire and all demonstrated a very high level of penicillin resistance. Widespread inadequate therapy and self-treatment with antibiotics from the marketplace are mentioned as possible contributing factors to the selection of resistant strains. The authors also believe that an important finding in this research is the amount of regional variation in resistance within Africa; the developing world is non-uniform and should not be overly aggregated.

Plummer, F.A.; D'Costa, L.J.; Nsanze, H.; Karasira, P.; MacLean, I.W.; Piot, P.; and Ronald, A.R. Clinical and microbiologic studies of genital ulcers in Kenyan women. *Sexually Transmitted Diseases* 12, 4 (Oct.-Dec. 1985) 193-197.

A study of 89 women attending a sexually transmitted disease clinic in Nairobi, Kenya, for treatment of genital ulcers. The clinic population is representative of the urban poor. Eligibility criteria were the presence of genital ulcers, no antibiotics in the prior week, and a willingness to be rechecked. All of the women were carefully examined and a clinical diagnosis was made at the initial visit before any laboratory test results were available. It was found that the value of the clinical diagnosis had distinct limitations; it was completely correct for only 60% of the women (the methods protocol unfortunately does not list the qualifications nor the number of examiners making the diagnoses). In one-third of the women, no microbiologic diagnosis could be found. The clinical picture for these women was compatible with chancroid and their lesions responded to therapy effective for H. Ducreyi.

Chancroid was the most frequent provable cause (48%); next was secondary syphilis (9%). Primary syphilis was quite rare, a situation attributed to unobserved and painless primary lesions occurring on the internal genitalia in women patients. Clinical findings which were the most reliable in differentiating chancroid and secondary syphilis were ulcer depth (excavated versus raised) and undermining of the edge. Distribution, induration, tenderness, and purulence were of little value, contrary to classical clinical descriptions.

Ratnam, A.V.; Din, S.N; Hira, S.K; Bhat, G.J.; Wacha, D.S.O.; Rukmini, A.; and Mulenga, R.C. Syphilis in pregnant women in Zambia. *British Journal of Venereal Disease* 58 (1982) 355-358.

During the five years prior to the publication of this paper, venereal syphilis was found to be quite common while no non-venereal syphilis was seen in over 60,000 patients at the dermatovenereology department of the University Teaching Hospital in Lusaka, Zambia. Preliminary studies found that 17.9% of women attending antenatal clinics had positive serologies for syphilis. Among infants under 3 months of age admitted to the hospital for any cause, congenital syphilis was also common (8.6%). The current research screened 202 antenatal patients, 340 pregnant women admitted for miscarriage or still birth, and 469 consecutive babies delivered at the hospital. Initial syphilis screening used the rapid plasma reagin test (RPR); positives were further evaluated with the Treponema pallidum hemagglutination test (TPHA). Confirmed positive syphilis serologies accounted for 12.5% of antenatal patients, 42% of women who aborted in the later half of pregnancy, and 6.5% of births (2 were stillborn and only 4 showed clinical signs of syphilis at birth). In all pediatric cases the blood samples from the mother were also positive.

The discussion emphasizes the need for more adequate screening and therapy of syphilis in African countries. The absence of significant differences in age, education, parity, and socioeconomic factors between women with positive and negative serologies points to a general lack of public awareness of the problem. Comparisons are made to the prevalence of prenatal and congenital syphilis in the pre-antibiotic era of the developed world in spite of the antibiotic availability and medical capabilities in Africa.

Ratnam, A.V.; Patel, M.I.; Mulenga, R.C.; and Hira, S.K. Penicillinase-producing gonococcal strains in Zambia. *British Journal of Venereal Disease* 58 (1982) 29-31.

In 1982, the majority of gonococcal strains in Lusaka, Zambia were at least partially resistant to penicillin. The authors attribute this pattern to the widespread inadequate treatment of gonorrhea with low penicillin dosages and long-acting forms. Self-medication with antibiotics from the marketplace is very common. Another factor may be free medications at clinics; which may contribute to a pattern of care providers tending to overprescribe antibiotics for minor conditions. All of these factors contribute to the selection of antibiotic-resistant gonorrheal strains. Penicillinase-producing strains of gonorrhea accounted for a third of all treatment failures (9/27 failures in 310 cases), though PPNG only represented 3.2% of 233 gonorrheal strains tested in Lusaka at the time of the article. The authors express concern about the developing trend toward absolute penicillin resistance since gonorrhea is so prevalent in Africa, alternatives to penicillin are so costly, and venereal disease programs have had such limited effect.

Verhagen, R. and Gemert, W. Social and epidemiological determinants of gonorrhea in an East African country. *British Journal of Venereal Disease* 48 (1972) 277-286.

Patients were drawn from a series of clinics in cities (Nairobi and Mombasa), provincial towns (Kisumu and Kericho), and rural areas (Kitui and Machakos). One of two clinics in Mombasa was specifically for prostitutes; all the others were for the general public. All those presenting with a history or exam suggestive of gonorrhea were investigated. Controls were obtained from other patients at the clinics. Gonorrhea was common in both urban and rural clinics. The most significant social factor correlated with gonorrheal disease was frequency of co-habitation with spouse; in cities less than half the male controls lived with their wives, compared to less than a quarter of the male VD patients.

Questions about extramarital intercourse showed that 95% of men with gonorrhea had extramarital sex during the fortnight before symptoms occurred and that half of those had four or more partners. The same figures for women with gonorrhea were 54% and 35%, respectively. Men sharing a regular life with their spouse were least likely to be involved with multiple partners outside of their marriage; 19% admitted such numerous extramarital contacts. Among women over 20 with VD most of the unmarried women had multiple partners, 10% of married women admitted extramarital sex with a single partner, and only 1% of married women had been with multiple partners.

In this set of interviews prostitution was defined as a short relationship in exchange for payment in cash or kind. Three quarters of the male gonorrhea patients had been with prostitutes, and a third of the women with gonorrhea acknowledged part or full-time prostitution. Characteristics of the prostitutes are described and it is noted that they were also present in rural areas. The historical influence of male labor migration is discussed as a determining factor in the pattern of gonorrhea in Kenya. The authors strongly caution against a perception of indiscriminate promiscuity in the community, ostracism of prostitutes or blaming a particular ethnic group.

Verhagen, A.R.; van der Ham, M; Heimans, A.L.; Kranendonk, O.; and Maina, A.N. Diminished antibiotic sensitivity of Neisseria gonorrhea in urban and rural areas in Kenya. *Bulletin of the World Health Organization* 45 (1971) 707-717.

Eight urban and rural clinics in Kenya yielded the 1,703 cases of suspected gonorrhea that were investigated in this study. Sensitivity tests were performed on 736 of the 902 positive cases. The authors found that over a half of gonorrheal strains showed relative resistance to penicillin and streptomycin in rural areas; in fact it was more common in rural than urban areas. The high rate of relative resistance in the average rural population means that the reservoir of resistant organisms is enormous - 90% of the country's population is rural.

It is noted that providers usually blamed the patients for treatment failures instead of considering resistant organisms, claiming that it was due to irresponsible promiscuity and reinfection. The failure of Kenyan clinics, even VD clinics to use adequate therapy is also pointed out as a contributing factor. Limits to adequate therapy are mentioned: time constraints on the busy practitioners, few laboratory services, and the cost of drugs, especially the ones needed to overcome increasingly resistant organisms.

Willis, R.G. Pollution and paradigms. *MAN* 7, 3 (Sept. 1972) 369-378.

This paper is a study of the causation of disease among the Fipa of south-western Tanzania. The author distinguishes social and "scientific" paradigms for illness. The social, or lay, paradigm emphasizes the willful contamination of food and drink by sorcery, a pollution of the sociability norms. The scientific, or healer, paradigm stresses disturbances of social relations manifesting as intrusions of ancestral spirits, territorial spirits or sorcery. It is pointed out that there is more congruence of social and scientific paradigms in Africa than the incongruence commonly noted in the West. Within Fipa symbolism, the loins and genitals are considered powerful but morally inferior. They are also thought to be the metaphoric equivalent of the wild bush. The intellect is correlated to the village. Properly the intellect should dominate the loins and genitals.

In a classificatory scale of illness danger, gonorrhea and syphilis are negligible to mild, roughly comparable to epilepsy, rheumatism and skin disease. Serious diseases include those that affect the middle and lower trunk, that are felt to be inside the body and those that are persistent. Among the really dangerous diseases is "incila", a condition due to contact with someone who has had clandestine adulterous sexual relations. The most vulnerable persons are the spouses of the adulterous partners. The explanation is the sexual pollution attacks the intellect, the center of one's being, and happens due to a lack of control over one's partner in a conjugal relationship. Ritual sex and masturbation and the kinds of pollution they are supposed to combat are described. In discussing traditional forms of therapy the author notes the frequent use of herbs and scarification.

BEHAVIORAL AND SOCIAL SCIENCE PAPERS ON AFRICA
from the
THIRD INTERNATIONAL CONFERENCE ON AIDS

A Selected Bibilography

Shelley Crandall*

The Third International Conference on AIDS was held June 1-5, 1987 in Washington, DC, under the sponsorship of the World Health Organization and the U.S. Public Health Service. The purpose of the conference, which included more than 1,000 papers, was to review and exchange information on AIDS; topics ranged from fundamental biological aspects of the disease, through issues of epidemiology and testing to those of public health, psychology, prevention and control. Relatively few papers were given by social scientists, particularly from the point of view of economic and cultural impact. **

Education, Prevention, Evaluation

Colebunders, Robert L.; A. Greenberg; P. Nguyen-Dinh; K. Ndoko; I. Lebughe; P. Piot *et al.* "Evaluation of a Clinical Case Definition of Pediatric AIDS in Africa." Projet SIDA, Kinshasa, Zaire.

De Cock, Kevin M.; R. Colebunders; N. Nzilambi; H. Francis; P. Piot; J.B. McCormick *et al.* "Evaluation of the WHO Case Definition of AIDS in Rural Zaire." Division of Viral Diseases, Centers for Disease Control, Atlanta, GA, USA.

---

* **Shelley Crandall,** a graduate of Carnegie-Mellon University, is a staff assistant to the Social Science Research Council, New York.
** While it is expected that most papers will be published, readers wishing to obtain advance copies may write to the first-named author at the institution given in the reference. Abstracts prepared for the conference may be consulted for further information. The Conference Secretariat, Fogarty International Center, Building 38A, Room B2N13, National Institute of Health, Bethesda, MD 20892, USA.

294

Lwegaba, A.M.T., Project Manager. "Use of Condoms for the Control of AIDS: a cross-section in Rikai District, Uganda." Uganda AIDS Programme, Kampala.

Ngugi, Elizabeth N.; F.A. Plummer; D.W. Cameron; M. Bosire; J.O. Ndinya-Achola et al. "Effect of an AIDS Education Program on Increasing Condom Use in a Cohort of Nairobi Prostitutes." Kenya Medical Research Institute, Nairobi, Kenya.

Worthington, George Marshall; L. de la Macorra; V. Prieto. "The Application of Social Marketing Principles to AIDS Prevention and Education Programs: implications and considerations drawn from a worldwide survey." Worthington and Associates Worldwide, New York, NY, USA.

Epidemiology

Allaire, J.M.; S. Chamaret; S. Farris; M. Barbier; A. Gindo; L. Montagnier et al. "Seroepidemiologic Evidence of HIV-2 Infection in Mali and Other West African Countries and of its Heterosexual Transmission." Unite d'Oncologie Virale, Institut Pasteur, Paris, France.

Antunes, F.; M.O.D. Ferreira; M.H. Lourenco; C. Costa; M. Pedro. "HIV Infections in Rural Areas of West Africa (Guinea-Bissau)." Institutio de Higiene e Medicina Tropical, Faculdade de Medicina de Lisboa, Lisbon, Spain.

Archibald, David W.; M. Essex; J. Sauk; M. Mann; H. Francis; T.C. Quinn et al. "Antibodies to HIV in Cervical and Oral Secretions of Female Prostitutes in Zaire." University of Maryland Dental School, Baltimore, MD, USA.

Ayehunie, Seyoum; S. Britton; T. Yemane-Berhan; T. Fehniger. "Prevalence of Human Immunodeficiency Virus (HIV) Antibodies in Prostitutes and their Clients in Addis Ababa, Ethiopia." Department of Biology, Addis Ababa University, Addis Ababa.

295

Barin, F.; A. Baillou; E. Petat; G. Guerois; P. Choutet; A. Goudeau *et al.* "HIV Antigenemia in Patients with AIDS or Related Disorders: a study in European and Central African populations." Laboratoire Virologie, CHU Bretonneau, Tours, France.

Bottiger, B.; I. Berggren; L.J. D'Costa; M. Marlene; L. Luzia; G. Biberfield. "Prevalence of HIV and HTLV-IV Infections in Angola." National Bacteriological Laboratory and Danderyds Hospital, Stockholm, Sweden.

Braddick, Michael; J.K. Kreiss; T.C. Quinn; J.O. Ndina-Achola; G. Vercauteren; F.A. Plummer *et al.* "Congenital Transmission of HIV in Nairobi, Kenya." University of Nairobi, Kenya.

Brink, Brian A.; R. Sher; L. Clausen. "HIV Antibody Prevalence in Migrant Mineworkers in South Africa during 1986." Chamber of Mines of South Africa, Johannesburg, South Africa.

Cameron, D. William; F.A. Plummer; J.H. Simonsen; J.O. Ndinha-Achola; L.J. D'Costa; P. Piot *et al.* "Female to Male Heterosexual Transmission of HIV Infection in Nairobi." University of Manitoba, Winnipeg, Manitoba, Canada.

De Cock, Kevin M.; N. Nzilambi; D. Forhal; R.W. Ryder; P. Piot; J.B. McCormick *et al.* "Stability of HIV Infection Prevalence Over 10 Years in a Rural Population of Zaire." Division of Viral Diseases, Centers for Disease Control, Atlanta, GA, USA.

De Lalla, F.; M. Galli; F. Ciantia; P.L. Zeli; G. Rizzardini; A. Saracco *et al.* "Rapid Spread of HIV Infection in a Rural District in North Uganda." Infectious Diseases Department, St. Anna Hospital, Como, Italy.

Delaporte, Eric; M.C. Dazza; S. Wain-Hobson; F. Brun-Vezinet; B. Larouze; A.G. Saimot *et al.* "HIV-Related Viruses in Pregnant Women in Gabon." CIRMF, Gabon.

Durand, J.P.; M. Merlin; R. Josse; G. Garrigue; L.K. Noche *et al.* "AIDS Survey in Cameroon." Centre Pasteur du Cameroun, B.P. 1274, Yaounde, Cameroon.

Fultz, Patricia N.; W.M. Switzer; C.A. Schable; R.C. Desrosiers; D. Silva; J.B. McCormick. "Serologic Evidence for Infection by HIV-2 in Guinea-Bissau in 1980." AIDS Program, Center for Infectious Diseases, Centers for Disease Control, Atlanta, GA, USA.

Gonzales, Jean P.; S.B. Etchebes; C.C. Mathiot; M.C. Georges-Courbot; A.J. Georges. "Malnutrition and HIV Antibody Prevalence in the Central African Republic." Institut Francais pour Recherche Scientifique pour le Developpement en Cooperation, ORSTROM, Bangui, Central African Republic.

Greenberg, Alan E.; P. Nguyen-Dinh; J.M. Mann; N. Kabote; R.L. Colebunders; T.C. Quinn *et al.* "The Association between HIV Seropositivity, Blood Transfusions, and Malaria in a Pediatric Population in Kinshasha, Zaire." Malaria Branch, Centers for Disease Control, Atlanta, GA, USA.

Gurtler, Lutz G.; G. Zoulek; G. Frosner; F. Deinhardt *et al.* "Prevalence of HIV-1 and HIV-2 Antibodies in a Selected Malawian Population." Max von Pettenkofer Institute, University of Munich, Federal Republic of Germany.

Kanki, Phyllis; J. Allan; F. Barin; M. Essex. "Absence of HTLV-IV in Central Africa." Harvard School of Public Health, Boston, MA, USA.

Kanki, Phyllis; S. Mboup; F. Barin; D. Ricard; F. Denis; M. Essex *et al.* "HTLV-IV and HTLV-III/HIV in West Africa." Harvard School of Public Health, Boston, MA, USA.

Katlama, Christine; M. Harzic; K. Kourouma; M.C. Dazza; F. Brun-Vezinet. "Seroepidemiological Study of HIV-1 and HIV-2 Infection in Guinea-Conakry." Hôpital Claude-Bernard, Paris, France.

Katzenstein, David A.; A. Latif; M.T. Bassett; J.C. Emmanuel. "Risks for Heterosexual Transmission of HIV in Zimbabwe." University of Zimbabwe School of Medicine, Harare, Zimbabwe.

Leonard, G.; F. Barin; A. Sangere; G. Gershy-Damet; J.L. Rey; P. Denis *et al.* "Prevalence of HIV and HTLV-III Related Human T-lymphotropic Retrovirus (HTLV-IV) in Several Populations of Ivory-Coast, West Africa." CHU Dupuytren, Limoges, France.

Lyons, Susan F.; B.D. Schoub; A.N. Smith; S. Johnson; G.M. McGillivray. "Absence of HIV Infection in Two Sentinel Cohorts of High-Risk Black South Africans." MRC Aids Virus Research Unit, National Institute for Virology, Private Bag X4, Sandringham 2131, South Africa.

Makuwa, M.; J. Miehakanda; J. Chotard; G. De The. "HIV Infections in the People's Republic of Congo." Public Health National Laboratory, Brazzaville, Congo.

Merlin, M.; R. Josse; E. Delaporte; J.P. Durand; C. Hengy; A.J. Georges. "Infection by HIV among Populations of Six Countries of Central Africa." OCEAC, Yaounde, Cameroon.

Mhalu, Fred; E. Mbena; U. Bredberg-Raden; J. Kiango; K. Nyamuryekunge; G. Biberfeld *et al.* "Prevalence of HIV Antibodies in Healthy Subjects and Groups of Patients in Some Parts of Tanzania." Muhimili Medical Centre, Dar Es Salaam, Bukoba Hospital, Tanzania.

Mpele, P.; A. Itoua-Ngaporo; M. Rosenheim; F. Yala; C. Bouramoure; M. Gentilini *et al.* "Sero-Prevalence of Anti-HIV Antibodies in Brazzaville (Congo)." Hôpital General, Brazzaville, Congo.

Ngaly, Bosenge; R.L. Colebunders; M. Mpania; M. Mussa; H. Francis; J.M. Mann *et al.* "HIV Seroprevalence Among Patients Hospitalized with Neuropsychiatric Illnesses in Kinshasa, Zaire." Projet SIDA, Kinshasa, Zaire.

Ngaly, Bosenge; K. Kayembe; J.M. Mann; R.W. Ryder; H. Mbesa; H. Francis *et al.* "HIV Infection in African Children with Sickle Cell Anemia." Projet SIDA, Kinshasa, Zaire.

Ngaly, Bosenge; R.W. Ryder; B. Kapita; H. Francis; T.C. Quinn; J.M. Mann *et al.* "Continuing Studies on the Natural History of HIV Infection in Zaire." Mama Yemo Hospital and Dept. of Public Health, Kinshasha, Zaire.

Nzilambi, Nzila; R.W. Ryder; F. Behets; H. Francis; E. Bayende; A. Nelson; J.M. Mann *et al.* "Perinatal HIV Transmission in Two African Hospitals." Projet SIDA, Kinshasa, Zaire.

Osei, William D.; E.T. Maganu; W. Manyeneng; R.K. Vyas; J. Van Dam; L. Mahloane *et al.* "Early Indications of Unidirectional Heterosexual

Transmission of AIDS in Botswana." Ministry of Health, Gaborone, Botswana.

Petersen, H.D.; B.O. Lindhardt; P.M. Nyarango; T. Bowry; A. Chemtai; K. Krogsgaard *et al.* "Prevalences of HIV Antibodies and PGL in Rural Kenya." Rigshospitalet, Copenhagen, Denmark.

Plummer, Francis A.; J.N. Simonsen; E.N. Ngugi; D.W. Cameron; P. Piot; J.O. Ndinya-Achola. "Incidence of Human Immunodeficiency Virus (HIV) Infection and Related Disease in a Cohort of Nairobi Prostitutes." Kenya Medical Research Institute, Nairobi, Kenya.

Quattara, A. "HIV-1 and 2 are Present in Ivory Coast in AIDS Patients." Groupe Ivoirien de Travail sur le SIDA, Pasteur Institute, Abidjan, Ivory Coast.

Ryder, Robert W.; W. Bertrand; R.L. Colebunders; B. Kapita; H. Francis; M. Lubaki. "Community Surveillance for HIV Infection in Zaire." Projet SIDA, Kinshasa, Zaire.

Sher, R.; E. Antunes; B. Reid; H. Palcke. "HIV Antibody Prevalence in Black Miners between 1970-1974." Department of Immunology, School of Pathology of the University of the Witwatersrand, Johannesburg, South Africa.

Taelman, H.; L. Bonneux; P. Cornet; G. Van Der Groen; P. Piot. "Transmission of HIV to Partners of Seropositive Heterosexuals from Africa." Institute of Tropical Medicine, Antwerp, Belgium.

Virology, Immunology, And Medicine

Anderson, David W.; K. Baird; A. Macher; A. Nelson; M. De Vinatea; D. Conner *et al.* "Malaria in African Patients with AIDS." Registry of AIDS Pathology, AFIP, Washington, DC, USA.

Biberfeld, Gunnel, J. Albert; U. Brederg; F. Chiodi; B. Bottiger; E. Fenyo; E. Norrby. "Serological Comparison of Human Retroviruses of West African Origin." Department of Immunology and Virology, National Bacteriological Laboratory, 105 21 Stockholm, Sweden.

Bonnaux, Luc; H. Taelman; P. Cornet; G. Van Der Groen; P. Piot. "Case Control Study of HIV-Seropositive versus HIV-Seronegative

European Expatriates in Africa." Institute of Tropical Medicine, Antwerp, Belgium.

Chermann, Jean-Claude; J.L. Becker; U. Hazan; B. Spire; F. Barre-Sinoussi; A. Georges *et al.* "HIV Related Sequences in Insects from Central Africa." Unite d'Oncologie Virale, Institut Pasteur, Paris, France.

De Wit, S.; P. Hermans; D. Roth; G. Zissis; N. Clumeck. "Disease Outcome among Heterosexual Africans with HIV Infection." Saint Pierre University Hospital, Brussels, Belgium.

Georges, Alain J.; D. Salaun; M. Merlin; J.P. Gonzales; F. Barre-Sinoussi; M.C. Georges-Corbut. "A Three Year Survey of Antibody Response to HIV Antigens in the Central African Republic." Institut Pasteur, B.P. 923, Bangui, Central African Republic.

Greenblatt, Ruth M.; S.L. Lukehart; F.A. Plummer; T.C. Quinn; C.W. Critchlow; L.J. D'Costa *et al.* "Genital Ulceration as a Risk Factor for Human Immunodeficiency Virus Infection in Kenya." University of Washington, Seattle, WA, USA.

Guyader, M; P. Sonigo; M. Emerman; F. Clavel; L. Montagnier; M. Alizon. "Nucleotide Sequence Analysis of the West-African AIDS Virus, HIV-2." Unite d'Oncologie Virale, Institut Pasteur, Paris, France.

Hermans, P.; F.K. Lee; M. Poncin; P. Van De Perre; A. Nahmias; N. Clumeck. "Possible Co-Factors of Human Immunodeficiency Virus (HIV) Infection among Central African Patients." Saint Pierre University Hospital, Brussels, Belgium.

Kitonyi, G.W.; T. Bowry; E.G. Kasili. "AIDS Studies in Kenyan Hemophiliacs." MRC Pathology, University of Nairobi, Kenya.

Mingle, Julius A.A.; M. Hayami; M. Osei-Kwasi, Y. Ishikawa; A.R. Neeguaye; V. Nettey *et al.* "Reactivity of Ghanaian Sera to Human Immunodeficiency Virus (HIV) and Simian T-Lymphotropic Virus III (STLV-III)." Institute of Medical Science, University of Tokyo, Japan.

Ndongala, Lubaki; J. Rowland; H. Francis; M.P. Duma; M. Kasali; T.C. Quinn *et al.* "Comparison of Six ELISA Assays for Detection of HIV Antibody in African Sera." Projet SIDA, Kinshasa, Zaire.

Nguyen-Dinh, Phuc; A.E. Greenberg; R.W. Ryder; J.M. Mann; N. Kabote; H. Francis *et al.* "Absence of Association between HIV Seropositivity

300

and *Plasmodium falciparum* Malaria in Kinshasa, Zaire." Malaria Branch, Centers for Disease Control, Atlanta, GA, USA.

Nzilambi, Nzila; R.L. Colebunders; J.M. Mann; H. Francis; K. Nseka; J.W. Curran *et al.* "HIV Blood Screening in Africa: are there no alternatives?" Projet SIDA, Kinshasa, Zaire.

Sension, Michael G.; N. Nzilambi; M.P. Duma; R.W. Ryder; T.C. Quinn; M. Linnan *et al.* "Does Concomitant HIV Infection in African Children Lead to Increased Morbidity and Mortality?" Johns Hopkins University School of Medicine, Baltimore, MD, USA.

Siegal, Frederick P.; C.Y. Wang; T. Hong; K. Shah; D. Imperato; J.C. Emmanuel. "Western Blot-Positive and -Negative Sera from Harare, Zimbabwe and New York, NY, USA are Identified Equally by a Synthetic Polypepide-Based Enzyme-Linked Immunoassy (ELISA)." Long Island Jewish Medical Center, New Hyde Park, NY, USA.

Simooya, Oscar O.; R.M. Mwendapole; S. Siziya; A.F. Fleming. "Relationship between *Plasmodium falciparum* Malaria and HIV Seropositivity at Ndola, Zambia." Tropical Disease Research Centre, Ndola, Zambia.

Vuillecard, E.; C.C. Mathiot; M.C. Georges-Courbot; A.J. Georges. "Diffuse Cervical Cellulitis Associated with HIV-1 Infection in Central Africa." Centre Nationale Hospitalier Universitaire, Bangui, Central African Republic.

Yourno, Joseph; S.F. Josephs; A.G. Fisher; D. Zagury; F. Wong-Stall; R.C. Gallo. "Structure/Function Studies of Cloned HTLV-III/LAV from Zairian and French Individuals." Laboratory of Tumor Cell Biology, National Cancer Institute, NIH, Bethesda, MD, USA.

RESOURCES FOR TEACHING ABOUT AIDS IN AFRICA: CURRICULAR AND FILMOGRAPHIC MATERIAL

Cathleen Church
Rikka Trangsrud*

Introduction

Much of the emphasis in North American educational programs about HIV/AIDS has been on the transmission and prevention of the spread of the virus. While there are quantities of these materials, little has yet been written for educational purposes on international and cross cultural implications of AIDS. In particular, there is a shortage of materials concerning Africa. Nevertheless, in searching of educational resources useful to instructors in public health and social science, it was found that some broader materials could be adapted for teaching about African AIDS. In particular, information available through private voluntary organizations, media and communications firms and health care associations are seen as useful. As indicated by the surveys of PVO/NGO activities elsewhere in this volume can be contacted for additional materials can be obtained through these organizations. In addition, publishers and distributors listed in this article also have other materials on HIV/AIDS that are not cited, or are in the process of planning or developing still further materials. Catalogues and publications lists are usually available from these organizations.

The following resources are suggested as a starting point for instructors and are divided into four sections:

    I. General Teaching Materials
    II. Bibliographies and Curricular Development Materials
    III. Film and video Materials
    IV. Materials for Adaptation to African Issues

---

* **Cathleen Church** is a graduate student in maternal and child health, School of Hygiene and Public Health, Johns Hopkins University. **Rikka Trangsrud** is a staff member of The Futures Group, Washington, D.C. Her graduate work included studies of public policy and health care administration at the University of Minnesota.

I. General Teaching Materials

A Basic Reader on AIDS: This report by the Academy for Educational Development provides an overview of the AIDS epidemic from a global perspective and addresses public policy issues, WHO policies, and prevention strategies. (Write AIDSCOM Project/AED, 1255 23rd Street, N.W., Washington, D.C., 20037; tel: 202-862-1900).

AIDS: A Global Challenge. This report developed by the Academy for Educational Development incorporates material from work underway through USAID contracts. A companion document *AIDS Education: Lessons from International Health* reviews AIDS problems and provides insights gained from other international health problems. An AIDS education approach is suggested (AIDSCOM Project, Academy for Educational Development, 1255 23rd Street, N W Washington D.C., 20037; tel. 202-862-1900.)

AIDS: A Global Perspective. Western Journal of Medicine (Special Issue), 1987, December, No. 147. This issue addresses international dimensions of the AIDS pandemic. Of particular interest are both the descriptions of global issues and of national AIDS programs in Uganda, Japan, France and The Philippines.

AIDS: A Public Health Crisis. Population Information Program, Johns Hopkins University, Baltimore: July 1986, reprinted June 1987. 35 pp. Discusses epidemiology, infection, transmission and education programs on a worldwide basis. Specific references are made to African cultural practices which inhibit and enhance the chance of infection. (PIP/JHU, 624 N. Broadway, Baltimore, MD 21205. $1.00).

AIDS: An International Bimonthly Journal. This journal, which seeks to further international cooperation, published its first volume in May, 1987. It receives contributions from epidemiology, virology, microbiology, immunology, addition, neurology, psychiatry, and general medicine. (Gower Academic Journals, 1 Cleveland St., London, W 1 P 5 FB, UK).

AIDS and the Third World (Panos Dossier 1). The Panos Institute. December 1986, revised March 1987, updated October 1987. 92pp. This is a comprehensive report of the AIDS situation worldwide which examines the impact of the epidemic on the developmental prospects of Third World countries and evaluates what is being done. It makes the point that AIDS is not just a health issue, but will effect all sectors of society. (In USA: The Panos Institute, 1409 King Street, Alexandria, VA 22314; 703-836-1302. (Head office, London, UK, see Haslegrave article below).

Confronting AIDS: Directions for Public Health, Health Care, and Research. This report is the result of an effort by the National Academy of Sciences and the Institute of Medicine to assess the extent of the problems arising from AIDS and to propose an appropriate national response. Chapter Seven deals specifically with International Aspects of AIDS and HIV infection and presents AIDS in Africa within the context of the world community. (Washington, D.C.: National Academy Press, 1986, for Institute of Medicine, National Academy of Sciences).

Consensus Statements on Transmission of Human Immunodeficiency Virus and Infection of Health Workers, *Epidemiological Bulletin*, Vol. 8, NO. 1-2, 1987. Includes statements from the Third Meeting of the WHO Collaborating Centers on AIDS, June 1987.

Development Communication Report, 1987. This report highlighted AIDS education and communication. Periodic future reports can be expanded, especially on use of media in education programs. (Available from Clearinghouse on Development Communication, 1255 23rd Street, N W, Washington, D.C. 20037; 202-862-1900.

304

Kulstad, Ruth, editor. *AIDS: Papers from Science, 1982-1985* is a collection of articles that appeared in *Science*, the publication of the American Association for the Advancement of Science organized by date of publication spanning the period 1982-1985. (Published in 1986 by AAAS, 1333 H Street, N W, Washington, D. C. 20005).

Quinn, Thomas C., *et al.*, "AIDS in Africa: An Epidemiological Paradigm." *Science*. 1986; 234:955-63.

Science, the publication of the American Association for the Advancement of Science dedicated a large portion of its February, 1988 issue to AIDS. The collection of articles is particularly useful in developing course materials for the college and university classroom. (Vol. 239, 5 February, 1988, pp. 533-696).

Slaff, James I and John K. Brubaker. *The AIDS Epidemic: How You Can Protect Yourself and Your Family - Why You Must*. Warner Books, 666 Fifth Avenue, New York, N Y 10103; 212-484-2900. This book covers what AIDS is, how it has spread to all population groups in other countries, why it is likely to follow the same pattern in the U. S., and how to protect both health and individual freedom while controlling the epidemic.

II. Bibliographies And Curricular Development Materials

AIDS Information and Education - A Resource Guide. This guide is intended to provide international health professionals with accessible sources of information on AIDS as well as AIDS education for both health workers and the general public. A primary focus is on developing countries. November 1987. (Available at Learning Resource Center, MAP International, Box 50, Brunswick, GA 31520; 912-265-6010).

Criteria for Evaluating an AIDS Curriculum. Some of the criteria listed in this document relate to curriculum content and some of curriculum development and evaluation. Developmental characteristics of students from grades 5-12 are listed, along with suggestions for appropriate approaches to AIDS education for each stage, 1987, 7 pp. (Available from the National Coalition of Advocates for Students, 100 Boylston St., Suite 737, Boston, MA 02116; 617-357-8507. $2.00).

Fifteen Ways to Talk Clearly About AIDS, AIDSCOM/AED. This document gives guidelines for developing accurate, clear, and compelling information about AIDS. (AIDSCOM/AED, see above address).

Fulton, Gere B., *et al.*, "AIDS: Resource Material for School Personnel," *Journal of School Health*. January 1987; 57(1):14-17.

Hillis, Susan and Marcia Angle. *An AIDS Curriculum for Family Planning Workers in Africa: Need, Design and Plans for Field Testing.* Paper prepared for the National Council for International Health Southern Regional Conference in October, 1987, University of North Carolina. (NCIH, 1101 Connecticut Ave., Washington, D. C. 20036, 202-833-5900.)

INTRAH: Training Module on AIDS for Nurse Midwives and Other Mid-level Service Providers. The program for International Training in Health (INTRAH) at the University of North Carolina School of Medicine has developed this module for use in Africa. It is currently in the field test stage and is expected to be published in 1988. (Contact INTRAH, University of North Carolina, School of Medicine, 208 North Columbia St., Chapel Hill, NC 27514; 919-966-5636).

Johnson, Ralph C. *Medical, Psychological and Social Implications of AIDS: A Curriculum for Young Adults.* 1987, 150 pp. This curriculum, designed for late high school and college courses in health or social studies consists of eight lessons of about two hours each. They cover such topics as basic facts about AIDS, AIDS in the human context, AIDS and sexuality, and the ethics of AIDS. (Available through SUNY AIDS Education Project,

SAHP, HSC-L2-052, SUNY, Stony Brook, NY 11794, 516-444-3242).

Kain, Edward L. "A Note on the Integration of AIDS into the Sociology of Human Sexuality." *Teaching Sociology*. July 1987; 15: 320-23. This article argues that the coverage of AIDS is an important priority for courses in human sexuality and sociology. Inclusion of material on this subject is profitable since it helps to illustrate a number of important sociological concepts and also underlies the crucial role played by social, historical and cultural factors in shaping social life. Specific reference is made to Africa.

Lareau, Annette P. and L. Hendrix. "The Spread of AIDs Among Heterosexuals: A Classroom Simulation." *Teaching Sociology*. July 1987; 15: 316-19. This article describes a classroom simulation designed to teach students about the transmission of the virus in the heterosexual population. It provides a visual image of a hidden social process by showing how a single person can be linked to a much larger network of sexual interaction. It is adaptable to many cultures or populations.

London School of Hygiene and Tropical Medicine, AIDS Bureau, Keppel Street, London WC1E 7HT, U.K., compiles and distributes an "AIDS Newsletter" and a monthly bibliographical update from their computerized database. The database is expected to be available in the U.S. through BRS Information Technologies.

National Library of Medicine has prepared an AIDS bibliography of over 200 pages from Medline, January 1986 through April 1987. (Available in paper or microfiche from the National Technical Information Service, Springfield, VA 22161; order number PB87-190716/GBB).

SIECUS. *Aids and Safer Sex Education: An Annotated Bibliography*. 1987. A list of current books, pamphlets, audio-visuals and curricula for AIDS education. (Available from Sex

Information and Education Council of the U.S., SIECUS, 32 Washington Place, NYU, New York, N Y 10003).

Schmidt, Nancy and Norman Miller. *The Social Impact of AIDS in Africa: A Working Bibliography.* J. Schmidt, Main Library E660. Indiana University, Bloomington, Indiana 47405, 812-335-1481, $2.00).

Strouse, Joan H. and John Phillips. Teaching About AIDS: A Challenge to Educators. *Educational Leadership.* April 1987; 44(7): 76-80.

III. Film And Video Materials

About AIDS (1986, 16mm or video, 15 mins). This film focuses on the medical issues of AIDS, but uses an approach that is informative for the general public [Pyramid, Box 1048, Santa Monica, CA 90406; 800-421-204 or 213-828-7577; Purchase $325 (16mm), $195 (video); rental $35].

AIDS Alert (1985, video, 23 mins). This video begins and ends with statements by Dr. Richard Keeling on AIDS and on the problems of transmission. Animation is used to answer questions from an audience of cartoon characters based on the male and female symbols. [Focus International, 14 Oregon Drive, Huntington Station, N Y 11746; 800-843-0305; 516-549-5320 (N Y only). Purchase $124.95].

AIDS: Challenge and Opportunity, features Dr. C. Everett Koop in a personal interview about the challenge presented to Christian health professionals and the Church by the AIDS crisis. Video produced by MAP International. (Available for $35.00 from AIDS Video, MAP International, Box 50, Brunswick, GA 31520; 912-265-6010).

AIDS-- The Killer Disease, (Zimbabwe, 1986, all video formats, 21 mins). This 21 minute documentary about AIDs in Zimbabwe was made for national television broadcasting in Zimbabwe at the request of the Ministry of Health and the National AIDS

Advisory Committee (who assisted in script development). The film explains the disease, discusses the means of transmission, and explains how to avoid getting AIDS. The video was produced by Edwina Spicer Productions Pvt. Ltd., a Zimbabwean firm, with assistance from Development Through Self-Reliance, Inc. This organization, with producer Steve Smith develops locally-made motion picture pieces on AIDS which are targeted for local general public audience and policy makers in Africa. (Further information and copies of the videos can be obtained by contacting Steve Smith, DRS Inc., PO Box 281, Columbia, MD 21045; 301-964-1647). Development Through Self-Reliance is also developing a 50 min. dramatic 16mm film to encourage behavior change and prevent AIDS transmission. It is designed for African general public audiences. (Completion date: mid 1988. Contact DSR, above).

AIDS: Our Worst Fears (1986, video, 57 mins). This program purports to separate fact from hysteria and from wishful thinking. It focuses on all types of people and explains what is known and not known about AIDS. It was originally shown on television in San Francisco. There are plans to update it in 1988. (Films for the Humanities, Inc., PO Box 2053, Princeton, NJ 08543; 800-257-5126).

The AIDS Dilemma: Higher Education's Response (1986, 90 min). Covers history and current development of the AIDS dilemma, information on diagnosis, treatment and prevention and recommendations on policy and appropriate actions for such institutions. It addresses statistics and patterns in Africa. (American College Health Association, 15879 Crabbs Branch Way, Rockville, MD 20855; 301-963-1100).

IV. Materials For Adaptation To African Issues

Instructional materials are available in a number of formats from national and international organizations. The following organizations are seen as examples of a growing number of institutions that are producing materials (see chapters in this volume on private volunteer organizations and non-governmental organizations by Edward Greeley, Ann Gowan, Marianne Haselgrave and their co-authors).

American Red Cross and U.S. Public Health Service. Materials are available from AIDS, Suite 700, 1555 Wilson Blvd., Rosslyn, VA 22209. Also contact local Red Cross offices or the American Red Cross, AIDS Education Office, 1730 D Street, N W, Washington, D C 20006; 202-737-8300.

Centers for Disease Control (U.S. Public Health Service). Provides scriptographic booklets, including "Why You Should Be Informed About AIDS," for health workers. (Available from the Office of Public Inquires, Centers For Disease Control, 1600 Clifton Road, Atlanta, GA 30333; AIDS hotline is 1-800-342-AIDS).

Health Education Resource Organization. HERO is a resource organization designed to provide facts about AIDS to the American public in the form of brochures, pamphlets, etc. (For information and publications, call 800-638-6262).

International Interdisciplinary AIDS Foundation. (P.O. Box 233. Decauter, GA 30031; 404-589-4997).

San Francisco AIDS Foundation distributes a catalogue entitled the "AIDS Educator," which lists brochures, pamphlets and other informational resources for public education on AIDS-related topics. (Contact SFAF, 333 Valencia Street, 4th Floor, San Francisco, CA 94110; 800-FOR-AIDS).

What Everybody Should Know About AIDS is a scriptographic booklet series on AIDS noted for easy reading and lively graphics. The texts include basic information on AIDS transmission and prevention and can be adapted for cross cultural use; English

310

and Spanish editions available. (Channing L. Bete Co., 200 State Road, South Deerfield, MA 01373; 1-800-628-7733).

What is AIDS? A Manual for Health Workers (1987), is a simply written guide with line drawings to inform health workers about AIDS. Also to be available in French, Spanish and Portuguese. The Christian Medical Commission, World Council of Churches, 150 Route de Ferney, 1211 Geneva 20, Switzerland.

RESOURCE GUIDE TO NON-GOVERNMENTAL ORGANIZATIONS CONCERNED WITH AIDS IN AFRICA BASED IN NORTH AMERICA

Ann Gowan
Priscilla Reining*

Introduction

Many non-governmental organizations based in North America have in recent years focused programs on HIV and AIDS. Some of these have had longstanding ties to Africa, particularly church-based and health-oriented groups or those who have worked on population, famine, refugee or child-care issues. Others currently involved in African AIDS issues have been concerned specifically with family planning, education, communications or broad developmental issues. Many in the latter group are, in fact, new to work on the continent. No one knows how many of these groups exist; one estimate is that there are over 2000 NGOs of all kinds working in Africa; some Kenya officials estimate there are 600 in that country alone, half international, half indigenous.

For nearly all organizations, the task of confronting the HIV/AIDS epidemic is fraught with difficulties. Many religious groups have reservations about dealing with sex-based issues; other groups are particularly sensitive to such issues as contraception and condom usage; still others are concerned about topics that take them directly into areas of government sensitivities. Experiences working on famine relief, emergency health care and refugee assistance, particularly in Ethiopia and the Sahel, have been sobering for most NGOs. Costs are high, political entry is difficult, far-flung communications are unsatisfactory and "competition" between groups an ongoing reality. When past projects are evaluated, hard assessments have had to be made. For many projects these include duplication and waste, local-level profiteering, local and national-level corruption, and

---

*Ann Gowan, who is a candidate for a Masters of Public Policy degree at Harvard University has worked on maternal child health and population issues for USAID in India. Priscilla Reining, Ph.D., is the Program Director, Office of International Science, American Association for the Advancement of Science. Shira Flax and Peggy Randall of the Social Science Research Council, New York, collected information on current NGO activity.

demoralization of personnel. Because of the human needs and the humanitarian challenge, these costs have often been borne quietly. Such experiences, however, do not promote immediate enthusiasm in the face of new problems such as those posed by AIDS.

AIDS is a difficult challenge for NGOs for other reasons. Long-term clients and supporters of an NGO may be very sensitive to new departures and activities. The disease in itself is so unyielding many feel little can be done except to work on prevention, yet "education, awareness and prevention" campaigns often have uncertain results, and are long-term, often ill-defined activities. There is also the very real problem of establishing policies for the protection of field personnel, and making policies that ensure such personnel do not unwittingly spread the virus. Strict working procedures concerning first-aid, trauma, surgery, blood handling techniques, use of syringes, and sterilization procedures are only a few examples.

The resource guide which follows is in four parts. The first surveys a specific NGO sector, that of the family planning organizations in the U.S. concerned with AIDS. The second section provides brief descriptions of some U.S.-based organizations concerned with AIDS. A third section focusses on the NGO organizations based in Canada. A final section provides a list of multi-national organizations plus governmental offices in Canada and the United States concerned with AIDS. These descriptions, it should be emphasized, are all based on a preliminary survey and are not intended to be exhaustive.

U.S.-Based Family Planning Organizations

As a logical extension of their ongoing work in family planning, several organizations have developed programs to address the AIDS epidemic. Some of these who have received funds in the past from the United States Agency for International Development (USAID) to carry out training and technical assistance in family planning have recently incorporated AIDS issues into their training courses. The depth of program involvement for each organization has been dependent largely on funding it has received and the extent to which the organization sees AIDS work as complementary to its ongoing mandate.

Funding is a crucial factor. While U.S. foundations and other private donors have contributed to AIDS programs, those organizations funded earlier for family planning by USAID have generally been the first to enter the AIDS arena. Even here, however, activities are very recent. USAID allocated 14 million dollars in fiscal year 1987 for AIDS control worldwide. These funds were mostly to support the WHO Special Program on AIDS (now Global Program on AIDS) and to secure additional condom supplies for countries that have so requested. In October, 1987, USAID began two major initiatives at the 43 million dollar level to assist developing countries in fighting the AIDS epidemic. The first, AIDSTECH, is via a contract awarded to Family Health International, a North Carolina organization, to provide technical assistance, training and applied research in third world countries. The second, AIDSCOM, a project headed by the Academy for Educational Development in Washington, D.C., is to provide communication support to developing countries to strengthen health promotion and AIDS prevention programs.

While other family planning organizations supported by USAID are sub-contractors to these two projects, USAID in early 1988 had little other funding to support AIDS containment programs. This is partly based on the current assessment that enough funds may already be flowing to AIDS programs from many sources and that the absorption capacity for the management of these funds may in fact have been reached in most nations. There is also a concern that non-governmental organizations engaged in family planning not feel compelled to divert money from their original family planning goals towards AIDS prevention.

Some problems mentioned earlier for all non-governmental organizations are particularly germaine to family planning organizations. Over-involvement with AIDS is a fear for some, because such activities could erode successes in family planning that have been won. Condoms, for example, are associated with prostitution in some parts of Africa, and family planning organizations have tried to disassociate themselves from prostitution. To promote condoms, some feel, will appear hypocritical.

Other groups fear that their messages will become complicated and confusing when associated with AIDS. For example, there is fear that programs could be discredited if information about the long latency period of HIV infection does not reach those they are trying to educate. If, for example, a few clients who began to use condoms were to develop AIDS through prior HIV infection, condoms could be branded as useless. The effect would be to hamper both family planning as well as AIDS prevention efforts.

One humanitarian aspect of AIDS does concern nearly all NGOs working in this area: how to develop policies concerning counselling and support for AIDS victims and their families. However, teaching health workers skills to deal with these situations rarely has been done, partly because field extension staffs are stretched so thin. In effect, many family planning organizations have found it easier to dwell on the positive messages about prevention, including the use of condoms, than to focus on the difficult issues of death and dying.

Non-Governmental Organizations Based In The United States

Those organizations indicated with an asterisk (*) are particularly concerned with family planning activities, and most have embarked on AIDS projects from this basis of expertise. Other organizations listed herein have multiple projects, many of them outside the AIDS sector. Both types of organizations may be contacted directly for further details.

African Medical and Research Foundation (AMREF)
420 Lexington Avenue
New York, New York 10170
(212) 986-1835

AMREF is a private voluntary organization that was founded in the United States in 1957. With its field headquarters in Nairobi, Kenya, AMREF works to improve the health of the rural people in East Africa. Its staff numbers more than 600, of which nearly 93% are African. Over 40 distinct projects are being carried out in the areas of public health, health training, clinical services, research, and health learning materials development. AMREF currently has projects in Kenya, Uganda, Sudan, Ethiopia, Somalia, and Tanzania. Additional services have been provided in Zambia, Malawi, Botswana, Zimbabwe, Lesotho, Zanzibar, and Swaziland. AIDS is a part of several new proposals.

Africare
440 R. Street, N.W.
Washington, D.C. 20001
(202) 462-3614

Although in preliminary stages, AFRICARE has planned an educational workshop on AIDS in Nigeria at the request of that government. AFRICARE is also working on issues of employment policies surrounding AIDS, particularly in Kenya, Rwanda and Uganda.

*AIDSCOM Project
Academy for Educational Development
1255 23rd Street, N.W.
Washington, D.C. 20037
(202) 862-1900

AIDSCOM is a 5 year, $15.4 million contract in public health communications which focuses on discouraging high-risk behavior. AIDSCOM will provide resident advisors to 15 emphasis countries and short-term consultation to others. It will plan media campaigns, provide training and counseling for those at high risk, and it will engage in targeted promotion of condoms.

*AIDSTECH Project
Family Health International
P.O. Box 13950
Research Triangle Park Branch
Durham, N.C. 27709
(919) 549-0517

AIDSTECH is a 5 year, $28 million contract for technical assistance. It will include surveillance, blood screening, and training for health workers. AIDSTECH will work directly with countries that request assistance to more fully develop and implement their national plans for AIDS containment.

American Friends Service Committee
1501 Cherry Street
Philadelphia, Pa. 19102
(215) 241-7000

AFSC is studying the possibility of a program concerning HIV/AIDS.

CARE
660 First Avenue
New York, N.Y. 10016.
(212) 686-3110

CARE has developed a policy regarding AIDS for its employees throughout the world and is in the process of developing a broad policy of action. Activities have included education programs, supplying of condoms and clean syringes, and coordination of its own activities with other agencies.

*Centre for Development and Population Activities (CEDPA)
1717 Massachusetts Avenue, N.W.
Washington, D.C. 20036
(202) 667-1142

CEDPA is involved in training in health and family planning for health managers in developing countries. CEDPA has incorporated information about AIDS into many of their training programs. They are also working on a joint project with AFRICARE to provide AIDS education to the Nigerian Ministry of Health and Education. In addition, CEDPA has formed an internal AIDS Task Force to discuss possible projects in this area.

Church World Service
475 Riverside Drive
New York, N.Y. 10027
(212) 870-2552

This organization's activities include an AIDS education campaign for schools.

*Development Associates
2924 Columbia Pike
Arlington, VA 22204-4399
(703) 979-0100

Development Associates works mostly in Latin America and the Caribbean to train nurses, community developers and other health sector personnel to train others in family planning. They have incorporated AIDS education into their training, and they have developed a special curriculum on AIDS and family planning for nurses and nurse/midwives. Their work has parallels to problems of AIDS in Africa.

*The Futures Group
1101 14th Street, N.W.
Washington, D.C. 20005
(202) 347-8165

The Group is involved in the social marketing of contraceptives, especially condoms, through an AIDS contract known as Social Marketing for Change, or SOMARC. They encourage condom use for both family planning and AIDS prevention by emphasizing generic messages such as "protection." They have also undertaken studies in several countries to see the effects that different promotional messages have on behavior change.

German Marshall Fund of the United States
11 Dupont Drive N.W.
Washington, D.C. 20036
(202) 745-3950

The German Marshall Fund participated in funding "AIDS, not just a Health Issue," under joint Overseas Development Council and Panos Institute auspices. The program officers of the Fund have, as an objective, stimulating and supporting younger Europeans to look at global issues in order to help in their solution. HIV/AIDS is one such issue.

International Society for AIDS Education
School of Public Health
University of South Carolina
Columbia, S.C. 29208
(803) 777-4845

This society was formed as the result of a conference on AIDS education held in 1987. A second conference, scheduled for mid 1988 focuses on the theme, "facilitating change and choice."

*John Snow, Inc. (JSI)
1100 Wilson Boulevard
Arlington, VA 22209
(703) 528-7474

JSI is involved in AIDS prevention in developing countries through two of its projects. One is the Family Planning Logistics Project which provides technical assistance to improve the implementation of family planning programs. One of the main aspects of the project has been forecasting population changes and contraceptive needs, and now it is trying to incorporate the AIDS epidemic into its forecasting. Another JSI project is the Enterprise Program which works in Asia, Latin America and Africa to promote family planning in the private sector, as well as to encourage businesses to offer their employees information about AIDS.

Overseas Development Council (ODC)
1717 Massachusetts Avenue N.W.
Washington, D.C. 20036
(202) 234-8701

A position paper in ODC's Policy Focus series, *AIDS and Poverty in the Developing World* was prepared by Kathryn Carovano.

*The Pathfinder Fund
9 Galen Street
Watertown, MA 02172-4501
(617) 924-7200

The Pathfinder Fund has developed its own policy on AIDS which recognizes its responsibility to prevent the spread of HIV. Its strategy focuses on increasing the awareness of AIDS, training family planning providers to educate and counsel others, and promoting sterile conditions and practices within the family planning setting. In addition, Pathfinder hopes to educate adolescents on the risks of AIDS.

*Population Communication Services (PCS)
The Johns Hopkins University
624 N. Broadway
Baltimore, MD 21205
(301) 955-7662

PCS works in the communication field to further family planning efforts. In addition to assisting with the AIDSCOM project, PCS has prepared manuals on AIDS for family planning workers in several Latin American countries. PCS also sponsored a workshop on AIDS for physicians in Nigeria.

*RONCO Consulting
1821 Chapel Hill Road
Durham, N.C. 27707
(919) 490-1103

RONCO's work in family planning takes place mainly in North Africa and the Middle East where the incidence of HIV infection is not yet high. However, RONCO has been innovative in its attempts to improve knowledge about the disease. A recent regional training session for midwives which was held in Turkey offered a thorough information session using films, pamphlets and lectures. The midwives then formed teams to develop strategies for incorporating AIDS prevention into their work.

Save the Children
54 Wilton Road
Westport, CT 06880
(203) 226-7271

This organization is interested in children with AIDS and is developing a prevention policy on the topic as well as a position paper for its own planning purposes.

Non-Governmental Organizations Based In Canada

Several non-governmental organizations in Canada report they are in the midst of designing programs dealing with AIDS. The IDRC listed below was seen by most as the key institution in Canada currently dealing with issues of global AIDS. A source for some of the information and data on other groups is *NGOs in Africa: Breakthrough at the UN Special Session in 1986*, (Resource Guide, Book III) United Nations, New York, N.Y.)

Canadian Council for International Cooperation
200 Isabella Street, Suite 300
Ottawa, Ontario K1S 1V7
(613) 236-4547

The CCIC is an information center for international development and a forum for 105 organizations. It publishes a monthly newsletter and a directory of Canadian NGOs. The CCIC is strictly an information source and does not have any specially designed programs dealing with AIDS.

Canadian Hunger Foundation
323 Chapel Street
Ottawa, Ontario K1N 7Z2
(613) 237-0180

The CHF supports rural development in Third World countries, with an emphasis on food production and water supplies, and stimulates Canadian understanding of global interdependence.

Canadian Lutheran World Relief
1820 Arlington Street
Winnipeg, Manitoba R2X 1W4
(204) 586-8558

This organization does not yet have any programs dealing with the AIDS issue, but their international organization in Geneva, the Lutheran World Federation, has initiated discussions on the topic of AIDS.

Canadian Public Health Association
210-1355 Carling Avenue
AIDS Education and Awareness Program
Ottawa K1Z 8N8
(613) 725-3769

This program coordinates AIDS education in Canada and works closely with the NGO sector on AIDS issues. As yet, they do not deal directly with the issue of AIDS overseas.

Canadian University Services Overseas (CUSO)
National Office
151 Slater Street
Ottawa, Ontario K1P 5H5
(613) 563-1242

CUSO disseminates print and audio materials for Africa and is now in the process of developing a program in East Africa to deal with the AIDS issue.

Carrefour de solidarite internationale
555 rue Short
Sherbrooke, Quebec J1H 2E6
(819) 566-8595

The Carrefour de solidarite internationale disseminates information to the public through the media, runs a resource centre, publishes a newsletter, provides training in international cooperation, and seeks the involvement of the public through information campaigns.

International Development Education
Resources Administration (IDERA)
2524 Cypress Street
Vancouver, British Columbia V6J 3N2
(604) 732-1496

IDERA provides educational resources on international and Canadian development concerns to residents of Western Canada. IDERA FILMS maintains an up-to-date and comprehensive film collection. They are beginning to develop publications dealing with the AIDs issue.

Partnership Africa-Canada
200 Isabella Street
Ottawa, Ontario K1N 8V5
(613) 234-8242

Partnership Africa-Canada is a coalition of NGOs committed to long-term development in Africa by supporting the work of African NGOs and developing an understanding of Africa.

International Development Research Centre
Health Sciences Division
250 Albert Street
Ottawa, Ontario K1G 3H9
(613) 236-6163

IDRC supports research designed to adapt science and technology to the needs of developing countries. They have over 150 monographs on technical aspects of research in agriculture, health, information and social sciences. IDRC is funding research on the AIDS issue in Brazil, Haiti, India, Kenya, Nigeria, Tanzania, Uganda, Zaire and Zambia.

National And Multi-National Agencies

The national and multi-national agencies based in North America or headquartered elsewhere with offices in North America, who are concerned with international AIDS issues, fall into three broad categories: Canadian Government agencies, United States Government agencies, and those in the United Nations systems.

CANADIAN AGENCIES

Canadian International Development Agency (CIDA)
200 Promenade du Portage
Hull, Quebec K1A 0G4
(819) 997-6202
Information Division: (819) 997-6899
Contact: Charles Morrow, Head of Social Dimensions

CIDA has a small section dealing with the AIDS issue. The Agency's focus is on third world development, and their Health and Population Sector is involved primarily in national efforts. It also works closely with the World Health Organization.

Africa 2000
200 Promenade du Portage
Hull, Quebec K1A 0G4
(819) 953-2817

Africa 2000 is a government project created to respond to the needs of African countries through the year 2000, featuring partnership with the private sector and international cooperation. This program is sponsored by the Canadian International Development Agency (CIDA). AIDS issues are dealt with through CIDA's Health and Population Sector.

Federal Center for AIDS
301 Elgin Street
Ottawa, Ontario K1A 0l3
(613) 957-1774
Contact: Joel Finley

The Federal Center for AIDS is part of the Canadian Ministry of Health and Welfare. Its involvement in research is primarily for Canada only.

UNITED STATES GOVERNMENT AGENCIES

African Development Foundation
1724 Massachussetts Avenue, N.W.
Suite 200
Washington, D.C. 20036
(202) 898-1320

An independent public corporation authorized by Congress in 1980, ADF focuses on direct support to indigenous African groups and individuals in farming, education, husbandry, manufacturing and water management. Publications: *Beyond Relief*, a quarterly newsletter.

Agency for International Development (AID)
320 21st Street, N.W.
Washington, D.C. 20523
Office of Public Liaison: (202) 647-4213
Bureau for Africa: (202) 647-9232

Peace Corps
806 Connecticut Avenue, N.W.
Washington, D.C. 20526
Public Affairs: (202) 254-6886

House Subcommittee on Africa
705 House Annex 1
Washington, D.C. 20515
(202) 226-3596
Chairman: Rep. Howard Wolpe
Staff Director: Steve Weisman
Information: Nancy Carmen

Subcommittee on Africa
Senate Foreign Relations Committee
Washington, D.C. 20510
(202) 224-4651
Chairman: Senator Paul Simon
Information: Nancy Stetson

UNITED NATIONS SYSTEM ORGANIZATIONS

**Int'l. Research and Training Institute for
the Advancement of Women (INSTRAW)**
Santo Domingo, Dominican Republic
(NY Liaison Office: Room S-2914F,
United Nations
New York, N.Y. 10017)

International vehicle for research, training and information to help
insure the integration of women into the mainstream of
development, particularly in developing countries.

UN Children's Fund (UNICEF)
866 UN Plaza
New York, N.Y. 10017
(212) 415-8000

Helps developing countries improve the conditions of children and
youth. It provides assistance for community-based service in areas of
primary health care, water supply, formal and non-formal education,
nutrition and emergency operations. Catalogue of publications,
slides, films, tapes, photo exhibits, and posters available upon
request.

UN Development Fund for Women (UNIFEM)
304 East 45th Street
Room 1120
New York, N.Y. 10017
(212) 906-6435

With contributions from governments and individuals, helps rural
and poor urban women obtain skills and resources for self-reliant,
long-term development.

UN Development Programme
One United Nations Plaza
New York, N.Y. 10017
(Division of Information: (212) 906-5300)

*UN Fund for Population Activities
220 E. 42nd Street
New York, N.Y. 10017
(212) 850-5600

The largest multilateral population agency.

UN High Commissioner for Refugees
1718 Connecticut Ave. N.W., 2nd Floor
Washington, D.C. 20009
(202) 387-8546
Provides legal protection to refugees and sometimes is asked by governments to provide emergency relief. Its assistance is primarily to promote durable solutions to the problems of refugees through voluntary repatriation, local integration or resettlement in another country. Publications: *Refugees*

World Health Organization
20, avenue Appia
1211 Geneva 27, Switzerland
(NY Liaison Office: Two UN Plaza, Room 0973
New York, N.Y. 10017 (212) 754-0973)

Works to attain the highest levels of health for all peoples. Cooperates with member states in development of health services, training of health professionals, disease prevention and control, and medical research. Publications: *World Health* (10/yr/$12.50, from Geneva). WHO is the key organization for the coordination, of Global HIV/AIDS projects, and coordination between the UN system and host governments.

RESOURCE GUIDE TO NON-GOVERNMENTAL ORGANIZATIONS CONCERNED WITH AIDS IN AFRICA BASED IN THE UNITED KINGDOM

Marianne Haslegrave*

Introduction

Africa has long been a major area of concern for development organizations and voluntary agencies based in the United Kingdom. While each organization pursues its own goals and objectives within its area of expertise, mechanism for cooperation do exist. Such cooperation usually occurs around specific issues, such as famine relief, refugee assistance and primary health care. This essay surveys recent developments among members of a new consortium in the United Kingdom concerned with AIDS in Africa and other parts of the third world.

Formation On An AIDS Consortium

In 1986, at the instigation of Oxfam, a number of organizations met to discuss their concerns about AIDS. From these discussions was formed the UK NGO AIDS Consortium for the Third World. The current membership of the Consortium, made up of over 30 organizations as of early 1988, includes several large organizations working in developing countries such as OXFAM, the International Planned Parenthood Federation (IPPF), Save the Children Fund (SCF), Christian Aid, and War on Want. A second group is comprised of organizations specializing in the dissemination of information, including the Panos Institute, which has a special AIDS and Development Unit, and the Appropriate Health Resources Technologies Action Group (AHRTAG) which publishes an international newsletter, *AIDS Action.* Another group of members have joined the consortium because of a concern with how AIDS will affect their own programs. The latter, for example,

* **Marianne Haslegrave**, BA Durham, (UK), MA Queens College, CUNY (USA) is a consultant on non-governmental organizations and women's issues. She has recently served as coordinater of the UK NGO AIDS Consortium for the Third World.

include The Baby Milk Action Coalition, and Help the Aged, an organization that works on problems related to the elderly in developing countries and whose concern includes the role grandparents will play where active wage-earning parents become ill or die of AIDS.

The initial work of the consortium has been to establish a means of information exchange on AIDS for its members, and to provide a link with AIDS programs including those in WHO, the Overseas Development Administration (British Aid), and the Narcotics Control and Drug Department of the Foreign and Commonwealth Office.

Given the rapid developments which have taken place in our knowledge of HIV infection and AIDS, one of the primary functions of the consortium has been to provide up to date technical information on the topic. This has been possible through the cooperation of the London School of Hygiene and Tropical Medicine which has provided briefings at consortium meetings.

The consortium has taken Africa as a priority area of concern and has begun to look at the economic impact of AIDS on the continent and its social and cultural implications. The overall concern is to encourage cooperation among those affiliated with the consortium.

This particular objective is pursued through the Consortium Newsletter, through regular exchanges of information and through periodic meetings.

Illustrative Activities Of Selected Consortium Members

Brief summaries of the activities currently under way in ten consortium members will serve as an illustration of the broad range of work concerning AIDS in Africa. Further information is available from the organizations themselves (see addresses below).

ActionAid. In its AIDS-related activities ActionAid is concentrating on three African countries: Kenya, Uganda, and The Gambia. In November 1987 the organization sponsored a study tour to the United Kingdom for two Ugandans, both of whom are active in helping AIDS sufferers and their families and have formed a group there to increase the support available to families. During the visit, arranged in conjunction with the Disabilities Study

Unit and the Department of Health and Social Security, they visited voluntary and statutory bodies involved with care for sufferers and support for families. They also attended a course on AIDS counselling.

Appropriate Health Resources and Technologies Action Group (AHRTAG). This organization publishes *AIDS Action*, an international newsletter focusing on the practical aspects of planning and running health education campaigns and counselling services on HIV infection and AIDS. Issues include a four-page insert produced by WHO which provides updated global overviews of AIDS prevention and control activities. The newsletter is similar in style and format to AHRTAG's other publications entitled *Dialogue on Diarrhoea*, and *ARI News* (Acute Respiratory Infections).

Baptist Missionary Society. As part of its activities the Baptist Missionary Society has provided scientific and technical statements on AIDS for its medical missionaries overseas, and has provided an emergency financial allowance for missionary healthmakers to draw on for education, prevention and diagnosis of AIDS.

British Life Insurance Trust For Health Education (Blithe)

Blithe Centre for Health and Medical Education has produced *Teaching AIDS for School Teachers* (now in its second edition). The organization also helped to design the first WHO training workshop on counselling and HIV infection held in Nairobi (September 1987). Blithe has also contributed to a counselling training manual to be published by the Scottish Health Education Group.

Christian Aid. This organization has provided a grant to the *Centre de Vulgarisation Agricole* in Zaire for the publication and dissemination of a 50-page booklet on AIDS. It is to be circulated within Zaire and in neighbouring countries, and extracts will be published in local newspapers and broadcast on radio and television.

In Uganda, Christian Aid has supported a seminar on AIDS (September 1987) for doctors, dispensary workers, clergy and other staff from the Church of Uganda. The meeting was attended by other local and international organizations and representatives of the Uganda Government. Further workshops are planned.

Equipment For Charity Hospitals Overseas (ECHO)

Among its activities, ECHO provides blood testing kits, low cost disposable needles, syringes, gloves, and vehicles for AIDS outreach programs and information on safe re-sterilization of equipment. Its relevant activities also include the supply of generic pharmaceuticals and maintenance of clinic and hospital equipment in developing countries.

International Broadcasting Trust (IBT)

Early in 1987, the British Broadcasting Corporation and the Independent Television Companies mounted a campaign against AIDS, with a week-long series of programs for the British audience. IBT, a non-governmental organization, has prepared two new programs of sequences from the AIDS Week material for use in Africa. The first program is "AIDS - Frankly Speaking"; the second is "AIDS - Young People Talking." Each program is introduced by Professor Kihumbu Thairu, Head of the Health Program of the Commonwealth Secretariat. IBT has also completed a program called "AIDS--An African Perspective," filmed in Zambia and Uganda and will be available on video.

International Planned Parenthood Federation (IPPF)

Following discussion of HIV and AIDS by IPPF's International Medical Advisory Panel (IMAP), an AIDS Prevention Unit was formed at IPPF with the support of the United Kingdom's Overseas Development Administration. The unit, activated in June 1987, is designed to serve the needs of Family Planning Association members around the world. IPPF has also provided visits to various countries, including Kenya Swaziland, Zaire and Zambia to assist FPAs in assessing their needs to respond to problems of AIDS.

Another project, with funding from the Swedish International Development Authority, (SIDA) is the preparation of a manual for field workers containing facts on HIV and AIDS. In addition, a manual is being produced to help FPAs consider a variety of responses to AIDS appropriate to the communities in which they work. A self-instruction module for health workers on AIDS is planned, as is a video tape for general use, particularly in Africa.

In other spheres, a new publication, *AIDS Watch*, has been launched as a supplement to the IPPF quarterly development journal, *People*. The aim of the new publication is to treat AIDS from a broad health and humanitarian viewpoint. It is produced in association with the Norwegian Red Cross and the Panos Institute and is funded by SIDA.

OXFAM

As part of its activities OXFAM has provided funding for research and social action on AIDS through Project Connaissida in Zaire which included a three- week training program on popular education for its workers. Further funding has subsequently been requested for AIDS workshops for women with multiple partners, which will attempt, at a later stage, to consider alternative sources of income for these women.

THE PANOS INSTITUTE

In November 1986, Panos, in association with the Norwegian Red Cross, published its first information dossier *AIDS and the Third World*. The third revised edition of the dossier will be available in mid-1988.

In 1987, Panos, in collaboration with WHO, the Swedish International Development Agency, (SIDA), and the American Foundation for AIDS Research, organized an international meeting in Talloires, France on AIDS and Development for representatives of bilateral, multi-lateral and the NGO donor agencies. A briefing paper entitled "Talloires Conclusion on AIDS and Development" is available.

332

A second dossier, "*Blaming Others: Racial and Ethnic Aspects of AIDS*," examines the global epidemic of blame which has accompanied the AIDS pandemic and the growing impact of HIV and AIDS in developing countries. The dossier, expected to be published in mid-1988, features articles from Third World researchers and scholars that reflect the concern of the developing world.

Save the Children Fund. As part of its work in AIDS prevention, this organization has been focusing on protection of their health workers in developing countries. Particular concerns are such measures as protective clothing and equipment. Other activities are in specific African countries. In The Gambia, the Fund has supported a training seminar for health staff. In Uganda it is providing research support to the National AIDS Programme. Through the provision of a Paediatrician AIDS Coordinator, assistance is also, planned for the Ugandan Health Education Campaign through the School Health Curricula. In Ethiopia it is anticipated that support will be given to the Ethiopian Health Education Program.

Catholic Fund for Overseas Development (CAFOD). This organization is an observer to the consortium. It is supporting the work of two hospitals in Uganda which have started a mobile care unit to help AIDS sufferers and their families. This pastoral care program involves health staff visiting sufferers in their homes and providing treatment for symptoms, while at the same time using the contact to provide education for the families and other contacts. CAFOD is helping with the costs of vehicles and drugs.

In December 1987 CAFOD hosted a conference in the United Kingdom for all the CARITAS agencies by representatives from over 40 countries. The main concern was the impact of AIDS in Africa, although discussion included South America and Asia.

MEMBERS AND ACTIVE OBSERVERS

Members and Active Observers of the UK NGO Consortium on AIDS in the Third World, as of January 1988, is appended. For further Information contact, Sue Lucas, Secretary, 1 London Bridge Street, London SE 19SG, UK.

ACORD
Francis House (3rd floor)
Francis Street
London SW1P 1DQ
01-828-7611

ACTION AGAINST AIDS
80 Cathcart Road
London SW10 9DJ
01-376-5651

ACTIONAID
Hamlyn House
Archway
London N19 5PG
01-281-4101

AHRTAG
Appropriate Health Resources & Technologies Action Group Ltd.
1 London Bridge Street
London SE1 9SG
01-486-4175

BABY MILK ACTION COALITION
34 Blinco Grove
Cambridge CB1 4TS
0223-210094

BLITHE
Centre for Health & Medical Education
British Medical Association
BMA House
Tavistock Square
London WC1H 9JP
01-388-1976

BRITISH RED CROSS SOCIETY
9 Grosvenor Cresent
London, SW 1 X 7EJ
01-235-5454

BMA COMMONWEALTH MEDICAL ASSOCIATION
Tavistock Square
London WC1H 9JP
01-387-4499

BUREAU OF HYGIENE 7 TROPICAL DISEASES
Keppel Street
London WC1E 7HT
01-636-8636

CAFOD (Observer)
2 Garden Close
Stockwell Road
London SW9 9TY
01-737-7900

CHRISTIAN AID
P.O. Box 100
London SE1 7RT
Inter-Church House
35 Lower Marsh
London SE1 7RL
01-620-4444

CHURCH MISSIONARY SOCIETY
157 Waterloo Road
London SE1 8UU
01-928-8681

ECHO
Ullswater Crescent
Coulsdon
Surrey CR3 2HR
01-660-2220

HELP THE AGED
St. James' Walk
London EC1R OBE
01-253-0253

INSTITUTE OF CHILD HEALTH
30 Guildford Street
London WC1N 1EH
01-242-9789

INTERNATIONAL BROADCASTING TRUST
2 Ferdinand Place
London NW1 8EE
01-482-2847

INTERNATIONAL CHRISTIAN RELIEF
PO Box 180
St. John's Hill
Sevenoaks, Kent TN3 3NP
0722-450250

INTERNATIONAL EXTENSION COLLEGE
Office D
Dales Brewery
Gwydier Street
Cambridge, CB1 2LJ
0223-353321

INTERNATIONAL PLANNED PARENTHOOD FEDERATION
Regents College
Inner Circle
Regents Park
London NW1 4NS
01-486-0741

LONDON SCHOOL OF HYGIENE & TROPICAL MEDICINE
Keppel Street
London WC'E 7HT
01-636-8636

METHODIST CHURCH OVERSEAS DIVISION
25 Marylebone Road
London NW1 5JR
01-935-2541 ext. 252

MISSIONARIES AND VOLUNTEERS HEALTH SERVICE
Mildmay Mission Hospital
Hackney Road
London E2 7NA
01-739-2331

OXFAM
274 Banbury Road
Oxford OX2 7DZ
0865-56777

OVERSEAS DEVELOPMENT ADMINISTRATION
Eland House
Stag Place
London SW1E 5DH

OVERSEAS MEDICAL AID TRUST
34 High Street
Aylesbury, Bucks

PANOS INSTITUTE
7 Alfred Place
London WC1 7EB
01-387-3601

QUAKER PEACE & SERVICE
Friends House
London NW1 2BJ
01-387-3601

SAVE THE CHILDREN FUND
17 Grove Lane
Camberwell, London SE5 8RD
01-703-5400

UK FOUNDATION FOR THE PEOPLES OF THE SOUTH PACIFIC
32 Howe Park
Edinburgh, EH10 7HF
Scotland
031-445-5010

MEMBERS OF BRITISH VOLUNTEER AGENCIES LAISON GROUP
UNA Ints
ternational Services Department
3 Whitehall Court
London SW1A 2 EL
01-930-0679

VOLUNTEER MISSIONARY MOVEMENT
Shenley Lane
London Colney
St. Albans, Herts AL2 1AR
0727-24853

WAR ON WANT
37-39 Great Guidford Street
London SE1 OES

WORLD IN NEED
318 St. Pauls Road
London N1 2LD
01-359-6408

STUDIES IN AFRICAN HEALTH AND MEDICINE

1. Norman Miller and Richard Rockwell (Eds.), **AIDS in Africa: The Social and Policy Impact**

2. Charles M. Good, **The Community in African Primary Health Care: Strengthening Participation and a Proposed Strategy**

3. C.K. Omari, **Socio-Cultural Factors in Modern Family Planning Methods in Tanzania**

Editors

Norman Miller, Ph.D., serves as President of The African-Caribbean Institute and concurrently holds appointments at Dartmouth College in Environmental Studies and in the Department of Community and Family Medicine of the Dartmouth Medical School. He is the author or editor of five books on Africa, including *Kenya: The Quest for Prosperity.*

Richard C. Rockwell, Ph.D., is an Executive Associate of the Social Science Research Council. A sociologist specializing in federal statistics and research methodology, he staffs the Council's program on the Global Social Consequences of the AIDS Epidemic and the Program in International Peace and Security Studies.